ACCESS YOUR ONLINE RESOURCES

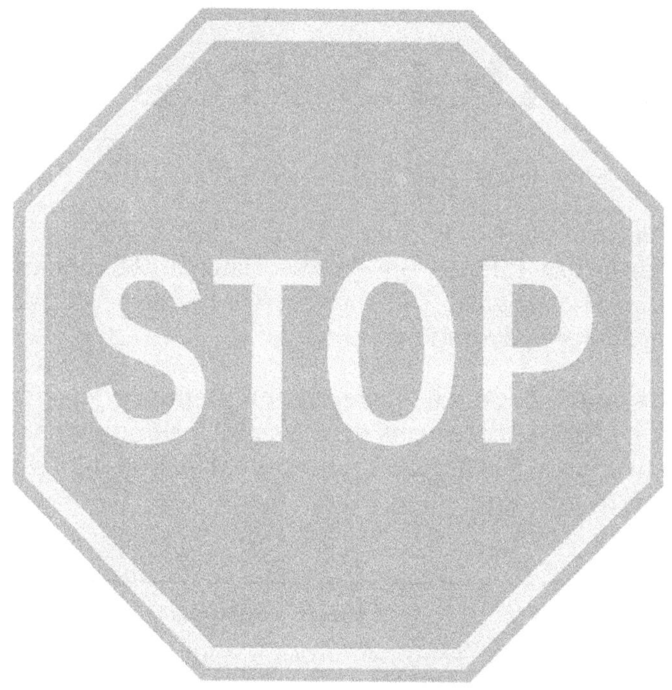

DON'T MISS OUT ON THE ONLINE RESOURCES INCLUDED WITH YOUR PURCHASE!

Your purchase of this product unlocks access to our Online Resources page. Elevate your study experience with our **interactive practice test interface**, along with all of the additional resources that we couldn't include in this book.

Flip to the Online Resources section at the end of this book to find the link and a QR code to get started!

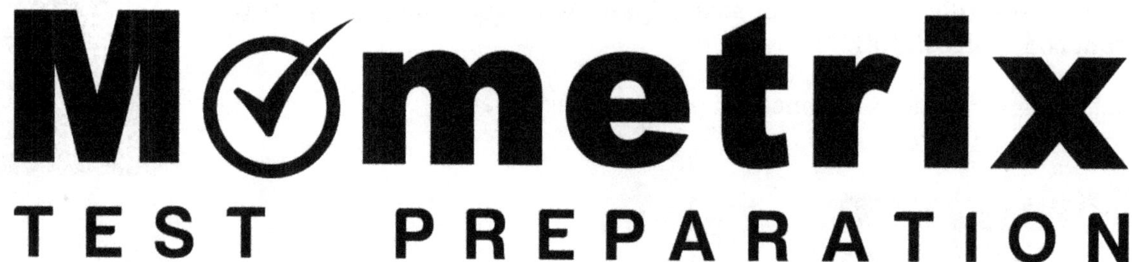

Certified Diabetes Educator Exam Secrets

Study Guide

Your Key to Exam Success

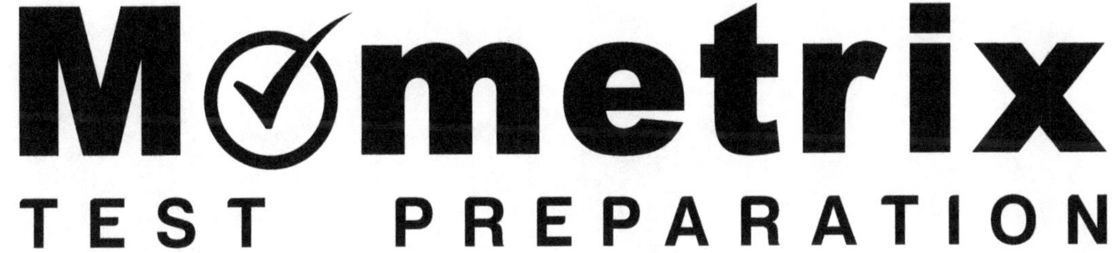

Written and edited by the Mometrix Diabetes Educator Certification Test Team

Paperback
ISBN 13: 978-1-60971-301-0
ISBN 10: 1-60971-301-X

Ebook
ISBN 13: 978-1-62120-418-3
ISBN 10: 1-62120-418-9

Hardback
ISBN 13: 978-1-5167-0552-8
ISBN 10: 1-5167-0552-1

Dear Future Exam Success Story

First of all, **THANK YOU** for purchasing Mometrix study materials!

Second, congratulations! You are one of the few determined test-takers who are committed to doing whatever it takes to excel on your exam. **You have come to the right place.** We developed these study materials with one goal in mind: to deliver you the information you need in a format that's concise and easy to use.

In addition to optimizing your guide for the content of the test, we've outlined our recommended steps for breaking down the preparation process into small, attainable goals so you can make sure you stay on track.

We've also analyzed the entire test-taking process, identifying the most common pitfalls and showing how you can overcome them and be ready for any curveball the test throws you.

Standardized testing is one of the biggest obstacles on your road to success, which only increases the importance of doing well in the high-pressure, high-stakes environment of test day. Your results on this test could have a significant impact on your future, and this guide provides the information and practical advice to help you achieve your full potential on test day.

Your success is our success

We would love to hear from you! If you would like to share the story of your exam success or if you have any questions or comments in regard to our products, please contact us at **800-673-8175** or **support@mometrix.com**.

Thanks again for your business and we wish you continued success!

Sincerely,
The Mometrix Test Preparation Team

Need more help? Check out our flashcards at:
http://MometrixFlashcards.com/certifieddiabeteseducator

Table of Contents

Introduction

Thank you for purchasing this resource! You have made the choice to prepare yourself for a test that could have a huge impact on your future, and this guide is designed to help you be fully ready for test day. Obviously, it's important to have a solid understanding of the test material, but you also need to be prepared for the unique environment and stressors of the test, so that you can perform to the best of your abilities.

For this purpose, the first section that appears in this guide is the **Secret Keys**. We've devoted countless hours to meticulously researching what works and what doesn't, and we've boiled down our findings to the five most impactful steps you can take to improve your performance on the test. We start at the beginning with study planning and move through the preparation process, all the way to the testing strategies that will help you get the most out of what you know when you're finally sitting in front of the test.

We recommend that you start preparing for your test as far in advance as possible. However, if you've bought this guide as a last-minute study resource and only have a few days before your test, we recommend that you skip over the first two Secret Keys since they address a long-term study plan.

If you struggle with **test anxiety**, we strongly encourage you to check out our recommendations for how you can overcome it. Test anxiety is a formidable foe, but it can be beaten, and we want to make sure you have the tools you need to defeat it.

Secret Key #1 – Plan Big, Study Small

There's a lot riding on your performance. If you want to ace this test, you're going to need to keep your skills sharp and the material fresh in your mind. You need a plan that lets you review everything you need to know while still fitting in your schedule. We'll break this strategy down into three categories.

Information Organization

Start with the information you already have: the official test outline. From this, you can make a complete list of all the concepts you need to cover before the test. Organize these concepts into groups that can be studied together, and create a list of any related vocabulary you need to learn so you can brush up on any difficult terms. You'll want to keep this vocabulary list handy once you actually start studying since you may need to add to it along the way.

Time Management

Once you have your set of study concepts, decide how to spread them out over the time you have left before the test. Break your study plan into small, clear goals so you have a manageable task for each day and know exactly what you're doing. Then just focus on one small step at a time. When you manage your time this way, you don't need to spend hours at a time studying. Studying a small block of content for a short period each day helps you retain information better and avoid stressing over how much you have left to do. You can relax knowing that you have a plan to cover everything in time. In order for this strategy to be effective though, you have to start studying early and stick to your schedule. Avoid the exhaustion and futility that comes from last-minute cramming!

Study Environment

The environment you study in has a big impact on your learning. Studying in a coffee shop, while probably more enjoyable, is not likely to be as fruitful as studying in a quiet room. It's important to keep distractions to a minimum. You're only planning to study for a short block of time, so make the most of it. Don't pause to check your phone or get up to find a snack. It's also important to **avoid multitasking**. Research has consistently shown that multitasking will make your studying dramatically less effective. Your study area should also be comfortable and well-lit so you don't have the distraction of straining your eyes or sitting on an uncomfortable chair.

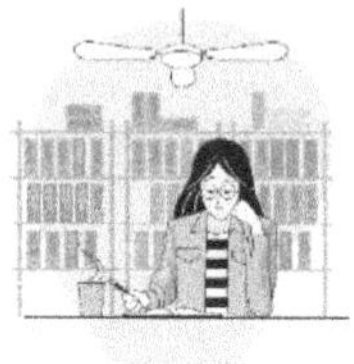

The time of day you study is also important. You want to be rested and alert. Don't wait until just before bedtime. Study when you'll be most likely to comprehend and remember. Even better, if you know what time of day your test will be, set that time aside for study. That way your brain will be used to working on that subject at that specific time and you'll have a better chance of recalling information.

Finally, it can be helpful to team up with others who are studying for the same test. Your actual studying should be done in as isolated an environment as possible, but the work of organizing the information and setting up the study plan can be divided up. In between study sessions, you can discuss with your teammates the concepts that you're all studying and quiz each other on the details. Just be sure that your teammates are as serious about the test as you are. If you find that your study time is being replaced with social time, you might need to find a new team.

Secret Key #2 – Make Your Studying Count

You're devoting a lot of time and effort to preparing for this test, so you want to be absolutely certain it will pay off. This means doing more than just reading the content and hoping you can remember it on test day. It's important to make every minute of study count. There are two main areas you can focus on to make your studying count.

Retention

It doesn't matter how much time you study if you can't remember the material. You need to make sure you are retaining the concepts. To check your retention of the information you're learning, try recalling it at later times with minimal prompting. Try carrying around flashcards and glance at one or two from time to time or ask a friend who's also studying for the test to quiz you.

To enhance your retention, look for ways to put the information into practice so that you can apply it rather than simply recalling it. If you're using the information in practical ways, it will be much easier to remember. Similarly, it helps to solidify a concept in your mind if you're not only reading it to yourself but also explaining it to someone else. Ask a friend to let you teach them about a concept you're a little shaky on (or speak aloud to an imaginary audience if necessary). As you try to summarize, define, give examples, and answer your friend's questions, you'll understand the concepts better and they will stay with you longer. Finally, step back for a big picture view and ask yourself how each piece of information fits with the whole subject. When you link the different concepts together and see them working together as a whole, it's easier to remember the individual components.

Finally, practice showing your work on any multi-step problems, even if you're just studying. Writing out each step you take to solve a problem will help solidify the process in your mind, and you'll be more likely to remember it during the test.

Modality

Modality simply refers to the means or method by which you study. Choosing a study modality that fits your own individual learning style is crucial. No two people learn best in exactly the same way, so it's important to know your strengths and use them to your advantage.

For example, if you learn best by visualization, focus on visualizing a concept in your mind and draw an image or a diagram. Try color-coding your notes, illustrating them, or creating symbols that will trigger your mind to recall a learned concept. If you learn best by hearing or discussing information, find a study partner who learns the same way or read aloud to yourself. Think about how to put the information in your own words. Imagine that you are giving a lecture on the topic and record yourself so you can listen to it later.

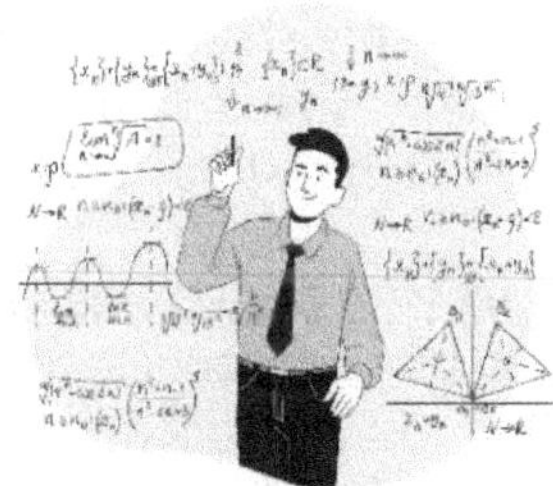

For any learning style, flashcards can be helpful. Organize the information so you can take advantage of spare moments to review. Underline key words or phrases. Use different colors for different categories. Mnemonic devices (such as creating a short list in which every item starts with the same letter) can also help with retention. Find what works best for you and use it to store the information in your mind most effectively and easily.

Secret Key #3 – Practice the Right Way

Your success on test day depends not only on how many hours you put into preparing, but also on whether you prepared the right way. It's good to check along the way to see if your studying is paying off. One of the most effective ways to do this is by taking practice tests to evaluate your progress. Practice tests are useful because they show exactly where you need to improve. Every time you take a practice test, pay special attention to these three groups of questions:

- The questions you got wrong
- The questions you had to guess on, even if you guessed right
- The questions you found difficult or slow to work through

This will show you exactly what your weak areas are, and where you need to devote more study time. Ask yourself why each of these questions gave you trouble. Was it because you didn't understand the material? Was it because you didn't remember the vocabulary? Do you need more repetitions on this type of question to build speed and confidence? Dig into those questions and figure out how you can strengthen your weak areas as you go back to review the material.

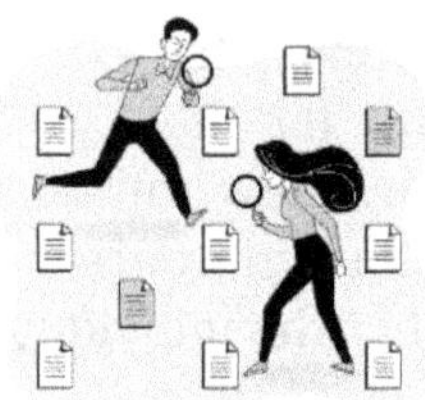

Additionally, many practice tests have a section explaining the answer choices. It can be tempting to read the explanation and think that you now have a good understanding of the concept. However, an explanation likely only covers part of the question's broader context. Even if the explanation makes perfect sense, **go back and investigate** every concept related to the question until you're positive you have a thorough understanding.

As you go along, keep in mind that the practice test is just that: practice. Memorizing these questions and answers will not be very helpful on the actual test because it is unlikely to have any of the same exact questions. If you only know the right answers to the sample questions, you won't be prepared for the real thing. **Study the concepts** until you understand them fully, and then you'll be able to answer any question that shows up on the test.

It's important to wait on the practice tests until you're ready. If you take a test on your first day of study, you may be overwhelmed by the amount of material covered and how much you need to learn. Work up to it gradually.

On test day, you'll need to be prepared for answering questions, managing your time, and using the test-taking strategies you've learned. It's a lot to balance, like a mental marathon that will have a big impact on your future. Like training for a marathon, you'll need to start slowly and work your way up. When test day arrives, you'll be ready.

Start with the strategies you've read in the first two Secret Keys—plan your course and study in the way that works best for you. If you have time, consider using multiple study resources to get different approaches to the same concepts. It can be helpful to see difficult concepts from more than one angle. Then find a good source for practice tests. Many times, the test website will suggest potential study resources or provide sample tests.

Practice Test Strategy

If you're able to find at least three practice tests, we recommend this strategy:

UNTIMED AND OPEN-BOOK PRACTICE

Take the first test with no time constraints and with your notes and study guide handy. Take your time and focus on applying the strategies you've learned.

TIMED AND OPEN-BOOK PRACTICE

Take the second practice test open-book as well, but set a timer and practice pacing yourself to finish in time.

TIMED AND CLOSED-BOOK PRACTICE

Take any other practice tests as if it were test day. Set a timer and put away your study materials. Sit at a table or desk in a quiet room, imagine yourself at the testing center, and answer questions as quickly and accurately as possible.

Keep repeating timed and closed-book tests on a regular basis until you run out of practice tests or it's time for the actual test. Your mind will be ready for the schedule and stress of test day, and you'll be able to focus on recalling the material you've learned.

Secret Key #4 – Pace Yourself

Once you're fully prepared for the material on the test, your biggest challenge on test day will be managing your time. Just knowing that the clock is ticking can make you panic even if you have plenty of time left. Work on pacing yourself so you can build confidence against the time constraints of the exam. Pacing is a difficult skill to master, especially in a high-pressure environment, so **practice is vital**.

Set time expectations for your pace based on how much time is available. For example, if a section has 60 questions and the time limit is 30 minutes, you know you have to average 30 seconds or less per question in order to answer them all. Although 30 seconds is the hard limit, set 25 seconds per question as your goal, so you reserve extra time to spend on harder questions. When you budget extra time for the harder questions, you no longer have any reason to stress when those questions take longer to answer.

Don't let this time expectation distract you from working through the test at a calm, steady pace, but keep it in mind so you don't spend too much time on any one question. Recognize that taking extra time on one question you don't understand may keep you from answering two that you do understand later in the test. If your time limit for a question is up and you're still not sure of the answer, mark it and move on, and come back to it later if the time and the test format allow. If the testing format doesn't allow you to return to earlier questions, just make an educated guess; then put it out of your mind and move on.

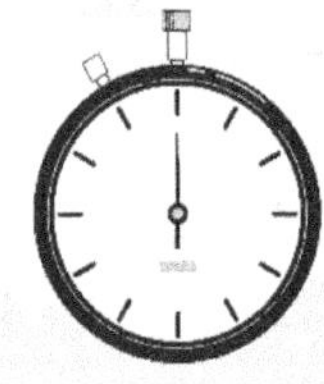

On the easier questions, be careful not to rush. It may seem wise to hurry through them so you have more time for the challenging ones, but it's not worth missing one if you know the concept and just didn't take the time to read the question fully. Work efficiently but make sure you understand the question and have looked at all of the answer choices, since more than one may seem right at first.

Even if you're paying attention to the time, you may find yourself a little behind at some point. You should speed up to get back on track, but do so wisely. Don't panic; just take a few seconds less on each question until you're caught up. Don't guess without thinking, but do look through the answer choices and eliminate any you know are wrong. If you can get down to two choices, it is often worthwhile to guess from those. Once you've chosen an answer, move on and don't dwell on any that you skipped or had to hurry through. If a question was taking too long, chances are it was one of the harder ones, so you weren't as likely to get it right anyway.

On the other hand, if you find yourself getting ahead of schedule, it may be beneficial to slow down a little. The more quickly you work, the more likely you are to make a careless mistake that will affect your score. You've budgeted time for each question, so don't be afraid to spend that time. Practice an efficient but careful pace to get the most out of the time you have.

Secret Key #5 – Have a Plan for Guessing

When you're taking the test, you may find yourself stuck on a question. Some of the answer choices seem better than others, but you don't see the one answer choice that is obviously correct. What do you do?

The scenario described above is very common, yet most test takers have not effectively prepared for it. Developing and practicing a plan for guessing may be one of the single most effective uses of your time as you get ready for the exam.

In developing your plan for guessing, there are three questions to address:

- When should you start the guessing process?
- How should you narrow down the choices?
- Which answer should you choose?

When to Start the Guessing Process

Unless your plan for guessing is to select C every time (which, despite its merits, is not what we recommend), you need to leave yourself enough time to apply your answer elimination strategies. Since you have a limited amount of time for each question, that means that if you're going to give yourself the best shot at guessing correctly, you have to decide quickly whether or not you will guess.

Of course, the best-case scenario is that you don't have to guess at all, so first, see if you can answer the question based on your knowledge of the subject and basic reasoning skills. Focus on the key words in the question and try to jog your memory of related topics. Give yourself a chance to bring the knowledge to mind, but once you realize that you don't have (or you can't access) the knowledge you need to answer the question, it's time to start the guessing process.

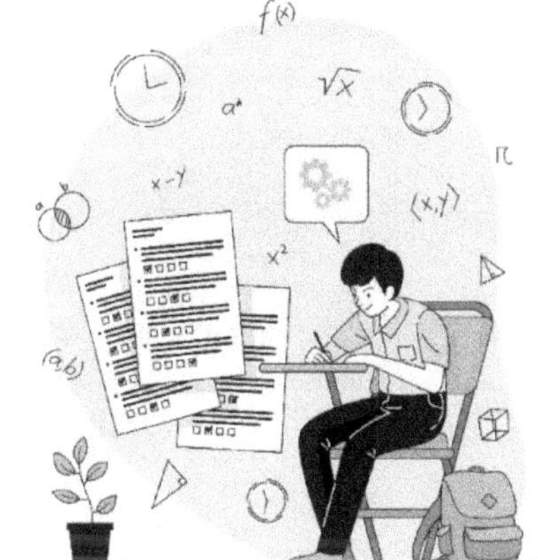

It's almost always better to start the guessing process too early than too late. It only takes a few seconds to remember something and answer the question from knowledge. Carefully eliminating wrong answer choices takes longer. Plus, going through the process of eliminating answer choices can actually help jog your memory.

Summary: Start the guessing process as soon as you decide that you can't answer the question based on your knowledge.

How to Narrow Down the Choices

The next chapter in this book (**Test-Taking Strategies**) includes a wide range of strategies for how to approach questions and how to look for answer choices to eliminate. You will definitely want to read those carefully, practice them, and figure out which ones work best for you. Here though, we're going to address a mindset rather than a particular strategy.

Your odds of guessing an answer correctly depend on how many options you are choosing from.

Number of options left	5	4	3	2	1
Odds of guessing correctly	20%	25%	33%	50%	100%

You can see from this chart just how valuable it is to be able to eliminate incorrect answers and make an educated guess, but there are two things that many test takers do that cause them to miss out on the benefits of guessing:

- Accidentally eliminating the correct answer
- Selecting an answer based on an impression

We'll look at the first one here, and the second one in the next section.

To avoid accidentally eliminating the correct answer, we recommend a thought exercise called **the $5 challenge**. In this challenge, you only eliminate an answer choice from contention if you are willing to bet $5 on it being wrong. Why $5? Five dollars is a small but not insignificant amount of money. It's an amount you could afford to lose but wouldn't want to throw away. And while losing $5 once might not hurt too much, doing it twenty times will set you back $100. In the same way, each small decision you make—eliminating a choice here, guessing on a question there—won't by itself impact your score very much, but when you put them all together, they can make a big difference. By holding each answer choice elimination decision to a higher standard, you can reduce the risk of accidentally eliminating the correct answer.

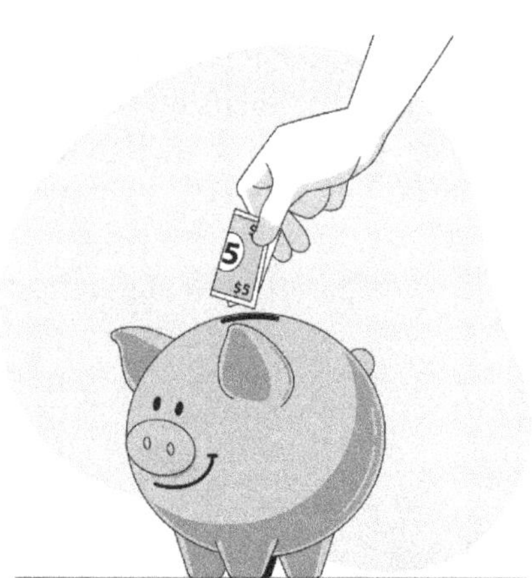

The $5 challenge can also be applied in a positive sense: If you are willing to bet $5 that an answer choice *is* correct, go ahead and mark it as correct.

Summary: Only eliminate an answer choice if you are willing to bet $5 that it is wrong.

Which Answer to Choose

You're taking the test. You've run into a hard question and decided you'll have to guess. You've eliminated all the answer choices you're willing to bet $5 on. Now you have to pick an answer. Why do we even need to talk about this? Why can't you just pick whichever one you feel like when the time comes?

The answer to these questions is that if you don't come into the test with a plan, you'll rely on your impression to select an answer choice, and if you do that, you risk falling into a trap. The test writers know that everyone who takes their test will be guessing on some of the questions, so they intentionally write wrong answer choices to seem plausible. You still have to pick an answer though, and if the wrong answer choices are designed to look right, how can you ever be sure that you're not falling for their trap? The best solution we've found to this dilemma is to take the decision out of your hands entirely. Here is the process we recommend:

Once you've eliminated any choices that you are confident (willing to bet $5) are wrong, select the first remaining choice as your answer.

Whether you choose to select the first remaining choice, the second, or the last, the important thing is that you use some preselected standard. Using this approach guarantees that you will not be enticed into selecting an answer choice that looks right, because you are not basing your decision on how the answer choices look.

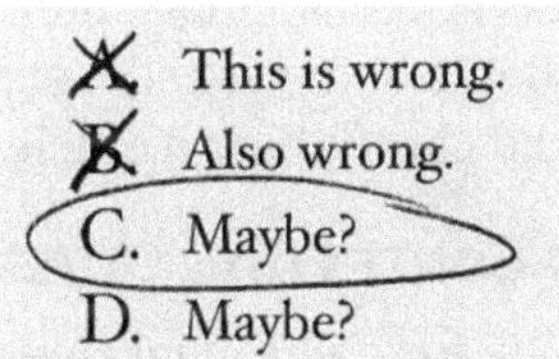

This is not meant to make you question your knowledge. Instead, it is to help you recognize the difference between your knowledge and your impressions. There's a huge difference between thinking an answer is right because of what you know, and thinking an answer is right because it looks or sounds like it should be right.

Summary: To ensure that your selection is appropriately random, make a predetermined selection from among all answer choices you have not eliminated.

Test-Taking Strategies

This section contains a list of test-taking strategies that you may find helpful as you work through the test. By taking what you know and applying logical thought, you can maximize your chances of answering any question correctly!

It is very important to realize that every question is different and every person is different: no single strategy will work on every question, and no single strategy will work for every person. That's why we've included all of them here, so you can try them out and determine which ones work best for different types of questions and which ones work best for you.

Question Strategies

✓ Read Carefully

Read the question and the answer choices carefully. Don't miss the question because you misread the terms. You have plenty of time to read each question thoroughly and make sure you understand what is being asked. Yet a happy medium must be attained, so don't waste too much time. You must read carefully and efficiently.

✓ Contextual Clues

Look for contextual clues. If the question includes a word you are not familiar with, look at the immediate context for some indication of what the word might mean. Contextual clues can often give you all the information you need to decipher the meaning of an unfamiliar word. Even if you can't determine the meaning, you may be able to narrow down the possibilities enough to make a solid guess at the answer to the question.

✓ Prefixes

If you're having trouble with a word in the question or answer choices, try dissecting it. Take advantage of every clue that the word might include. Prefixes can be a huge help. Usually, they allow you to determine a basic meaning. *Pre-* means before, *post-* means after, *pro-* is positive, *de-* is negative. From prefixes, you can get an idea of the general meaning of the word and try to put it into context.

✓ Hedge Words

Watch out for critical hedge words, such as *likely, may, can, often, almost, mostly, usually, generally, rarely*, and *sometimes*. Question writers insert these hedge phrases to cover every possibility. Often an answer choice will be wrong simply because it leaves no room for exception. Be on guard for answer choices that have definitive words such as *exactly* and *always*.

✓ Switchback Words

Stay alert for *switchbacks*. These are the words and phrases frequently used to alert you to shifts in thought. The most common switchback words are *but, although*, and *however*. Others include *nevertheless, on the other hand, even though, while, in spite of, despite*, and *regardless of*. Switchback words are important to catch because they can change the direction of the question or an answer choice.

⊘ Face Value

When in doubt, use common sense. Accept the situation in the problem at face value. Don't read too much into it. These problems will not require you to make wild assumptions. If you have to go beyond creativity and warp time or space in order to have an answer choice fit the question, then you should move on and consider the other answer choices. These are normal problems rooted in reality. The applicable relationship or explanation may not be readily apparent, but it is there for you to figure out. Use your common sense to interpret anything that isn't clear.

Answer Choice Strategies

⊘ Answer Selection

The most thorough way to pick an answer choice is to identify and eliminate wrong answers until only one is left, then confirm it is the correct answer. Sometimes an answer choice may immediately seem right, but be careful. The test writers will usually put more than one reasonable answer choice on each question, so take a second to read all of them and make sure that the other choices are not equally obvious. As long as you have time left, it is better to read every answer choice than to pick the first one that looks right without checking the others.

⊘ Answer Choice Families

An answer choice family consists of two (in rare cases, three) answer choices that are very similar in construction and cannot all be true at the same time. If you see two answer choices that are direct opposites or parallels, one of them is usually the correct answer. For instance, if one answer choice says that quantity *x* increases and another either says that quantity *x* decreases (opposite) or says that quantity *y* increases (parallel), then those answer choices would fall into the same family. An answer choice that doesn't match the construction of the answer choice family is more likely to be incorrect. Most questions will not have answer choice families, but when they do appear, you should be prepared to recognize them.

⊘ Eliminate Answers

Eliminate answer choices as soon as you realize they are wrong, but make sure you consider all possibilities. If you are eliminating answer choices and realize that the last one you are left with is also wrong, don't panic. Start over and consider each choice again. There may be something you missed the first time that you will realize on the second pass.

⊘ Avoid Fact Traps

Don't be distracted by an answer choice that is factually true but doesn't answer the question. You are looking for the choice that answers the question. Stay focused on what the question is asking for so you don't accidentally pick an answer that is true but incorrect. Always go back to the question and make sure the answer choice you've selected actually answers the question and is not merely a true statement.

⊘ Extreme Statements

In general, you should avoid answers that put forth extreme actions as standard practice or proclaim controversial ideas as established fact. An answer choice that states the "process should be used in certain situations, if..." is much more likely to be correct than one that states the "process should be discontinued completely." The first is a calm rational statement and doesn't even make a definitive, uncompromising stance, using a hedge word *if* to provide wiggle room, whereas the second choice is far more extreme.

✓ Benchmark

As you read through the answer choices and you come across one that seems to answer the question well, mentally select that answer choice. This is not your final answer, but it's the one that will help you evaluate the other answer choices. The one that you selected is your benchmark or standard for judging each of the other answer choices. Every other answer choice must be compared to your benchmark. That choice is correct until proven otherwise by another answer choice beating it. If you find a better answer, then that one becomes your new benchmark. Once you've decided that no other choice answers the question as well as your benchmark, you have your final answer.

✓ Predict the Answer

Before you even start looking at the answer choices, it is often best to try to predict the answer. When you come up with the answer on your own, it is easier to avoid distractions and traps because you will know exactly what to look for. The right answer choice is unlikely to be word-for-word what you came up with, but it should be a close match. Even if you are confident that you have the right answer, you should still take the time to read each option before moving on.

General Strategies

✓ Tough Questions

If you are stumped on a problem or it appears too hard or too difficult, don't waste time. Move on! Remember though, if you can quickly check for obviously incorrect answer choices, your chances of guessing correctly are greatly improved. Before you completely give up, at least try to knock out a couple of possible answers. Eliminate what you can and then guess at the remaining answer choices before moving on.

✓ Check Your Work

Since you will probably not know every term listed and the answer to every question, it is important that you get credit for the ones that you do know. Don't miss any questions through careless mistakes. If at all possible, try to take a second to look back over your answer selection and make sure you've selected the correct answer choice and haven't made a costly careless mistake (such as marking an answer choice that you didn't mean to mark). This quick double check should more than pay for itself in caught mistakes for the time it costs.

✓ Pace Yourself

It's easy to be overwhelmed when you're looking at a page full of questions; your mind is confused and full of random thoughts, and the clock is ticking down faster than you would like. Calm down and maintain the pace that you have set for yourself. Especially as you get down to the last few minutes of the test, don't let the small numbers on the clock make you panic. As long as you are on track by monitoring your pace, you are guaranteed to have time for each question.

✓ Don't Rush

It is very easy to make errors when you are in a hurry. Maintaining a fast pace in answering questions is pointless if it makes you miss questions that you would have gotten right otherwise. Test writers like to include distracting information and wrong answers that seem right. Taking a little extra time to avoid careless mistakes can make all the difference in your test score. Find a pace that allows you to be confident in the answers that you select.

⊘ Keep Moving

Panicking will not help you pass the test, so do your best to stay calm and keep moving. Taking deep breaths and going through the answer elimination steps you practiced can help to break through a stress barrier and keep your pace.

Final Notes

The combination of a solid foundation of content knowledge and the confidence that comes from practicing your plan for applying that knowledge is the key to maximizing your performance on test day. As your foundation of content knowledge is built up and strengthened, you'll find that the strategies included in this chapter become more and more effective in helping you quickly sift through the distractions and traps of the test to isolate the correct answer.

Now that you're preparing to move forward into the test content chapters of this book, be sure to keep your goal in mind. As you read, think about how you will be able to apply this information on the test. If you've already seen sample questions for the test and you have an idea of the question format and style, try to come up with questions of your own that you can answer based on what you're reading. This will give you valuable practice applying your knowledge in the same ways you can expect to on test day.

Good luck and good studying!

Assessment

Physical and Psychosocial

General Health History

Components of a general health history include:

- Reason for seeking care
  - Sometimes referred to as the **chief complaint**
  - Allows client to state his or her priorities and objectives
- Past health history, including duration of diabetes
- Concurrent medical problems
- Family health history
- Allergies to food and medicine
- Immunizations, such as flu and pneumonia vaccines
- Medications (name, dosage, frequency), including over-the-counter and homeopathic medications
- Nutrition history, such as dietary recall and personal/cultural preferences in addition to screening for food insecurity
- Habits, such as alcohol, tobacco, caffeine, and recreational drug use
- Exercise and activity patterns
- Rest and sleep patterns
- Stress level and coping mechanisms
- Social support systems
- Cultural preferences with regard to healthcare practices, family support, and food preferences

Physical Health Status

Physical health can affect a person's ability to engage in self-care behavior.

- An acutely ill person may not be ready to learn and may be unable to concentrate on education.
- Chronic illness can interfere with the ability to meet the challenges of diabetes self-care on a day-to-day basis. Complex medication regimens may need to be addressed and the potential for drug interactions considered.
- People who are acutely or chronically ill may need shorter teaching sessions, and recommendations may need to be modified or adapted. For example, the exercise recommendation may need to be modified or adapted for people who have neuropathy or hypertension.
- Visual impairment can affect the ability to safely self-administer medications or insulin. Adaptive equipment, such as talking blood glucose meters and syringe magnifiers, is available for those with visual impairment.

Functional Challenges

Many people who have physical limitations will need to learn how to do self-care tasks within those limitations, and support is available to them for that process:

- Occupational therapists are trained to help people perform activities of daily living as independently as possible.
- Adaptive devices are available for testing blood sugar and for drawing and injecting insulin.
- Social and family support is important, as significant others may be needed to pre-draw insulin syringes. The diabetes educator may be called upon to teach insulin preparation and care to families and caregivers of stroke victims.
- Patients who have had amputations need support in dealing with limited mobility. Education on exercise as an integral part of diabetes management will need to be modified. Wheelchair users can be encouraged to move as much as possible and to use light handheld weights or soup cans to exercise the upper body.

Functional Assessment for Visual Impairment

Assess ability to read printed information and medication labels:

- Effect of print size
- Effect of lighting
- Use of magnifying devices

Assess ability to read syringe markings:

- Effect of syringe size and size of syringe markings
- Effect of lighting
- Use of syringe magnifier
- Request demonstration of drawing insulin into syringe to correct amount and/or evaluate cost/benefit of using insulin pen, premixed insulin, or prefilled syringes as needed.

Assess ability to self-monitor blood sugar:

- Request demonstration
- Assess need and cost/benefit of using talking meter as needed

Assess ability to verbalize correct timing, frequency, and dose of prescribed insulin.

Assess ability to correctly inject insulin and request demonstration.

Assess understanding of causes, prevention, recognition, and treatment of hypoglycemia and ability to respond to low blood sugar.

Assessment Data for Newly Diagnosed Clients

Initial diabetes education should begin as soon as feasible. This may be in the hospital or outpatient setting. Before beginning initial education, it is important to assess:

- Current health status
- Baseline understanding of the diabetes diagnosis and its implications
- Attitudes and beliefs about diabetes and self-care
- Emotional response to diagnosis and readiness to learn
- Current level of knowledge and skill related to diabetes self-care

- Age
- Functional status
- Preferred learning style
- Home/social situation and identification of helpers
- Cultural influences and language

Reassessment is recommended at later stages to evaluate adjustment and assimilation of self-care behavior.

Differentiating Between Presentation of Type 1 and 2 Diabetes

The patient with type 1 diabetes often presents with abrupt onset of illness. Symptoms of hyperglycemia include polyuria, polydipsia, extreme hunger, weakness, and recent history of unexplained weight loss. If ketoacidosis is present, symptoms may include dehydration, tachycardia, orthostatic hypotension, and abdominal pain. The patient may also present with fruity acetone breath. Patients who present with type 1 diabetes are often younger than the age of 30 with a lean body type.

Typically, patients are over the age of 40 when diagnosed with type 2 diabetes, but onset in children and young adults is increasingly common. The patient may exhibit no signs of hyperglycemia, as the diagnosis is often an incidental finding. Family history of diabetes, excess body weight, and sedentary lifestyle are risk factors for type 2 diabetes. Certain ethnic groups have higher incidence of type 2 diabetes, namely Native Americans, Alaska Natives, Hispanics, and African Americans.

Comprehensive Foot Assessment

According to the American Diabetes Association, the components of a complete foot assessment include:

- Inspection for injury, skin breakdown, fungal infections, blisters, red marks from ill-fitting shoes, deformities, dryness or cracking, and condition of the toenails.
- Assessment of foot pulses and other signs of circulation.
- Testing for loss of protective sensation (LOPS) with a monofilament and by assessing any one of the following:
    - Vibration sensation
    - Pinprick sensation
    - Ankle reflexes
    - Vibration perception threshold

Foot assessment should also include screening for peripheral artery disease, determining history of intermittent claudication, and possibly performing an ankle-brachial index. History should include asking about high-risk conditions for amputation, including:

- Tobacco use
- Previous foot ulcer or amputation
- Neuropathic symptoms
- Visual impairment
- Poor glycemic control

The Wound Ischemia Foot Infection (WIFI) staging system has proven increasingly useful, not only in the assessment of PAD, but also for predicting risk for foot ulcers and predicting wound healing.

Monofilament Test

The American Diabetes Association recommends a thorough foot exam by a healthcare provider at least once a year. This includes testing for loss of protective sensation (LOPS) with a 10-gram monofilament.

This noninvasive procedure uses a flexible bristle to touch the sole, or plantar surface, of the foot, testing the client's ability to detect injury to the foot. People who cannot feel the monofilament are at higher risk for undetected foot injury and amputation.

The procedure involves having the client remove shoes and socks and sitting with eyes closed. The provider touches the plantar surface of each foot in several spots and asks the client to indicate each time the monofilament is felt. If the client does not feel the monofilament, he or she is at increased risk for serious foot problems. This client should be counseled on good foot care practices including checking his or her own feet each day for injury.

Ankle Brachial Index

The ankle brachial index (ABI) is a test for peripheral artery disease (PAD). Peripheral artery disease is a serious condition that is common in people with diabetes; it is often asymptomatic.

Clients with symptoms of PAD, such as intermittent claudication, should have a diagnostic ABI. Intermittent claudication is described as lower extremity pain that occurs during physical activity such as walking and subsides with rest. Other criteria for performing an ABI on people with diabetes include age over 50, smoking/e-cigarette use, hypertension, dyslipidemia, or diabetes duration of more than 10 years.

The ABI measures blood pressure in the ankle and at the arm while the client is at rest, and then is repeated 5 minutes after walking on a treadmill. Ankle pressure is measured using a standard cuff placed around the calf and a Doppler. Normally, the pressure at both areas should be approximately the same. In PAD, ankle pressures are lower than arm pressures, indicating narrowing of the arteries.

Assessment of Acanthosis Nigricans

Acanthosis nigricans is a skin condition that occurs in up to 90% of children with type 2 diabetes. It is an indicator of hyperinsulinemia and insulin resistance. Acanthosis nigricans is most commonly found in obese dark-skinned children, occurring about 25% more frequently in African American children than in those of other ethnicities.

Acanthosis nigricans is characterized by raised, dark brownish to black patches that are velvety to the touch. It most commonly occurs on the back of the neck and other body folds. It can occur at other areas of increased body friction, such as knees and elbows. It can sometimes appear as ring around the neck. Parents or caregivers may mistake the dark coloration for dirt or poor body hygiene and may try to scrub it off.

The condition usually resolves when the underlying insulin resistance is addressed.

Insulin Injection Site Assessment

The client's insulin injection technique should be reviewed periodically. Clients should understand the importance of proper site selection and rotation. Site rotation prevents hypertrophy, a thickening of the fatty tissue that results from overuse of the same site.

Injection site assessment includes inspection for signs and symptoms of infection, such as puffiness or redness. Excessive bruising may indicate a bleeding disorder or improper injection technique. Redness may indicate that the client is using impure insulin or is sensitive to something, such as latex or an additive to the insulin. Insulin allergies are rare with the use of human insulin, which is highly purified. Rotating sites also reduces local irritation.

Tissue atrophy can result from impure insulin and appears as a pitting of the fatty tissue at the injection site. This problem has become less common with the use of human insulin.

Assessing for Alcohol Abuse

Alcohol can affect blood sugar and impair the judgment needed for good self-care. It can also be dangerous when used with medications to treat diabetes, such as sulfonylureas, metformin, and insulin. When taken with insulin or a sulfonylurea, alcohol can trigger hypoglycemia. If taken with metformin, it can cause lactic acidosis.

Assessment of alcohol abuse can be challenging because many people are inaccurate or dishonest in their reporting due to shame, denial, or fear of reprisal from the healthcare provider.

Clients under the influence of alcohol may exhibit staggering gait, slurred speech, irritability, and mental confusion. These symptoms are also seen with hypoglycemia.

Excessive alcohol consumption may also mimic ketoacidosis, producing fruity breath, drowsiness, and coma.

Assessment of alcohol intake includes asking the client how much he or she drinks. This can include asking about how much is consumed in a typical week and the largest amount consumed at one time. Since increased tolerance is a sign of addiction, it is important to ask how much the person needs to become intoxicated.

Pediatric Assessments

Toddlers with Diabetes

Naps and other sleep patterns of a toddler may interfere with regular feedings. Nighttime feedings are often required to prevent nocturnal hypoglycemia. Normal toddler behaviors, such as defiance, can increase the challenges of checking blood sugar, taking insulin, and eating properly. Assessment should include an exploration of how the parents negotiate these behaviors. Toddlers also often have erratic eating patterns and specific food preferences. They usually require three meals and at least three snacks per day. The timing of these meals and snacks is important for a child using insulin.

Activity level can be sporadic. Frequent rest periods are counteracted by bursts of intense activity. Extra snacks may be needed to prevent hypoglycemia.

Toddlers are at a high risk for dehydration. Assessment of a parent's ability to prevent, detect, and respond to this is important.

Toddlers may not be able to detect hypoglycemia. Toddlers may exhibit hypoglycemia with staggering gait, uncoordinated movements, or inactivity. Parents of toddlers may have to test blood sugar frequently to detect hypoglycemia because normal toddler behaviors, such as irritability or defiance, may mask hypoglycemic symptoms.

Adolescents with Diabetes

Puberty in adolescence can be delayed due to poor glycemic control. Physical characteristics of puberty onset are:

- Girls: breast buds, pubic hair, menses (normally at 10–11 years of age)
- Boys: pubic hair, enlargement of testicles (normally at 12–16 years of age)

Due to hormonal changes in puberty, glycemic control deteriorates during this time, even with higher insulin doses.

Psychosocial issues of adolescence include:

- Independence from parents
- Increased awareness of body image
- Increased importance of peer group
- More challenges within the parent-child relationship
- More risk-taking behavior
- Increased sexual awareness and development of sexual relationships

An adolescent with diabetes may struggle more with body image issues related to checking blood sugar, using insulin, and being labeled as "a diabetic." Risk-taking behavior may interfere with good self-care practices. Independence may be hampered by parents wanting or needing to remain actively involved in diabetes management.

Pregnancy prevention is of utmost importance and the elevated risks of unplanned pregnancy in diabetes must be discussed.

Family Assessment

Social Support and Family Dynamics

Assessment of social support is important because research shows that active family support improves diabetes outcomes for children and adults alike. Conversely, people who do not have a strong social support system are less motivated to engage in self-care. However, social dynamics can also hinder a person's diabetes self-management if significant others downgrade its importance. Therefore, assessment of social and family dynamics must explore the positive and negative effects of the social environment on the individual.

Assessment of family dynamics can include inviting family members to attend appointments and diabetes education programs with the person who has diabetes. This allows for observation of how family members interact and problem-solve together.

It is important to question clients about their support system. They can be asked who helps them with their diabetes management and what they find most helpful from others. It is also important to explore what barriers others present and how the person with diabetes would like things to be different.

Influence of Family and Social Support on Diabetes Self-Care

Diabetes self-care pervades all aspects of the person's life and much of it takes place within a social context. Family and friends can have a significant impact on a person's self-care behavior.

- The major social influence on children is parents.
- The major social influence on adolescents is peers.
- The major social influences on adults are spouses, friends, co-workers, and family members.

Social influences can enhance self-care if significant people are supportive. People are more likely to engage in positive self-care behavior when supported by their social network. Social influence can have a negative impact if others are not supportive or undermine self-care efforts.

Social assessment includes finding out:

- Who helps with diabetes management?
- Who hinders diabetes management?
- What is needed for feeling supported?
- Where can additional support be found?
- How can the healthcare provider help increase social support resources?

Data to Collect in the Family Assessment of a Child with Diabetes

Determine the normal developmental level of the child. Assess if diabetes is interfering with the child's age-appropriate tasks. Ascertain if the child is at a developmental level appropriate for performing self-care procedures such as checking blood sugar or administering an insulin injection.

Identify how the tasks of diabetes management are distributed. Ask who is responsible for each of the management areas and at what times. Studies indicate that a child is at risk for poor glycemic control when there is disagreement among family members with regard to the delegation of these tasks.

The psychological response of family to diagnosis should be explored. Anxiety and depression are common in parents, especially in the first year after diagnosis. Other common reactions are parental guilt and anger toward the child. Parents may also be fearful of hypoglycemia and the child's risk for long-term complications.

Other assessment data includes:

- Family's understanding of diabetes diagnosis, significance, and treatment
- Parents' perceptions of child's ability to participate in diabetes management
- Child's eating habits
- Child's activity patterns
- Child's social adjustment to diabetes (i.e., effect on peer relationships and activities)
- Immunizations

Assessment of Economic Factors

People with diabetes pay about three times more for out-of-pocket medical expenditures than those without diabetes. Poverty can affect the person's ability to have the food, shelter, and other resources necessary for proper self-management. A comprehensive assessment includes asking the patient directly if he or she has the resources needed to practice diabetes self-care.

Community resources may include:

- Government medical programs such as Medicare and Medicaid
- Government food programs such as SNAP benefits and WIC
- Local groups, such as the Lions Club, that may help those with visual impairment
- Low-cost or free diabetes education programs in the community
- Community food banks
- State vocational training resources

Mental Health Well-Being

Depression

While depression is a common problem in the general population, its incidence is roughly three times higher among people with diabetes. It is estimated that depression affects 15–20% of people with diabetes.

Depression can cause impairment in personal, social, and occupational functioning, and can significantly affect the self-care behaviors necessary for diabetes management. It is a condition in which the person experiences persistent feelings of sadness and/or a lack of pleasure or interest in almost all activities. Other symptoms may include feelings of guilt or worthlessness, sleep disturbance, low energy, hopelessness, and difficulty making decisions.

Impact of Depression on Diabetes Self-Management

Diabetes educators can screen for depression by asking a series of questions. The 2026 ADA Standards recommend annual screening for depression in clients with diabetes, particularly in the older adult population that are especially prone towards depression, in individuals with a history of depression, in individuals struggling to meet their goals in diabetes self-management, and in individuals experiencing complications secondary to diabetes.

Screening questions for depression include:

- Do you feel sad much of the day, on most days?
- Have you gained or lost weight without trying?
- Do you have trouble falling asleep or do you sleep too much?
- Do you feel anxious most days?
- Are you low on energy most days?
- Have you lost interest or pleasure in things that you usually like?
- Do you feel guilty or worthless?
- Are you having trouble concentrating or making decisions?
- Do you think about death and dying a lot?
- Have you thought about suicide or made any such plans?

Assessing for Fears Associated with Diabetes

It is important to assess the client for diabetes-related fears, since anxiety and phobias can interfere with treatment adherence and self-care behavior.

Asking clients how they feel about common diabetes-related fears can be helpful in establishing trust and can provide an opportunity to help them deal with anxieties. Observing nonverbal behavior and body language can uncover fears that the client is harboring. If a client resists blood glucose monitoring, he or she may be afraid of blood, needles, or invasive procedures. If a client is resistant to using insulin or certain medications, he or she may have a fear of hypoglycemia.

Common diabetes-related fears include:

- Fear of blood
- Fear of needles
- Fear of hypoglycemia
- Fear of rotating injection sites
- Fear of complications
- Fear of weight gain

Validated assessment tools for diabetes-related fears are available. These include:

- Hypoglycemia Fear Survey
- Diabetes Fear of Injecting and Self-Testing Questionnaire
- Fear of Progression in Chronic Disease

CHANGE THEORY

HEALTH BELIEF MODEL, LOCUS OF CONTROL THEORY, AND SELF-EFFICACY THEORY

Health belief model: People are more likely to engage in health behaviors if they perceive that the benefits of taking action outweigh the costs. In addition, this model suggests that people are more likely to adhere to self-care practices if they believe that their condition is serious enough to warrant behavior change and that they are susceptible to poor outcomes if they do not practice these behaviors.

Locus of control theory: People with an internal locus of control are more likely to make health behavior changes than those with an external locus of control. People with an internal locus of control believe that their health outcome is dependent upon their own actions rather than the actions of others or chance.

Self-efficacy theory: People who feel confident that they can perform health behaviors are more likely to engage in these behaviors than people who lack this confidence.

Each of these models helps educators assess the belief systems that determine adoption of health behaviors and adherence to diabetes self-care practices.

COMPONENTS OF THE HEALTH BELIEF MODEL

Components of the health belief model include:

- **Perceived benefits:** People who feel that they will reap benefits from engaging in self-care behaviors will be more likely to learn and apply these skills.
- **Perceived costs:** Costs include financial expense, time spent and energy invested. People who perceive that the benefits outweigh the costs are more likely to engage in the learning process and make the necessary changes.
- **Severity of diabetes and complications:** Disability, illness, and loss of productivity are markers of disease severity. People who believe that diabetes is a serious condition are more likely to accept education.
- **Susceptibility:** Those who perceive that the negative consequences of diabetes can happen to them are more willing to engage in education. Those who feel they have "borderline" or "mild" diabetes may not believe that education is necessary for them.

According to research, perceived susceptibility and disease severity are the strongest predictors for behavior change.

Review Video: What is the Health Belief Model?
Visit mometrix.com/academy and enter code: 954833

Transtheoretical Model of Behavior Change

Stages of change according to the transtheoretical model of behavior change:

1. **Precontemplation:** The person is not actively thinking about making any behavioral changes. This may be due to believing that the changes are not important or achievable or that the costs of change outweigh the benefits. If asked, the person would say that they are not planning to make any changes in the next 6 months.
2. **Contemplation:** The person is thinking about making changes within the next 6 months, but has not made any changes yet.
3. **Preparation:** The person has decided to change and is making plans to do so. For example, he or she has begun researching weight loss programs but has not yet started.
4. **Action:** The person has started making the changes within the past 6 months.
5. **Maintenance:** The person has made the changes and maintained them for 6 months or more.

The progression through these stages is not always linear and relapse is common. Recycling is a term used when a person goes back to a previous stage after relapse.

Intervention Strategies Based on the Client's Stage of Change

Intervention strategies based on stage of change:

Precontemplation

- The person may actively resist change.
- Help client identify feelings and beliefs in a supportive way.

Contemplation

- The person may be ambivalent about change.
- Build confidence and support efforts.

Preparation

- Patient begins to visualize future self.
- Help with setting short- and long-term goals.
- Provide encouragement and resources.

Action

- Patient is practicing new behaviors.
- Help strengthen client's commitment to the new behavior.
- Assist with problem-solving.

Maintenance

- The person has engaged in the new behavior for 6 or more months.
- Continue to support behaviors and self-efficacy.

Relapse

- The person has returned to any of the other earlier stages of change.
- Help client overcome feelings of failure.
- Avoid showing signs of disappointment or annoyance.
- Explore causes of relapse.
- Encourage movement to the next stage of change.

VARIABLES THAT INFLUENCE BEHAVIORAL CHANGE

The transtheoretical model describes stages of psychological readiness that a person goes through in the behavior change process. This model stipulates that there are two major variables that affect the decision to make change.

- **Decisional balance** involves weighing the pros and cons of making the change. If the person perceives that the benefits and rewards of a behavior outweigh the costs and disadvantages, he or she is more likely to make the change.
- **Self-efficacy** is the person's self-confidence that he or she can actually initiate and maintain the proposed behavior change. The higher the self-efficacy, the greater the chance the person will make the change. Studies have indicated that self-efficacy is an important variable in diabetes self-management behaviors.

SELF-EFFICACY AND DIABETES MANAGEMENT

Self-efficacy refers to a person's level of confidence in his or her ability to perform a behavior or set of behaviors. Studies show that people with diabetes who have high self-efficacy tend to be more active in self-care, have better emotional health, and maintain better glycemic control than those with low self-efficacy. Assessing self-efficacy can help target areas of educational need. The Diabetes Empowerment Scale (DES) is a 28-item questionnaire that measures diabetes self-efficacy.

Informal assessment of self-efficacy can include asking clients how confident they feel in performing specific diabetes-related behaviors such as checking blood sugar, eating the right amount of carbohydrate, or responding to low blood sugar. Using a scale of 0–10 is recommended when asking the client to rate confidence (i.e., 0 = not all confident; 10 = very confident).

Self-Management Behaviors and Knowledge

EATING HABITS AND PREFERENCES

NUTRITIONAL ASSESSMENT

Obesity and history of weight gain are common findings during a nutrition assessment in type 2 diabetes. Asking the patient for a dietary recall can help identify poor food choices. Dietary recall can be done by asking the patient to remember what they have eaten in the past 24–48 hours or by asking them to keep a food diary.

Nutritional assessment includes measurement of height and weight and calculation of body mass index (BMI). BMI should be measured annually in patients who are obese or overweight, along with an additional measurement of body fat.

Assessment of the client's level of physical activity helps evaluate energy expenditure. The healthcare provider should make note of the daily food patterns and the proportional intake of all major food groups.

Other nutritional assessment items should include:

- Regularity and spacing of meals
- Timing of meals (Does the client eat breakfast? Does the client eat most calories at the end of the day?)
- Methods of food preparation
- Recent blood sugar patterns
- Cultural practices with regard to food and food preparation
- Exposure to food insecurity

Evaluating Effectiveness of Diet and Lifestyle Changes on Blood Glucose

Behavior changes include medical nutrition therapy, exercise, and stress management. The **effects of behavior changes** are usually evaluated at 6 weeks to 3 months following implementation. If blood glucose targets have not been achieved by this time, further changes in nutritional therapy and/or the addition of medication to the regimen are needed.

Educators should avoid the words "diet failure" as the client may interpret this as a personal failure when, in fact, there may be a physiologic need for medication.

As diabetes is a progressive disorder, it is expected that therapy will intensify over time as beta cell function declines. Therefore, evaluation of the therapeutic regimen must be ongoing.

Assessing Knowledge Regarding Carbohydrate Intake

When assessing the client's current understanding regarding the impact of carbohydrates on diabetes, consider the following:

- Assess the client's understanding that carbohydrate is the type of food with the greatest effect on postprandial blood glucose levels.
- Ask the client to give examples of carbohydrate foods, ensuring that starch, sugar and sweet foods, fruits, and milk are all included.
- Ensure that the client understands that healthy carbohydrates such as whole grain, fat- free or low-fat dairy products, fruits, and vegetables should not be eliminated from the diet due to concerns about their effect on blood glucose.
- Assess if the client is consuming a consistent amount of carbohydrate from day to day.
- Check to see if the client understands the appropriate amount of carbohydrate that he or she should consume at each meal and each snack.
- Review records of blood glucose monitoring and food diaries to assess the effect of carbohydrate choices and portion sizes.

According to 2026 ADA Standards, evidence shows that there is not an ideal percentage of intake that carbohydrates, protein, and fat should make up of the total calories consumed. Rather, it is acknowledged that diets should be specifically targeted at each individual. The 2026 recommendations stress the importance that carbohydrates, when consumed, should be high in fiber (14 g per 1000 kcal).

Assessing Nutritional Practices of a Person with Type 1 Diabetes

Since people with type 1 diabetes depend upon exogenous insulin, the amount of carbohydrate consumed must closely match insulin dosing.

For those on a fixed insulin dose regimen, consistency in carbohydrate consumption is important. Assess regularity of meals and consistency of carbohydrate portions from day to day.

For clients who adjust their pre-meal insulin doses or use a pump, the educator should assess the client's understanding and application of the prescribed carbohydrate-to-insulin ratio. A common carbohydrate-to-insulin ratio is 15:1, meaning that the client injects 1 unit of rapid or short-acting insulin for each 15 grams of carbohydrate to be consumed. Provide practice exercises to assess the client's ability to adjust the insulin dose for different situations, such as a large meal, a special party, or a late dinner.

Clients with type 1 diabetes are at a higher risk for hypoglycemia. The educator should periodically assess the client's understanding of its prevention and treatment. This includes ensuring that the client is aware that a carbohydrate snack may be needed prior to exercise.

Food Diaries

The food diary is a record kept by the client of everything that he or she eats in a given period of time. It should include the foods eaten, the approximate amounts, time of day, and the situation in which eating occurred. It can be kept for any specified amount of time, such as one full week, one day each week, a few days a month, or a longer amount of time. A complete food diary will also include a record of exercise.

The food diary helps in evaluating food choices and identifying where changes are needed. It is also very useful in correlating blood glucose results with food intake. Issues that can be identified by a food diary include inconsistent eating patterns, inappropriate portion sizes, undesirable food choices, and amount of carbohydrate consumed. Recording the circumstances under which a person eats raises awareness of unconscious consumption and eating to fulfill emotional needs. For those who have already begun medical nutrition therapy, diaries help in evaluating the client's progress toward making the recommended changes.

Activity Habits and Preferences

Assessing Knowledge of Safety Precautions Related to Exercise

When assessing the client's understanding of safety precautions surrounding exercise, consider the following:

- Clients who use insulin and sulfonylurea medication should know that they are at substantial risk for hypoglycemia. Those using insulin should be aware of how to adjust insulin prior to planned exercise. They should also know how to increase carbohydrate intake at times of unplanned exercise. All clients at risk for hypoglycemia should check blood glucose prior to exercise and carry a fast-acting source of carbohydrate during activity.
- Assess clients' adherence to recommendations for using proper footwear and understanding the importance of hydration.
- Ensure that clients know to avoid vigorous exercise in hot, humid conditions and when air quality is poor.

- Clients who use a beta blocker should know that this medication can impair awareness of hypoglycemia and that they should take special precautions to monitor for it and to prevent it.

Assessing Insulin Adjustment During Exercise

Ensure that clients who use insulin understand that they are at significant risk for exercise-induced hypoglycemia. Hypoglycemia can occur during exercise, immediately after exercise, or after a longer period of time. It is important to assess their knowledge and practices with making insulin adjustments for exercise.

Questions to ask include:

- Do you reduce rapid or short-acting insulin prior to exercise? If so, by how much?
    - Reducing by 30–50% effectively decreases risk of hypoglycemia
- Do you reduce intermediate-acting insulin when you are planning to exercise? If so, by how much?
    - Reducing by 10% is recommended
- Do you check your blood glucose before and after exercise?
    - Checking provides feedback on results of insulin adjustment and can signal when blood glucose is becoming too low

Also assess insulin injection technique, ensuring that injections are subcutaneous, not intramuscular.

Assessing Exercise Intensity

For best results, exercise intensity should be sufficient that the client's heart rate is 60–85% of their age-adjusted maximum heart rate. A precise target heart rate can be calculated from the results of an exercise stress test. Alternatively, the following equation can be used to estimate age-adjusted maximum heart rate:

$$220 - \text{Client's age} = \text{Estimated age-adjusted maximum heart rate}$$

The **rating of perceived exertion** can also be used to assess exercise intensity. This is a subjective measure in which the client rates how intense the exercise feels on a scale of 0–10. Zero means there is no effort at all and 10 corresponds with extremely strong or maximal feelings of exertion. An exertion level of 2 (weak) to 5 (strong) is recommended, depending upon the fitness level of the individual.

Medication Practices and Preferences

Medication Assessment

When performing a medication assessment, first ask for a complete list of all of the medications the client is currently taking. Alternatively, the client can bring all of his or her current medications to the appointment. A current medication history includes all prescription and nonprescription medicines, herbal and homeopathic remedies, and vitamins. Patients often forget to include nonprescription medications in their reporting if they are not prompted.

Ask if the client has any known allergies to medication. If the client reports a medication allergy, obtain specific information about the effect of the medication. Be aware that a drug reaction may not be a drug allergy. Sometime patients perceive medication side effects as allergic reactions. Interactions with concurrent medications may also be reported as drug allergies.

Find out what medications the client has used for diabetes in the past. Evaluate if they were effective and how they were tolerated by the client.

Assessing Insulin Injection Technique

Assess patient adherence to the following elements of the insulin injection procedure:

- Washes hands before starting
- Checks insulin vial for type, expiration date and ensures that the insulin is free of sediment, frosting, or other signs of contamination
- Cleanses top of insulin vial with alcohol
- Injects air into the insulin vial equal to the amount of insulin to be injected
- Measures and draws the appropriate amount of insulin
- Selects appropriate site for subcutaneous injection and has a site rotation system
- Administers injection subcutaneously (For most people, this involves lightly grasping a fold of skin and injecting at a 90-degree angle. If very thin, the client should inject at a 45-degree angle to avoid injecting the insulin into muscle.)
- Follows appropriate technique for disposing of sharps waste

Assessing Medication Adherence

When assessing a client's medication adherence, consider the following:

- Is the medication taken on a regular schedule?
- Does the client know the right time to take the medication? For example, glipizide works best when taken 30 minutes before the meal. Other medications, such as metformin, are best taken with food to reduce gastrointestinal upset. Statin medications are most effective when taken at bedtime.
- What does the client do if he or she misses a dose? The client should know not to double the dose of medication when a dose is missed.
- Is the client taking the dose that was prescribed?
- Is the client up to date on laboratory testing of liver and kidney function, as appropriate?
- If using a sulfonylurea or insulin, what is the client's eating pattern and spacing of meals? Meals should be no more than 4–5 hours apart to prevent hypoglycemia.
- What does the client do when blood sugar is low (if applicable)?

Monitoring and Data Collection

Troubleshooting Self-Monitored Blood Glucose Results

A comprehensive analysis of factors affecting blood glucose includes:

- Food:
    - Questions: What did I eat? How much? When?
    - The client should pay particular attention to the amount and type of carbohydrate consumed.
- Exercise:
    - Questions: How much exercise or physical activity have I had? Was it more or less than usual?
    - The client should understand that the blood glucose-lowering effects of exercise can be immediate or prolonged, affecting blood glucose for a period of up to 48 or more hours.

- Medication:
  - Questions: When did I take my diabetes medication (including insulin)? Did I take it at the right time in relation to meals? Did I take the correct dose? Did I properly prepare my insulin (i.e., by rolling the vial of NPH insulin)? Is my medication expired?
- Stress:
  - Questions: Am I under a lot of emotional stress? Am I ill? Do I have an infected sore?
- Blood Glucose Testing:
  - Questions: Did I perform the procedure correctly? Is my meter coded correctly? Are my test strips expired or damaged?

Blood Glucose Monitoring Results Based on Whole Blood or Plasma

Whole blood consists of plasma, red blood cells, white blood cells, and platelets. The **blood glucose** level of whole blood is lower than the blood glucose level of plasma.

Laboratory tests of blood glucose measure glucose in the plasma only, as it can be separated out in the laboratory.

Home blood testing always uses a drop of whole blood. However, most meters are programmed to calibrate results to conform to plasma values. This allows for better comparison between laboratory and home results. A meter that is programmed to report results as plasma values will be close to results reported from a laboratory test.

However, some meters still report results as a whole blood measurement. In this case, results of home glucose monitoring will be lower than if a plasma-calibrated meter had been used. The results of whole blood testing are about 10–15% lower than results of plasma glucose.

Recordkeeping of Self-Monitored Blood Glucose

Good recordkeeping is an essential first step in utilizing the important self-management tool of blood glucose monitoring (BGM).

Although most blood glucose testing meters have an electronic memory function, records of BGM should also be kept on paper. Instruct clients that the electronic memory is an optional convenience for use in writing down results at a later time.

Clients can keep effective records in printed logbooks, on computer spreadsheets, or on notebook paper. A chart indicating blood glucose results corresponding to specific times of day, fashioned in lines or columns, can help to identify patterns. These patterns can then be used to adjust food, exercise, or medication. Clients should distinguish between pre-meal and postprandial results to help interpret the effect of food on blood glucose. They can also keep notes of foods eaten, medications taken, and exercise patterns.

Some clients may prefer to record results as a graph or download graphs of their blood glucose using computer programs. This is an acceptable alternative method of recordkeeping.

USE OF TECHNOLOGY FOR SELF-MONITORING

Self-management technology that is available for the self-monitoring of diabetes includes:

- **Glucometers and continuous glucose monitoring (CGM) systems**: Glucometers remain the most common glucose measuring device, but increasingly CGM systems are used for continuous monitoring of glucose levels. CGM systems alert individuals to high and low glucose levels. CGM systems must be frequently calibrated and sensors changed to ensure accuracy. Training on CGM use should be offered upon initiating and routinely to ensure proper use.
- **Insulin pumps**: Battery-powered devices that deliver pre-set doses of insulin at specific times during the day. Individuals can provide a manual bolus based on eating or to correct hyperglycemia.
- **Smart insulin delivery systems**: Combinations of a CGM system with an insulin pump (known as an automated insulin delivery [AID] system) that, using a software algorithm, adjust insulin administration according to glucose levels read by the CGM. The ADA considers the AID system the standard of care for individuals with diabetes (type 1 or type 2) on insulin and is considered a closed-loop ("artificial pancreas") system.
- **Insulin pens**: Reusable insulin injectors that contain multiple doses of a specified insulin. New needles are attached for each administration and then disposed of.
- **Smart insulin pens**: Reusable insulin injector pens that use a software application and smart phone to adjust insulin dosage automatically based on blood glucose level.
- **Software applications**: Mobile apps to log and track glucose levels, meals, medications, and exercise in one place. Other apps provide databases of calories, carbohydrates, and other nutritional data about foods. Apps can also send reminders regarding medications or glucose testing.
- **Online education**: Online courses, information, and videos for individuals, families, and caregivers. For instance, YouTube videos demonstrate use of various forms of diabetic technology, and UCSF's *Diabetes Education Online* provides information for newly diagnosed individuals and others. Topics vary widely, and include type 1 and type 2 diabetes and living with diabetes. Online education platforms also include resources in a learning library and short classes (lasting 2–4 days) and workshops both in person and online. The ADA provides links to virtual diabetes education programs.
- **Individual portals**: These portals allow individuals access to their electronic health records, including laboratory testing results, and allow easy communication and collaboration with healthcare providers. Individuals can book appointments and request prescription reordering through the portal.

ASSESSING QUALITY OF LIFE IN INDIVIDUALS WITH DIABETES

"Quality of life" is a somewhat ambiguous term, but there is general agreement that it encompasses the client's subjective appraisal of his or her emotional, psychosocial, and physical well-being. Improving quality of life is a primary goal of diabetes self-management education and support (DSMES). Certain aspects of diabetes have been shown to decrease quality of life, such as insulin dependence, retinopathy, and comorbid conditions.

There are several diabetes-specific tools for measuring quality of life. These include:

- Diabetes Quality of Life Measure (DQOL)
- Diabetes Treatment Satisfaction Questionnaire
- Diabetes-Specific Quality of Life Scale (DSQOLS)

Examples of domains measured by these tools include:

- Satisfaction with diabetes treatment
- Impact of treatment, such as experience with hypoglycemia and adherence to dietary guidelines
- Impact of diabetes on social, physical, and vocational functioning
- Psychological aspects, such as worry about future health

Simply asking the client how diabetes is affecting his or her life is an informal and expedient way to assess quality of life.

Barriers to Self-Management in the Older Adult

Functional limitations in the elderly that may affect diabetes self-management include hearing loss, loss of vision, decline in mobility, and cognitive decline. Other challenges may include chronic illness, depression, economic hardship, and lack of social support.

Assessment of functional status includes assessing fine motor skills. This includes observing the client's ability to open pill bottles, use a blood glucose meter, and draw insulin into a syringe. Other functional motor skills to assess are the person's ability to move around, shop and prepare meals.

Assessment of cognitive status includes orientation, memory, and recall. While older people can still learn, assimilating new information takes longer. Information should be presented in a paced or step-wise fashion. Verbal feedback from the client and return demonstration of skills can be used to assess comprehension.

Economic hardship can result in the inability to purchase proper food or medical supplies or to pay for increasing medical bills. The 2026 ADA Standards emphasize the consideration of this barrier when prescribing medications to older adults in order to reduce cost-related noncompliance. Income and resources must be assessed and the client should be connected to community resources whenever possible.

Learning

Elements of a Learning Needs Assessment

Elements of a learning needs assessment include:

- Previous learning, current level of knowledge, and health beliefs about diabetes: "Tell me what you already know about diabetes."
- Patient's goals: "What would you like to learn?"; "What goals do you have for various health measures such as blood pressure, blood sugar, lipid values and bodyweight)?"
- Attitudes and feelings about diabetes and the educational program: "How important is education to you?"; "How can education help you?"
- Preferred learning styles: "How do you prefer to learn (e.g., video, reading, listening, hands-on, etc.)?"; "Do you have any conditions that could affect how you learn (e.g., hearing loss, vision loss, low reading level, second language)?"
- Psychological status: "How are you feeling mentally?" Assess for depression, anxiety, stress, or other factors that could get in the way of learning.
- Social and cultural factors: "Who else should learn with you?"
- Readiness and willingness: "On a scale from 1 to 10, how ready are you to learn (0 = not at all ready; 10 = as ready as I could possibly be)?"

Impact of the Locus of Control on Perceived Learning Needs

Locus of control refers to one's belief about who or what controls health outcomes. The **locus of control** theory provides three possible orientations for this belief system:

Internal locus of control

- The person believes that he or she holds most of the power in determining the outcome of a health event. A person with diabetes who has an internal locus of control will feel that his or her actions make a difference.

External locus of control

- Also known as the "powerful other" orientation
- The person believes that others have the most power in determining their outcome. Healthcare providers are often perceived as powerful others. Those having this orientation may believe that their doctor plays the most important role in their healthcare. Other significant people in the person's life can be perceived as the powerful other.

Chance orientation

- The person believes that fate, luck, or chance determines his or her outcome.

Assessing locus of control can help identify those who do not recognize the important role that self-management plays in positive diabetes outcomes.

Characteristics of the Adult Learner

The adult learner:

- Is self-directed. The adult prefers to have a say in the learning agenda. It is helpful to start by asking the client what he or she would like to learn.
- Needs a reason to learn. The adult wants information that is useful. Teaching content should focus on specific problems rather than comprehensive subject matter.
- Prefers information that is personalized and relevant. Curriculums for adult education should incorporate past experiences of participants. Time should be spent on discussing problems that the participant has identified.
- Is an active learner. Programs should include plenty of opportunity for sharing and problem-solving.

Teaching and Learning Strategies for Adult Learners

Group discussions allow learners to be active participants in their learning. These also make the program more relevant by allowing group members to select content that is important to them. Group discussion provides a forum for practicing problem-solving skills. Group leaders need to be able to keep the group focused and prevent one or two members from dominating.

Demonstration is a preferred strategy for tactile learners. Skills such as blood glucose testing and injecting insulin can be learned by demonstration. The participant should provide a return demonstration to assess learning and receive feedback.

Audiovisual aids help to hold interest by engaging multiple senses and learning styles. Examples include food models, slide show presentations, flip charts, and videos. Audiovisual aids with few or no written words can be especially useful for clients with low literacy.

Role-playing engages learners and allows them to be active in the learning process. Role-plays are helpful in practicing problem-solving skills.

Common Learning Styles and Preferences

Most people have one or two predominant **learning styles**. Assessing a person's preferred learning style can help in tailoring a program to the individual's needs.

- **Visual learners** prefer to see the material being presented. Programs should make use of graphics, charts, models, pictures, books, videos, and demonstrations.
- **Auditory learners** prefer to hear the material being presented. Programs for auditory learners include audio tapes and discussions.
- **Tactile learners** like a hands-on approach. Demonstrations, return demonstrations, and other show-and-tell methods will appeal to this learner.
- **Social learners** learn best in a group environment. These learners will benefit from group classes and workshops where interaction and sharing occur. Referral to community resources can also be beneficial.
- **Solitary learners** prefer to learn 1:1 or independently. Providing reading material and web-based resources are best for these learners.
- **Low literacy clients** present challenges as traditional education normally involves reading material. Programs can be adapted for people with low literacy by using pictorial handouts, videos, and demonstrations. Individual teaching sessions may be necessary for the person with low literacy.

Low Literacy

Assessment can be difficult, as many people with low literacy are ashamed. Building trust is key. Approach the client in a way that normalizes the situation. For example, begin by saying "I have had a lot of clients who had trouble reading the handouts they were given. How are you doing with those?"

Ask clients what the best learning methods are for them. Do they prefer videos, 1-on-1 discussions, or handouts with lots of pictures?

Start with modest goals for learning, focusing on the most important and basic information first. Work up to material that is more complex.

Personalize the content, using phrases such as "your meal plan" and "your diabetes."

Use repetition freely and periodically ask the client to recall what has been discussed.

Use visual aids, mnemonic devices, and analogies to help the client mentally organize the material.

Considerations Related to Learning

Cultural Sensitivity

Cultural sensitivity involves understanding and accepting that others may have differing views of healthcare than the educator. Education that is culturally sensitive is more relevant to the client and promotes a more trusting relationship with the educator.

A thorough assessment includes gathering information about how clients view diabetes and their care from a cultural standpoint.

Cultural perspectives to be included in the assessment:

- Food preferences, including everyday foods, celebratory foods, and foods used for religious purposes
- Role of fasting, if applicable
- Perceived cause of diabetes
- Perceived significance of diabetes
- Fears related to having diabetes

The educator cannot be expected to be an expert on every culture, but is expected to be sensitive that differences exist. The educator should be honest with clients in sharing that he or she would like to learn more about their cultures.

Teaching Methods for the Older Adult

Normal changes in aging can affect the ability to assimilate new information. In addition, comorbidities, such as sensory loss and chronic medical conditions, are common in the elderly client. Teaching sessions should be adapted to these variables.

- The pace of teaching should be reduced to accommodate a slower processing time. A needs assessment is important in identifying priorities. Teaching sessions should focus on 1 or 2 main points and remain brief.
- Reading material should be in print that is easy to read. Blue and green print is often difficult for older people to distinguish. A magnifier should be available for those who need it.
- Audio material and verbal instructions should be clear and concise. Use gestures and visual aids to reinforce verbal instructions. Do not assume a hearing-impaired person is mentally confused.
- Memory aids can help with medication and blood glucose testing adherence. Pill boxes, alarms, calendars, and reminder systems can all be employed.
- Significant others and caregivers should be involved in education whenever possible.

Language Barriers

Body language is often universal. Voice quality, tone, facial expression, and mannerisms all communicate something to the client. The educator should keep his or her voice tone friendly, smile appropriately, and create a relaxed environment for the client.

- The client should be addressed by name and the educator should introduce him- or herself. The voice should be kept at normal tone and volume. Talking loudly may be perceived as shouting.
- Pictorials and visual aids are very helpful in overcoming language barriers. Printed-word resources are available online in many different languages. Medical phrase books are also available in many languages.
- It is best to simplify the material and use one-syllable, common words. Discuss one topic at a time and use short sentences. Gesture and pantomime where appropriate.
- Make use of any translator services available. Beware of using family members as translators. They may pass on their own interpretation of the material, leaving out information they do not want their family member to hear or adding something that they believe should be included.

Indications of a Lack of Understanding Amidst Language Barriers

Lack of effective communication may be exhibited by certain **nonverbal cues** on the part of the client. The client may be nonresponsive when a question is asked. Conversely, he or she may ask questions that are off topic or about something that was already covered. Attempts to change the subject may also signify that the client does not understand the current topic and is attempting to switch to something more understandable.

Clients who do not understand due to a language barrier may also demonstrate lack of participation or engagement in the teaching session. They may close their eyes, sit passively, or fail to ask any questions.

Clients who demonstrate inappropriate laughter or jesting may be trying to cover embarrassment about not understanding the language. On the other hand, a blank expression can also mean that the material is not being communicated. It is important to realize, however, that certain cultures, such as some Asian and Native American cultures, perceive direct eye contact as impolite.

Care and Education Interventions

Disease Process and Approach to Treatment

Diagnostic Criteria for Diabetes

According to the American Diabetes Association, diabetes is diagnosed if any of the following criteria are met:

- HbA1c ≥6.5%
- Fasting plasma glucose (FPG) ≥126 mg/dL. **Fasting** means no caloric intake for 8 or more hours.
- 2-hour plasma glucose ≥200 mg/dL during an oral glucose tolerance test (OGTT). The test should be performed using a glucose load of 75 grams and performed as described by the World Health Organization. Additionally, at least 150 g/day of carbohydrates should be eaten for the three days prior to the OGTT.
- Random plasma glucose ≥200 mg/dL when patient presents with classic symptoms of hyperglycemia, such as polydipsia and polyuria.

If the presence of hyperglycemia is not unequivocal on the HbA1c, FPG, or OGGT, repeat testing is indicated. Repeat testing can be same day using a different test type, or retesting on another day using the same test.

Classification of Risk for Diabetes

Impaired fasting glucose (IFG) and impaired glucose tolerance (IGT) are categories of **increased risk for diabetes**, collectively known as **prediabetes**. They represent an intermediate category where blood glucose levels are elevated above normal, but not high enough to be classified as diabetes. Both conditions are associated with obesity, increased abdominal fat, dyslipidemia, and hypertension.

The American Diabetes Association stipulates that these are not true diagnostic categories, but represent a condition of elevated risk for the development of both diabetes and cardiovascular disease.

- IFG is characterized by fasting plasma glucose levels of 100–125 mg/dL.
- IGT is manifested by 2-hour oral glucose tolerance test values of 140–199 mg/dL.

As of 2026, American Diabetes Association guidelines recommend that one of three criteria can be used to define prediabetes/risk for diabetes in nonpregnant individuals: an HbA1c level of 5.7–6.4%, a fasting plasma glucose of 100–125 mg/dL, or a 2-hour plasma glucose of 140–199 mg/dL during a 75-g oral glucose tolerance test.

Type 1 Diabetes

Pathophysiology of Type 1 Diabetes

Type 1 diabetes is the result of an autoimmune attack on the **beta cells** of the pancreas.

Although hyperglycemic symptoms, and even ketoacidosis, may appear abruptly, the disease begins to develop long before it becomes apparent.

While there is a genetic predisposition, many people with genetic risk do not develop the disease. An environmental or viral trigger is believed necessary for the disease to express itself in predisposed individuals.

Islet cell antibodies appear early in the course of type 1 diabetes and direct their attack against the beta cells. While there are several different islet cell antibodies, a high titer of glutamic acid decarboxylase (GAD) is considered the best immunologic predictor for the development of type 1 diabetes.

The onset of illness is usually abrupt, followed by a "honeymoon period" in which beta cells are in a compensatory phase and temporary normoglycemia results. Ultimately, continued beta cell destruction leads to acute loss of glycemic control, resulting in the permanent need for exogenous insulin.

Causes of Type 1 Diabetes

Causes of pancreatic beta cell destruction other than autoimmune causes include:

- Genetic defects of beta cells can lead to maturity-onset diabetes of the young (MODY), manifested by the onset of hyperglycemia in young people, usually younger than age 25.
- Genetic defects of insulin action result in abnormalities of the insulin receptors, leading to insulin resistance and hyperglycemia.
- Diseases, conditions, and events that can lead to the onset of diabetes include pancreatitis, trauma, infection, cancer, hemochromatosis, and cystic fibrosis.
- Excessive production of hormones that are antagonistic to insulin can cause diabetes. These hormones include growth hormone, cortisol, glucagon, and epinephrine.
- Drugs that can impair insulin secretion and precipitate diabetes in insulin-resistant people include nicotinic acid, glucocorticoids, alpha-interferon, thiazides, and Dilantin.
- Viral infections such as congenital rubella, coxsackievirus B, cytomegalovirus, and mumps have been known to induce diabetes.
- Other genetic syndromes associated with diabetes onset include Down syndrome, Klinefelter syndrome, and Turner syndrome.

Characteristics of Type 1 Diabetes

Characteristics of type 1 diabetes include:

- Caused by autoimmune destruction of the beta cells of the pancreas.
- Leads to an absolute deficiency of endogenous insulin.
- Usually involves rapid destruction of beta cells in children and slower destruction in adults.
- Children and adolescents sometimes present with ketoacidosis as the first sign of the disease.
- Absence of endogenous insulin secretion is manifested by low C-peptide levels.
- Causes include genetic predisposition and environmental factors.
- Patients are usually lean, but normal or overweight status does not preclude diagnosis.
- Patients are also prone to Hashimoto's thyroiditis, Addison's disease, vitiligo, celiac sprue, autoimmune hepatitis, pernicious anemia, and myasthenia gravis.

Review Video: Diabetes Mellitus
Visit mometrix.com/academy and enter code: 501396

Type 2 Diabetes

Pathophysiology of Type 2 Diabetes

Three key concepts related to type 2 diabetes include:

- **Relative insulin deficiency:** Insulin production by the beta cells of the pancreas is insufficient for the body's needs. There is a 50% reduction in beta cell mass in people with type 2 diabetes.
- **Insulin resistance:** Insulin receptors, found mostly on muscle and liver tissue, have developed a resistance to the biological activity of insulin. Insulin resistance is present years before the onset of hyperglycemia.
- **Overproduction of glucose by the liver:** Normally, increased insulin levels in the blood suppress hepatic glucose production. In type 2 diabetes, insulin resistance of hepatic receptors results in continued hepatic glucose production despite circulating insulin levels.

Characteristics of Type 2 Diabetes

Characteristics of type 2 diabetes include:

- Pathophysiology involves insulin resistance and relative insulin deficiency.
- Treatment with exogenous insulin is not needed for immediate survival.
- Unlike type 1 diabetes, there is no autoimmune destruction of pancreatic beta cells.
- Obesity or increased body fat in abdominal region increases the risk.
- Ketoacidosis is rare.
- Often goes undetected for years.
- Hyperglycemia develops gradually in earlier stages of disease and is usually asymptomatic.
- Occurs with higher incidence in people who have hypertension and dyslipidemia.
- Risk factors include increased age, obesity, sedentary lifestyle, positive family history, and personal history of gestational diabetes.
- Genetic predisposition is a significant risk factor.

Maturity-Onset Diabetes of the Young (MODY)

Maturity-onset diabetes of the young (MODY) is a rare type of secondary diabetes associated with inherited genetic defects on chromosomes 7, 12, and 20. Due to these chromosomal defects, beta cell function is impaired, which leads to early onset of mild hyperglycemia. While insulin secretion is impaired, insulin action and sensitivity are unaffected.

Although MODY affects young people, it should not be confused with type 2 diabetes in youth.

Since there is no way to ameliorate the cause of MODY, treatment relies on the traditional cornerstones of therapy for diabetes: medical nutrition therapy, exercise, and medication.

The Honeymoon Period

The honeymoon period is a remission phase that occurs early in the natural course of type 1 diabetes. It is characterized by a temporary improvement in endogenous insulin secretion and a decreased need for injected insulin.

The temporary increase in endogenous insulin production is due to a decrease in the inflammation of the Islets of Langerhans that was caused by the original autoimmune assault. When exogenous insulin is started, inflammation of the beta cells subsides and the beta cells resume insulin production. As the autoimmune disease progresses, these revived cells eventually lose their function and the need for injected insulin resumes or increases.

The honeymoon period typically lasts between 3 and 12 months and is more common in young adults with type 1 diabetes than in younger children with the disease.

During the honeymoon period, insulin doses are decreased to prevent hypoglycemia.

Clients should be prepared for the honeymoon period so that they do not question the diagnosis of type 1 diabetes. If necessary, they should be supported emotionally as the need for insulin inevitably increases.

The Dawn Phenomenon

The dawn phenomenon refers to normal hormonal fluctuations that trigger the liver to release excessive glucose in the latter part of the nightly sleep cycle. It is often responsible for elevated fasting glucose levels in the person with diabetes.

People who do not have diabetes produce the additional insulin needed to maintain normal glucose levels during sleep. People with type 2 diabetes often see higher blood glucose results in the morning due to the dawn phenomenon. Metformin can be an effective medication to address the dawn phenomenon because it decreases glucose production by the liver.

People who require exogenous insulin need to adjust the dose and timing of their medication to provide for a greater insulin need during the pre-waking hours. Long-acting insulin and insulin pump therapy are especially helpful in regulating the variable blood glucose pattern produced by the dawn phenomenon.

People who work rotating shifts or suffer from jet lag require careful adjustment of insulin therapy to accommodate the dawn phenomenon.

The Somogyi Phenomenon

The existence of the Somogyi phenomenon is controversial. However, some people believe it may be a rare cause of fasting hyperglycemia. Theoretically, the Somogyi phenomenon is a rebound effect of nocturnal hypoglycemia. As the blood glucose level drops during prolonged fasting, the counter-regulatory hormones cause an excess release of glucose from the liver as a compensatory mechanism.

Continuous glucose monitoring (CGM) can detect if this phenomenon is causing morning hyperglycemia. Alternatively, sometimes patients are asked to awaken during the night to check their blood glucose to determine if hypoglycemia is triggering the Somogyi effect. This is often not practical as it is difficult to determine the precise time to awaken for the test.

Basal insulin, such as NPH or glargine, usually affects the morning blood glucose. Regardless of the cause of early morning hyperglycemia, adjustment of these insulins is often indicated to offset the rise in blood glucose.

Hypoglycemic Unawareness

Normally, low blood glucose triggers the release of counter-regulatory hormones such as glucagon and epinephrine. Among other things, these hormones are responsible for producing the physical symptoms of hypoglycemia, such as palpitations, sweating, and anxiety.

In **hypoglycemic unawareness**, however, the body fails to release or only produces a small amount of counter-regulatory hormones. As a result, the hypoglycemic patient may experience no symptoms and remain unaware that he or she needs to take action to prevent subsequent coma.

Alternately, symptoms of hypoglycemia may occur at much lower glucose levels than usual, substantially decreasing the window of opportunity for prompt action. Hypoglycemic unawareness clearly presents a serious safety issue, especially for patients with diabetes who require insulin.

In the past, autonomic neuropathy was believed to be the sole cause of hypoglycemic unawareness. However, recent findings suggest that it is largely due to a lack of adaptation by the body to previous episodes of hypoglycemia. Longer duration of diabetes and a history of frequent hypoglycemic episodes increase the risk for this condition.

Management and Education Considerations

The first step in management of hypoglycemia unawareness is usually liberalization of glycemic goals to prevent hypoglycemia. For the patient with hypoglycemic unawareness on a basal bolus insulin regimen, greater use of long-acting insulin and smaller boluses are recommended.

Although a longer duration of diabetes increases the risk for developing hypoglycemic unawareness, repeated episodes of hypoglycemia increase the risk further. To delay the onset of this condition, care should be taken to prevent hypoglycemia in the earlier stages of diabetes treatment. This presents a challenge and a barrier to optimizing glycemic control. In some cases, the normal counter-regulatory response can be restored with treatment programs to prevent hypoglycemia, especially in those who do not have autonomic neuropathy.

Clients with hypoglycemic unawareness and their significant others require education about careful insulin dosing, increased home glucose monitoring, caution while driving, and wearing diabetes medical identification.

Fuel Metabolism

Normal Fuel Metabolism in the Fasting, Fed, and Post-Absorptive States

During the **fasting state**, blood glucose levels are maintained primarily through hepatic sources. Hepatic sources of glucose include those made by the liver (gluconeogenesis) and those stored in the liver as glycogen, which are then converted into glucose (glycogenolysis).

When carbohydrate is ingested, circulating glucose increases significantly and phase 1 of fuel metabolism is initiated. In this **fed state**, plasma insulin levels are high and insulin acts to transport glucose from the blood. At the same time, glucagon levels are low. Since the main role of glucagon is to stimulate gluconeogenesis by the liver, glucagon activity significantly declines during the fed state.

Phase 2 of fuel metabolism is also known as the **post-absorptive state**, which occurs 4–16 hours after food is consumed. During this time, plasma insulin levels decrease as glucagon levels increase. Blood glucose during this time is maintained from hepatic sources.

Role of Insulin and Amylin in Fuel Metabolism

Insulin and amylin are both glucoregulatory hormones secreted by the pancreatic beta cells in response to an increase in blood glucose. Initially, they are secreted into the portal vein before being released into the general circulation. They work in a complementary fashion to regulate the arrival and departure of glucose in the blood.

- **Insulin** is taken up by receptors in the peripheral and hepatic tissue, resulting in the transport of glucose from the blood. Insulin also inhibits glucose production from the liver and inhibits the release of glucagon from the alpha cells of the pancreas.

- **Amylin** is secreted along with insulin from the pancreatic beta cells. Like insulin, it inhibits glucagon secretion. It also regulates the appearance of glucose in the blood by slowing gastric emptying and possibly by suppressing the appetite.

Risk Factors for Diabetes

Modifiable Risk Factors

Modifiable risk factors for diabetes include the following:

- **Diet:** Decreasing calories and total dietary fat, especially saturated fat, is recommended to reduce risk for type 2 diabetes. In addition, increasing the intake of dietary fiber and whole grains is recommended.
- **Body weight:** Results of the Diabetes Prevention Program (DPP) showed that when high-risk overweight subjects lost 5–7% of their initial body weight, risk for developing diabetes was reduced by 58%.
- **Waist circumference:** Men with a waist circumference greater than 40 inches and women with a waist circumference greater than 35 inches are at higher risk for diabetes. Waist circumference has been found to be a stronger predictor for diabetes risk than both BMI and body weight.
- **Sedentary lifestyle:** Exercise boosts both carbohydrate metabolism and insulin sensitivity. The DPP showed that subjects who participated in approximately 150 minutes of moderate intensity exercise per week, in addition to implementing healthy eating choices, significantly reduced their risk for type 2 diabetes.

Risk Factors for Type 2 Diabetes in Children

Children who are overweight and have any TWO of the risk factors listed below should be tested for type 2 diabetes, beginning at age 10 or at onset of puberty if puberty occurs at an earlier age. These risk factors are:

- Family history of type 2 diabetes in first- or second-degree relatives
- Native American, African American, Hispanic/Latino, Asian American, Pacific Islander
- Signs of insulin resistance, such as acanthosis nigricans, hypertension, dyslipidemia, small-for-gestational-age birth weight, or polycystic ovary syndrome
- Maternal history of gestational diabetes during child's gestation
- Overweight

Overweight is defined as:

- BMI >85th percentile for age and sex.
- Weight for height >85th percentile.
- Weight >120% of ideal weight for age.

According to 2026 ADA Standards, fasting plasma glucose should be tested in at-risk children every 2 years after initial screening (if the initial screening results are normal), or more frequently if their BMI is increasing.

Lifestyle Modifications to Minimize Modifiable Risk

The Diabetes Prevention Program (DPP) was a large multicenter study that demonstrated that the onset of diabetes can be prevented or delayed in high-risk subjects when certain lifestyle modifications are implemented. The at-risk population was identified as those with glucose intolerance. Many of the participants came from high-risk minority groups.

It was shown that healthy eating and increasing physical activity, which led to weight loss, decreased the risk for developing diabetes by 58%. Based on the findings from this study, the following recommendations for lifestyle modification are recommended to prevent or delay the onset of type 2 diabetes:

- Weight loss recommendations vary from 7–10% of baseline for individuals with prediabetes to a more aggressive recommendation of up to 15% of baseline weight for individuals with obesity and type 2 diabetes
- A diet low in fat and calories but high in fiber
- Moderate exercise (brisk walking) for 150 minutes per week

If lifestyle modifications are insufficient for weight control, ADA guidelines recommend considering pharmacotherapy to help manage weight, prevent cardiovascular complications, and slow the progression of prediabetes/diabetes. ADA guidelines also consider the infusion of teplizumab to delay the onset of symptoms in individuals with type 1 diabetes (ages 8 years and older with stage 2 diabetes).

Individualized Education Plan

Consideration of Client Characteristics

Because people with diabetes are a heterogeneous group, educational programs should be relevant to the individuals being served. This involves tailoring the program content to meet the characteristics of the learner while recognizing that participants have the right and responsibility to set their own educational and behavioral goals.

All aspects of the educational program, including learning objectives, teaching content, methodology, and communication style, should be personalized. Individualization is considered an appropriate and viable option for both individual and group education programs.

Individual characteristics to consider when developing an individualized teaching plan include:

- Learning styles
- Culture
- Educational level and literacy
- Psychosocial status
- Cognitive status
- Functional limitations
- Readiness to learn and make behavior change
- Baseline knowledge
- Age and developmental level
- Personal and metabolic goals
- Access to resources

Diabetes Education Plan Individualized to the Acutely Ill Patient

Acutely ill patients may be distracted by pain or other types of physical discomfort. The direct effects of the illness or medications may induce lethargy or impair cognitive functioning and memory. Therefore, the teaching plan for these patients should focus on basic "survival skill" information. Assessment of specific problems the patient is having helps the educator to prioritize and focus teaching content.

Patient safety should be assessed, and information to promote safety should be considered a priority. This may include such things as medication instruction or the prevention, recognition, and treatment of hypoglycemia. Observation of body language can be used to assess patient response and can help in determining the amount and type of information that the patient is able to assimilate. Involvement of caregivers and family members is important.

It is important to make arrangements for follow-up with the acutely ill patient so that education that is more detailed can be provided at a later time.

Learning Objectives vs. Behavioral Objectives

Both learning and behavioral objectives are developed based on individual assessment and in collaboration with the client. Both types of objectives are written as measurable outcomes so that the results of education can be evaluated.

- **Learning objectives** assess knowledge in an indirect way, since learning cannot actually be witnessed. Behavioral objectives are a more direct assessment since behavior is something that can be observed. The purpose of learning objectives is to spell out the intended content of education. An example of a learning objective is: *Describe the effect of carbohydrate on blood glucose.*
- **Behavioral objectives** provide the client with a plan for taking specific actions that he or she feels have value and are feasible. An example of a behavioral objective is: *Walk for 20 minutes during lunch break 5 days a week for the next 2 weeks.*

Considerations for The Sequence of Information to Present

The empowerment approach to diabetes education recognizes that the person with diabetes holds the primary rights and responsibilities for his or her own self-care. In diabetes education programs, the **sequence of information** should take into account the priorities of the client.

One of the first messages that participants should hear in a program is that diabetes is a self-managed condition.

Client priorities can be assessed by asking what they would like to learn and by showing a list of possible topics from which to select.

Psychosocial issues should be addressed early in the program. Educators should remember that having diabetes is not an academic exercise, but a situation that affects the daily lives of clients. Therefore, a physiology lesson on diabetes is less important than learning how to eat the right foods.

Another important factor in prioritizing program content is safety. Learning to use insulin or to prevent and manage hypoglycemia are examples of high-priority topics that may need to be covered first when time is limited.

Instructional Methods

Computer Programs

Computer programs, apps, and online resources are appropriate choices for self-directed learners and those who are comfortable with technology. While many older adults are proficient in the use of the computer, lack of experience or functional limitations may make this an inappropriate choice for some.

People who prefer to learn independently and at their own pace may prefer computerized education or an app. This type of learning often provides an opportunity for interactive learning as well.

Clients with unusual hours, limited time, or inflexible schedules may benefit from the 24-hour access provided by computers and apps.

Clients of lower socioeconomic status may not own a computer. Computers are available for public use at most public libraries, though the time one is allowed to remain at the computer is limited. With apps now available on smartphones, this possibility may also be explored with those without access to a computer.

Clients who consult internet sites for information on diabetes self-management should be cautioned that not all sources of information are reliable. Sites hosted by major authoritative bodies, such as the American Diabetes Association, or by government bodies and universities are usually most appropriate.

Group Discussion

Group discussion supports the empowerment approach to diabetes education by allowing participants to direct the content of education and practice decision-making in a supportive environment. This method allows clients to seek and acquire the information that is most important to them. The role of the educator in the discussion group is to provide guidance and support and to keep exchanges focused on learning objectives and within time constraints.

Group discussion is an appropriate methodology for adult learners as it is an active, self-directed approach that is relevant to the individual. An example of an appropriate topic for group discussion is to share blood glucose logs and share suggestions for how to interpret and respond to results.

A limitation of group discussions is that the educator has less control over program content than in traditional lecture programs. In addition, some group members may monopolize the discussion, leaving others with unmet needs. Group discussions may not be appropriate for clients with impaired hearing or language barriers.

Demonstration

Demonstration as an instructional method allows for an active hands-on learning experience. It is appropriate for teaching diabetes self-management skills such as using a monitor to test blood glucose, drawing and injecting insulin, and calculating insulin dosages.

Demonstration has the benefit of allowing the educator to directly observe behaviors that can indicate that learning has taken place. Likewise, it can help identify areas that require additional instruction.

A limitation of demonstration is that it can be difficult to do effectively in large groups, as participants may not be able to see the instructor's demonstration and the instructor may not be able to observe a return demonstration by each member. Demonstration can also be a time-consuming instructional method.

Role-Playing

Role-playing is an interactive teaching method appropriate for a variety of age groups, including children, teens, and adults. It provides an opportunity to practice problem-solving, explore feelings, and practice new behaviors. It can be equally effective in both individual and group education programs.

Appropriate topics for role-playing include practicing asking for support from significant others or learning to respond assertively to peers who ask questions about having diabetes or using insulin.

Facilitating effective role-plays requires skill on the part of the educator. Some people may not be comfortable being asked to "act" and should be allowed to be an observer. Assessment of hearing, language, and culture are all important before deciding to implement role-playing as an instructional method.

Group Teaching

Reading, writing, listening, watching, and doing are examples of preferred **learning styles**. Many people have a combination of preferred learning styles.

Literacy includes the level at which one reads and writes, as well as the ability to speak, compute, and solve problems.

Group classes usually include people with varying learning styles and degrees of literacy. To meet a wider variety of needs, instructional methods should include a variety of formats. Videos are an example of a format that appeals to a wide variety of learners. Group discussions and role-plays are also appropriate for heterogeneous groups, as clients can learn through problem-solving and brainstorming with others who have diabetes.

Reading materials written at a lower reading level are often preferred by clients regardless of their literacy or educational level.

Instructional Methods for Various Age Groups

Preschool children learn best from simple question-and-answer sessions based on age-appropriate experiences. Props, such as puppets and dolls, are often used to appeal to the child's developmental level.

School-aged children learn best through games and puzzles as well as age-appropriate videos and interactive computer programs.

Teens are motivated by peer influence. Therefore, same-age group classes and discussions are most appropriate. At this age, learning to make decisions and solve problems are important components of diabetes education. Diabetes camps can be very valuable learning experiences for this age group.

Adults prefer learning content that is relevant to their day-to-day living. Practical content that addresses everyday problems is most appropriate for adults. Adults also prefer self-directed learning. Therefore, collaboration on educational objectives is appropriate with this population.

Setting Goals with the Client

Behavioral Goals

Behavioral goals for diabetes education are based on an individualized assessment of client needs. They are based on knowledge gaps identified during assessment and on identified client preferences.

Behavioral goals are developed in collaboration with the client, with the client initiating the direction of the goals. Collaboration with the multidisciplinary team provides the information and guidance needed for informed decision-making on the part of the client.

Tools that the educator can use to help facilitate goal setting include behavioral change theory, the patient empowerment approach, and patient-centered communication.

A self-directed approach to goal setting empowers clients and keeps them involved in the learning process. In addition to providing information for informed decision-making, the educator's role in goal setting includes promoting confidence or self-efficacy, facilitating effective problem-solving, developing coping skills, and identifying strategies to overcome barriers.

Finally, goals should include metrics for success that are developed in collaboration with the client.

SMART Behavioral Goals

Behavioral goals should be individualized and developed in collaboration with the client. They represent a planned change in behavior that reflects the values of the client. In order to be successful, the clients should select goals that they feel will reap benefit, that they are interested in doing, and that they are able to do.

The acronym **SMART** is often used in developing behavioral goals:

- S – Specific: describes what the client will do
- M – Measurable: indicates how much, how often, or how many
- A – Achievable: is something the client is capable of doing
- R – Relevant: has a direct impact on the client's health and well-being
- T – Time bound: includes a time period after which the behavior will be evaluated

An example of a **SMART goal**:

I will check my blood sugar twice a day, before breakfast and before dinner, every day for 2 weeks.

Person-Centered Education on Self-Care Behaviors: Nutrition Principles and Guidelines

ADA Nutrition Recommendations for Prevention of Diabetes

The Diabetes Prevention Program and other studies have demonstrated that type 2 diabetes can be prevented in high-risk, overweight people through intensive lifestyle modification. Nutrition recommendations and interventions for the prevention of type 2 diabetes include:

- Weight loss of at least 5–7% of body weight
- 150 minutes of moderate physical activity per week and limitation of sedentary time (prolonged sitting should be interrupted every 30 minutes)
- Dietary reduction of fat and calories; Mediterranean diet with low carbohydrates is specifically recommended
- Dietary fiber intake of 14 g/1,000 kcal, with one-half of grain intake coming from whole grains

There are no nutritional recommendations for the prevention of type 1 diabetes.

Data for preventing diabetes in youth is unavailable. However, the ADA proposes that the same measures demonstrated to be effective in adults would be appropriate for children as long as growth and developmental needs are met.

ADA Medical Nutrition Therapy (MNT) Recommendations

Team Approach

Nutrition recommendations and interventions for diabetes are published by the American Diabetes Association (ADA) to provide science-based information to people with diabetes and their healthcare providers. Medical nutrition therapy (MNT) is appropriate at all levels along the diabetes care continuum, from primary prevention of diabetes to prevention and management of complications and prevention of morbidity and mortality.

The ADA recommendations stipulate that the person with diabetes is central to the nutritional management team and plays an active role in decision-making. While supporting the goals of MNT is considered a team effort, it is recommended that a registered dietitian play the leading role. At the same time, other healthcare providers, such as doctors and nurses, should be knowledgeable about these guidelines and play an active role in their implementation. 2026 ADA guidelines recommend the incorporation of inclusive food-based (rather than nutrient-based) eating patterns into MNT.

General Tenets

There is not a single "diabetic diet." Medical nutrition therapy (MNT) is a process provided by a registered dietitian to assess and diagnose a client's nutritional status and to make individualized dietary recommendations.

The general **principles of the meal plan for diabetes** include:

- If overweight, start by losing 3–7% of body weight. Even modest weight loss can produce significant results in glucose and lipid levels. For overweight clients, achieving weight loss shares priority status with achieving glycemic control.
- Eat consistent amounts of carbohydrates from day to day and distribute them evenly throughout the day. While eating sugar is not forbidden, the daily intake of carbohydrates should be monitored and controlled.
- Limit sodium, particularly sodium from processed foods.
- Practice portion control.
- Limit fats in the diet, especially saturated fats and trans fats.
- Engage in 150 minutes of moderate intensity physical activity every week.

Utilize blood glucose monitoring results to evaluate the effect of food type, portion size, timing of meals, and physical activity on blood glucose level.

Goals for Individuals with Diabetes

Medical nutrition therapy (MNT) is an integral part of diabetes management throughout the continuum of care.

According to the American Diabetes Association, the **goals** of MNT for diabetes are to:

- Achieve and maintain glycemic control
- Achieve and maintain a lipid profile that will reduce the risk for cardiovascular disease
- Achieve and maintain blood pressure at target level

- Prevent or delay long-term complications of diabetes
- Individualize nutritional needs based on personal and cultural preferences and willingness to change eating habits
- Integrate the meal plan with the insulin regimen if the patient uses insulin
- Maintain eating as a pleasurable activity with limitations based on scientific evidence
- Meet the concurrent nutritional needs of people with diabetes at different times in the lifecycle, such as youth, pregnancy, lactation, and old age
- Safely coordinate nutritional recommendations with risk for hypoglycemia

Implications of Sodium

As part of the metabolic syndrome, **hypertension** is a common finding in clients with diabetes. People with diabetes also tend to be more salt-sensitive than the general population, meaning that reductions in sodium intake are more likely to have a beneficial effect on blood pressure. As a population, African Americans tend to have a high degree of sodium sensitivity.

Moderate sodium intake is considered 2,300 mg/day. People with diabetes are recommended to limit sodium consumption to less than 2,300 mg/day. For diabetic patients with hypertension, a reduction to 1,500 mg/day is often recommended.

Clients should be instructed to look for the sodium content of foods on food labels. It is listed as mg of sodium per serving. For single-serving foods, 400 mg or less of sodium is recommended. For an entrée, less than 800 mg of sodium is recommended. A food labeled "low sodium" has 140 mg or less of sodium per serving.

A teaspoon of salt contains 2,300 mg of sodium.

Micronutrient Requirements

There is no evidence that specific vitamin or mineral supplements benefit people with diabetes. Getting adequate micronutrients from natural foods and a healthy, well-balanced diet is encouraged. Multivitamin supplementation may be appropriate in elderly clients, strict vegetarians, and those on calorie-restricted diets, as well as in pregnant and lactating women.

The American Diabetes Association (ADA) has stated that further research is needed on micronutrients such as chromium and vitamin D to determine whether they should be recommended for diabetes management.

The benefit of antioxidant supplementation in people with diabetes has been studied because diabetes is a state of increased oxidative stress. So far, there is no evidence that antioxidant therapy improves glycemic control or reduces the risk of long-term complications. In fact, there is evidence that supplementation with vitamin E, carotene, and other antioxidants is potentially harmful.

Carbohydrate, Protein, Fat, Sodium, and Fiber Requirements

Carbohydrates, protein: According to the ADA's most recent standards update, evidence suggests that there is no ideal amount or percentage of daily calories that should come from the macronutrients carbohydrates and proteins. Rather, diet plans and servings should be individualized to the patient's preferences, eating patterns, and goals. 2026 guidelines recommended a focus on food-based eating patterns when considering nutrition therapy in individuals with diabetes.

Fat: Total fat intake is individualized, and 2026 ADA Standards emphasize that each individual's lifestyle, eating patterns, and preferences be considered when accounting for fat in the diet. Less than 7% of calories should come from saturated fat, and when possible, saturated fat should be replaced with unsaturated fat (not carbohydrates). Daily intake of trans fats should be zero.

Sodium: Sodium intake should be limited to 2,300 mg/day. For hypertension, reduction to 1,500 mg/day is recommended. One teaspoon of salt contains 2,300 mg of sodium.

Fiber: Fiber intake should be at least 14 grams of fiber per 1,000 calories. Some studies show that larger amounts have a beneficial effect on glycemic control.

Dietary Carbohydrates

Dietary carbohydrate is the major determinant of postprandial blood glucose excursions. While carbohydrate limitation is beneficial, carbohydrates cannot be eliminated from the diet as they are an important source of fiber, vitamins, and minerals.

Below is a summary of the ADA nutrition recommendations for carbohydrates in diabetes management:

- A balanced diet including carbohydrate from fruit, vegetables, whole grains, legumes, and low-fat milk is encouraged. These are nutrient-dense carbohydrates.
- People with diabetes should monitor carbohydrate intake by a method such as carbohydrate counting, food exchanges, or visual estimation.
- Use of the glycemic index may be an appropriate supplement to monitoring total carbohydrate intake.
- Although a specific value for fiber intake has not been determined for people with diabetes, a diet rich in fiber is recommended.
- Non-nutritive sugar substitutes and sugar alcohols are safe when used within guidelines established by the Food and Drug Administration, but water is preferred.
- Beverages sweetened with sugar should be replaced with water as much as possible.

Carbohydrate Counting

In carbohydrate counting, the client keeps track of the total amount of carbohydrate being consumed. Done properly, it can provide a healthy, balanced diet with controlled portions of carbohydrate. One carbohydrate serving equals 15 grams of carbohydrate. The client selects the correct number of carbohydrate servings to meet their recommended allowance.

Examples of 15-gram carbohydrate servings include:

- 1 small piece of fruit
- 1/3 cup cooked rice
- 1/2 cup cooked pasta
- 1 cup milk
- 3/4 cup yogurt
- 1 slice bread
- 1 small potato

Nonstarchy vegetables contain approximately 5 grams of carbohydrate per cup. If eaten in moderate amounts, they are usually not counted in the allowance. If a large amount is eaten, nonstarchy vegetables should be counted. "Free foods," which contain less than 20 calories and fewer than 5 grams of carbohydrate per serving, are not counted. These include pickles, salsa, many condiments, and sugar-free gelatin.

READING FOOD LABELS FOR CARBOHYDRATE COUNTING

Clients who are carbohydrate counting should be taught to prioritize the information they find on the Nutrition Facts **food label.**

The first thing to determine is the serving size. All other values on the label are based on the specified serving size.

Next, the client should look at the total carbohydrate value. This reports the total number of grams of carbohydrates from sugar, starch, and fiber that corresponds with the serving size. Clients should compare this to the 15-gram carbohydrate serving used in the carbohydrate counting meal plan. Many clients need to be instructed to ignore the grams of sugar reported on the label, as this is already included in the total carbohydrate figure.

Lastly, clients should check the food label for fiber content. If a food has more than 5 grams of fiber per serving, they can subtract that amount from the total carbohydrates and use the difference when figuring their carbohydrate intake.

TYPICAL MEAL PLAN FOR CLIENTS WITH TYPE 2 DIABETES USING CARBOHYDRATE COUNTING

For carbohydrate counting, the client is given an allowance of how many carbohydrate choices are allowed for each meal and snack.

A **typical carbohydrate counting meal plan** allows 3–4 carbohydrate choices per meal. Each carbohydrate choice, or serving, equals 15 grams. Examples of serving sizes are 1 small piece of fruit, 1 slice of bread, or 1/3 cup of cooked rice. Some clients also receive an additional allowance of 1–2 carbohydrate choices for snacks each day.

Clients select, or mix and match, the carbohydrates of their choice to equal the allowance for the meal. The type of carbohydrate is not specified, only the amount. Consistent carbohydrate intake, no matter the source, helps stabilize the blood glucose. Care should be taken to limit carbohydrate choices that are high in fat and calories.

The carbohydrate allowance recommendation is based on factors such as gender, physical activity level, and medications. Blood glucose logs help in evaluating results and optimizing the recommendation.

GLYCEMIC INDEX

Many factors influence the postprandial glucose response to carbohydrate ingestion. These factors include the type of starch (amylase versus amylopectin), degree of processing, the composition of the meal, method of cooking, the ripeness of the plant consumed, and the insulin availability or sensitivity of the individual.

The **glycemic index** compares the postprandial response of carbohydrate-containing foods. The glycemic response of a food is compared to the glucose response of a reference food, such as white bread or rice. The glycemic index is the rise in blood glucose at 2 hours following ingestion of a 50-gram carbohydrate portion. Low glycemic index foods include oats, legumes, pumpernickel bread, apples, and oranges.

Research results conflict on the efficacy of the glycemic index in diabetes management, and methodological problems exist. How a food is processed or where it is grown can cause variability in the glycemic index of the same type of food. The ripeness of a fruit or vegetable can also cause variability among the same foods.

Sucrose and Fructose

There is strong evidence that, in equal caloric amounts, dietary **sucrose** does not increase blood glucose more than starch does. Therefore, the intake of sugar and sweet foods is not forbidden to people with diabetes. Sucrose can be substituted for equivalent amounts of starch without a significant difference in the effect on glycemia. However, clients should be cautioned to avoid excessive caloric intake of sweets and to possibly increase insulin or other glucose-lowering medication when sugar is added to the diet.

Fructose has a lower glycemic index than either sucrose or starch. However, adding fructose as a sweetening agent is not recommended because of its adverse effect on plasma lipids. Naturally occurring fructose in fruits and other foods does not need to be eliminated from the diet if these foods account for only 3–4% of total energy intake.

Sugar Alcohols and Non-Nutritive Sweeteners

Sugar alcohols are FDA-approved reduced-calorie sweeteners such as isomalt, maltitol, sorbitol, xylitol, and hydrogenated starch hydrolysates. When ingested, these substances have reduced glycemic effect when compared to sucrose and glucose. They contain about half the calories of sucrose, but are also less sweet, which may result in more use. When counting the carbohydrates of a food containing sugar alcohols, it is appropriate to subtract half of the sugar alcohol grams from the total carbohydrates. Sugar alcohols are associated with decreased risk for dental caries. Side effects of consuming sugar alcohols are abdominal discomfort and diarrhea. Currently, little evidence exists on the benefit of sugar alcohol use in individuals with diabetes.

There are five non-nutritive sweeteners approved by the Food and Drug Administration. All have undergone rigorous testing and have been determined safe for human consumption, including people with diabetes and pregnant women. The approved non-nutritive sweeteners are acesulfame potassium, aspartame, neotame, saccharin, and sucralose.

Fiber

While there is not a specific recommendation for fiber intake in the management of diabetes, a diet high in fiber is encouraged. People with diabetes are encouraged to at least strive for a dietary intake of fiber that matches the USDA recommendation for the general population, which is 14 grams/1,000 kcal. Research indicates that a high-fiber diet (approximately 50 grams of fiber per day) is associated with reduced glycemia in people with type 1 diabetes and reduced glycemia and lipemia in people with type 2 diabetes.

Foods containing at least five grams of fiber per serving are considered rich in fiber and should be encouraged. Examples include legumes, fiber-rich cereals, and many whole grain products. Barriers to adhering to a high-fiber diet include gastrointestinal side effects, palatability, and limited food choices.

Dietary Fats

Dietary fats can be broken down into the following categories:

- **Saturated fats** raise LDL-C levels. While 2026 ADA Standards emphasize that a universal ideal percentage of calories from fat does not exist, it is agreed that saturated fats should be limited. Sources include animal fat and coconut, palm, and hydrogenated vegetable oils.
- **Trans fatty acids**, a form of saturated fats, are found in processed foods, such as boxed dinners and baked goods. Their intake should be restricted.

- **Polyunsaturated fats** lower total cholesterol but have a mixed effect on HDL-C levels. Sources are corn and sunflower oils and walnuts. Intake should be less than 10% of daily calories.
- **Monounsaturated fats** lower total cholesterol but do not lower HDL-C. They are more beneficial to the lipid panel than polyunsaturated oils. Sources include nuts and canola, olive, and peanut oils.
- **Omega-3 polyunsaturated fats** lower serum triglycerides and have an antiplatelet-clotting effect. Sources include fatty fish such as salmon, herring, and sardines as well as flaxseed and walnuts.
- **Dietary cholesterol** raises cholesterol levels in some people more than others. Intake should be less than 200–300 mg/day. Sources are egg yolks, organ meats and dairy fat.

Impact of Fat on Cardiovascular Risks

Since cardiovascular risk is high in people with diabetes, a primary goal in their dietary management is to limit saturated fats, trans fatty acids, and cholesterol. Saturated fats and trans fatty acids are the fats that affect the LDL-C level.

The effects of diets containing specific percentages of saturated fats, trans fatty acids, and cholesterol on people with diabetes have not been adequately studied. Therefore, recommendations are based on the guidelines for people with pre-existing cardiovascular disease, since the risk among the two groups is relatively equivalent. A **Mediterranean diet** is recommended because it is rich in healthy fats (monounsaturated and polyunsaturated), which have been proven to enhance glucose metabolism and decrease cardiovascular risk more than a low-fat diet.

The ADA recommendations for dietary fat and cholesterol management are:

- Limited saturated fats in diet
- Minimal intake of food containing trans fat
- Dietary cholesterol intake <200 mg/day
- Two or more servings of fish per week (excluding commercially fried fish filets)

Dietary Protein

The recommended dietary intake of protein for people with diabetes is the similar to that for the general population and generally does not exceed 20% of daily energy intake. Examples of good-quality protein sources include meat, poultry, fish, eggs, milk, cheese, and soy.

Although some studies indicate that a high-protein diet may have a positive effect on glycemic control and can reduce appetite, these diets are not recommended for people with diabetes, even those having normal kidney function, due to lack of adequate evidence regarding their safety and efficacy.

ADA recommendations for protein in the management of diabetes are summarized as follows:

- Protein intake by a person with diabetes who has normal renal function should be similar to that of the general population.
- Protein intake for older adults with diabetes should be at least 0.8 g/kg of body weight per day.
- Protein is not effective in treating hypoglycemia and should not be used to prevent nighttime hypoglycemia because it can increase insulin response without increasing plasma glucose.
- High-protein diets are not recommended for weight loss, even in patients with normal renal function.

Impact of Protein on Blood Glucose

Although 50–60% of ingested protein converts to glucose, it is not known for certain where this glucose goes. Researchers have suggested that it is probably stored in the liver or muscle as glycogen. In those with poor glycemic control, gluconeogenesis following protein consumption can happen rapidly and cause an increase in blood glucose. For those with type 2 diabetes in good control, protein consumption does not increase plasma glucose levels.

Contrary to popular belief, consuming protein simultaneously with carbohydrate does not slow the blood glucose response to carbohydrate or have an effect on its peak activity. Consuming protein following treatment of a hypoglycemic episode does not prevent recurrence of the hypoglycemia. Similarly, consuming protein at bedtime or prior to exercise has not proven beneficial in preventing nocturnal hypoglycemia. The current recommendation for insulin users is to reduce insulin dose or consume a snack, either carbohydrate alone or with protein, prior to bedtime.

Protein Restriction for Chronic Kidney Disease

The progression of the microvascular complications of diabetes may be moderated by restricting protein in the diet, along with attaining glycemic control and lowering blood pressure.

The usual dietary intake of protein for Americans is 1.0–1.5 g/kg of body weight per day, or approximately 15–20% of daily energy. 2026 ADA guidelines recommend 0.8 g/kg of body weight per day for individuals with CKD stages 3 or higher and increasing that to 1.0–1.2 g/kg of body weight per day for individuals with CKD on dialysis.

For microalbuminuria: Studies show that reducing protein to 0.8–1.0 g/kg of body weight per day has a beneficial effect on renal function.

For clinical nephropathy: Reducing the amount of protein consumed to 0.8 g/kg of body weight per day improves measures of renal function.

Reducing protein intake to less than 0.8 g/kg of body weight per day is controversial. Limitation of protein should not preclude maintaining adequate nutritional status of the patient with CKD.

Guidelines for Alcohol Use in Individuals with Diabetes

While some people with diabetes can safely drink alcohol in moderation, abstinence is advised for those who are pregnant, have a history of alcohol abuse, or have liver disease, severely elevated triglycerides, or other contraindicating medical conditions.

Moderation means drinking less than one alcoholic beverage per day for women and less than two a day for men. One serving of alcohol equals 12 oz beer, 5 oz wine, or 1.5 oz distilled spirits.

When consumed with food, alcohol has minimal immediate effect on glycemia. When ingested with carbohydrate, it can raise blood glucose. For those taking insulin or insulin secretagogues, alcohol can cause hypoglycemia. ADA guidelines for alcohol use are summarized as follows:

- People with diabetes who choose to use alcohol should do so in moderation.
- Alcohol should be consumed with food to reduce the risk for nocturnal hypoglycemia in people using insulin and glucose-lowering oral agents.
- Drinks mixed with carbohydrate, such as juice or soda, should be avoided to prevent high blood glucose.
- People with diabetes who choose to use alcohol should be educated on the symptoms and management of delayed hypoglycemia after drinking alcohol.

Integrating Food and Insulin into the Diabetes Treatment Plan

For people using insulin and oral glucose-lowering medications, the treatment plan should integrate the medication with food intake and the physical activity pattern. The approach to this depends upon the individual's medication, preferred meal pattern and physical activity pattern.

For those on basal bolus insulin regimens, the individual will count carbohydrates and inject the corresponding amount of rapid-acting insulin prior to the meal according to the established insulin-to-carbohydrate ratio. This applies to clients on either an insulin pump or multiple daily injections.

For clients on fixed insulin doses and oral glucose-lowering medications, daily carbohydrate consumption should remain consistent.

For planned exercise, decreasing the insulin dosage is recommended to prevent hypoglycemia. For unplanned exercise, carbohydrate intake will need to be increased to prevent hypoglycemia. Clients taking oral insulin secretagogues may need to lower the daily dose when undertaking an ongoing and consistent pattern of increased physical activity.

Descriptive Terms Commonly Used on Food Labels

Descriptions of food products, such as "fat free" and "no sugar added," are regulated by law. In order for manufacturers to make such claims, a food must comply with its intended definition.

Examples of some descriptive terms and their meanings:

- Fat free: 1/2 gram or less per serving
- Low fat: 3 grams or less per serving
- Reduced fat: at least 25% less fat than the regular version of a food
- Sugar free: 1/2 gram or less per serving
- No sugar added: no sugar or fruit juice added during processing
- Reduced sugar: less than 25% of the sugar in the regular version
- Light or lite: 50% less fat or 1/3 fewer calories than the regular version

Certain health claims on food packaging must be approved by the Food and Drug Administration. Examples:

- If a food is high in fiber, the package can claim that it helps reduce risk for cancer and heart disease.
- The label for a food low in sodium can claim that it helps prevent hypertension.

WEIGHT MANAGEMENT

CLASSIFICATION OF OVERWEIGHT AND OBESITY

The **body mass index (BMI)** is a commonly used screening tool to identify weight problems and associated health risks. ADA guidelines recommend screening annually for overweight and obesity using BMI in addition to another measurement of body fat. Calculated from a person's height and weight, BMI is highly correlated to obesity or fat mass and risk for disease. The BMI classifications according to the National Heart, Lung, and Blood Institute are:

- Normal: 18.5–24.9 kg/m^2
- Overweight, increased risk for disease: 25.0–29.9 kg/m^2
- Obese, high risk: 30.0–34.9 kg/m^2
- Very high risk: 35.0–39.9 kg/m^2
- Extremely high risk: ≥40 kg/m^2

Waist circumference is a measure of visceral body fat. This is useful because excessive abdominal fat is a risk factor for type 2 diabetes, hypertension, dyslipidemia, and cardiovascular disease (CVD). Excess waist circumference with associated health risk is identified as:

- Men: >40 inches
- Women (non-pregnant): >35 inches

Other anthropometric measures to consider when evaluating weight include the waist-to-hip ratio and/or the waist-to-height ratio.

ADA RECOMMENDATIONS FOR WEIGHT LOSS IN INDIVIDUALS WITH DIABETES

There is strong evidence that moderate weight loss increases insulin sensitivity in overweight and obese people with insulin resistance. ADA recommendations for weight loss include:

- Moderate (5-7%) weight loss for overweight or obese people who have diabetes or who are at risk for diabetes.
- Weight loss can be achieved through calorie-restricted diets followed for up to one year.
- Exercise and behavior modification are essential components of any weight loss plan.
- Weight loss medications (GLP-1 RA-based therapy) may be appropriate for some overweight or obese people with diabetes if combined with lifestyle modification.
- Metabolic surgery may be appropriate for some obese people with type 2 diabetes and a BMI ≥30 kg/m^2, or for Asian American patients, a BMI of ≥27.5 kg/m^2.
- Lipid profiles and renal function should be monitored for those on low-carbohydrate diets. Protein intake should be monitored in patients with nephropathy who are on a low-carbohydrate diet. Low-carbohydrate diets should be adjusted for prevention and treatment of hypoglycemia.

EFFECTIVENESS OF WEIGHT LOSS IN THERAPY FOR TYPE 2 DIABETES

There is a strong correlation between overweight or obesity and type 2 diabetes. Much of this is due to an association between excess body fat and insulin resistance. Several major studies have concluded that even a modest amount of weight loss can prevent the development of diabetes in high-risk people, while more aggressive weight loss (10% or greater) could possibly result in remission in those already diagnosed with type 2 diabetes and obesity.

Weight loss, through healthy eating and exercise, can improve glycemic control and decrease the need for medication in people with type 2 diabetes. On the other hand, progressive loss of beta cell function over time can result in the need for medication despite changes in lifestyle. At minimum, healthy lifestyle choices leading to weight loss improve glycemic control and reduce the risk for cardiovascular disease and a host of other health problems.

Maintaining weight loss can be one of the most challenging aspects of diabetes self-management. Clients can become frustrated and require emotional support as much as education. Correlating weight loss and improved HbA1c can help boost confidence and motivate patients.

Factors Necessary for Long-Term Weight Management

Scientific evidence demonstrates that certain factors are necessary for successful long-term weight management. Components of the most successful programs are:

- Structured and intensive lifestyle modification
- Participant education
- Individualized counseling
- Calorie restriction (500–1,000 fewer calories than estimated as necessary for weight maintenance) when weight loss is needed
- Regular physical activity
- Frequent participant contact

Participants in this type of program have demonstrated an average weight reduction of 5–7% of body weight and successful long-term maintenance of their weight loss. Unfortunately, delivering this type of program is challenging since it is labor and time intensive. Most third-party payers do not cover medical nutrition therapy visits adequately enough to achieve weight loss goals through this type of program.

Risks and Benefits of Low-Carbohydrate Diet for Weight Loss

The recommended daily allowance for digestible carbohydrate is 130 grams/day. This is based on the estimated need for glucose as fuel for the brain and to meet the dietary needs for fiber, vitamins, and minerals found in carbohydrate foods. People on diets too low in carbohydrate are missing important nutrients that come from a balanced diet.

Two studies showed that subjects on low-carbohydrate diets lost more weight at 6 months than those on low-fat diets. However, at 1 year, weight loss between the two groups was roughly the same, with both demonstrating modest weight loss at that point.

Other studies demonstrate that low-carbohydrate diets have a favorable effect on triglycerides and HDL-C and are associated with a greater decrease in HbA1c in subjects with type 2 diabetes. On the other hand, LDL-C was significantly higher in these subjects.

The American Diabetes Association (ADA) recognizes the conflicting findings of this research and states that more study is needed to determine the long-term safety and efficacy of low-carbohydrate diets in people with diabetes.

Nutritional Considerations for Diabetes During Pregnancy

Nutritional goals during pregnancy include achieving normoglycemia and preventing ketosis. Tight glycemic control during pregnancy reduces the risk for serious perinatal complications and improves maternal health-related quality of life.

Weight loss during pregnancy is generally not recommended. Hypocaloric diets in obese women with gestational diabetes (GDM) can result in ketosis. However, a carefully monitored, moderate reduction in calories to achieve glycemic control is sometimes appropriate.

The diet for gestational diabetes is carbohydrate-controlled while meeting the nutritional needs for maternal and fetal health. The diet is individualized based on body weight, glucose levels, ketone levels, and use of insulin. The daily carbohydrate allowance during pregnancy should be at least 175 grams distributed throughout the day in 3 small-to-moderate meals and 2–4 snacks. Evening snacks are sometimes required to prevent ketosis overnight. If the patient uses insulin, carbohydrate intake must be consistent to avoid hypoglycemia.

Regular physical activity can help lower plasma glucose concentrations and prevent excessive weight gain during pregnancy.

Person-Centered Education on Self-Care Behaviors: Physical Activity

Evaluating a Client Prior to Exercise Program Recommendation

It is generally safe to recommend a physical activity program of brisk walking to most people with type 2 diabetes without having them undergo cardiac stress testing. Those with predisposing risks such as severe neuropathy, either autonomic or peripheral, and preproliferative or proliferative retinopathy require more thorough evaluation.

For patients who plan to start an exercise program more vigorous than brisk walking, an **assessment of cardiovascular risk factors** is advised. The recommendation about when to perform exercise stress testing is controversial. American Diabetes Association (ADA) guidelines suggest that the clinical judgment of the healthcare provider should guide the decision about whether to perform cardiac stress testing. Examples of patients appropriate for the test include:

- Previously sedentary individuals with moderate to high risk for cardiovascular disease
- Those with concurrent autonomic neuropathy, peripheral vascular disease, or microvascular disease
- Those with type 2 diabetes for longer than 10 years
- Those with type 1 diabetes for longer than 15 years if age 35 years or older

Benefits of Physical Activity to Individuals with Diabetes

Exercise improves glycemic control and lowers risk for cardiovascular disease and mortality. It can also prevent or delay the onset of diabetes in people at high risk.

Specific benefits of exercise include:

- Decreases insulin resistance
- Lowers fasting and postprandial glucose concentrations
- Improves uptake of glucose by muscle tissue
- Increases fat metabolism
- Increases cardiac output
- Helps with weight loss and maintenance of weight loss*
- Reduces BMI
- Decreases blood pressure by about 5–10 mmHg
- Modestly increases HDL cholesterol

- Modestly decreases triglyceride level
- Helps alleviate stress, depression, and anxiety

*Following weight loss, regular exercise has been shown to be the primary predictor of maintaining the loss.

Beneficial Effect of Exercise on Insulin Sensitivity

During the post-exercise period, there is increased uptake of glucose by the muscles mediated by increased insulin sensitivity of the muscular receptors. While insulin secretion decreases during exercise, the increased insulin sensitivity more than compensates for this, resulting in a lowering of the blood glucose concentration. This often results in decreased need for medications by people with diabetes who exercise regularly.

The favorable effect of exercise on insulin sensitivity is additive when exercise is performed daily. Depending on the duration and intensity of the activity, the insulin-sensitizing effect lasts for 24 – 72 hours following an exercise session. Therefore, to optimize the benefits of exercise, it is recommended that no more than 2 days pass between sessions.

Both aerobic and resistance exercise affect insulin sensitivity to about the same degree. There is evidence that insulin sensitivity following resistance exercise may last somewhat longer.

Aerobic Exercise in Type 2 Diabetes

Aerobic exercise has been shown to decrease HbA1c values in people with type 2 diabetes regardless of weight loss. Increased aerobic fitness is also associated with significantly lower rates of cardiovascular disease and mortality.

While the recommendation for an activity program should be individualized, a target of at least 150 minutes of moderate aerobic activity per week is advised for most adults with diabetes. Children with type 2 diabetes should participate in physical activity for at least 60 minutes each day in addition to bone- and muscle-strengthening exercises at least three times a week. Those who are already active can gain further benefits by increasing the intensity of their exercise. The exercise should be distributed over at least 3 days per week and no more than 2 consecutive days should elapse between exercise sessions. For individuals with sedentary lifestyles, sedentary periods should be interrupted every 30 minutes with standing or walking to reap benefits reflected in blood glucose levels.

Greater reduction in cardiovascular risk can be attained by performing at least 4 hours of moderate to vigorous aerobic and/or resistance exercise per week. Larger amounts of such exercise are also associated with maintenance of weight loss over the long-term.

Resistance Training in Type 2 Diabetes

Resistance training is a recommended part of the fitness program for people with type 2 diabetes. This type of exercise increases insulin sensitivity to the same degree as aerobic activity. It is especially beneficial to older adults, who are at risk for decline in muscle mass. Studies show that a resistance training regimen can lower HbA1c values in people with type 2 diabetes.

There is insufficient evidence to conclude that resistance exercise increases the risk for stroke, myocardial ischemia, or retinal hemorrhage in people with type 2 diabetes. The American Diabetes Association (ADA) has concluded that high-intensity resistance training is safe for these individuals, even those with cardiovascular risk factors.

ADA recommendations call for resistance exercise 3 times per week (on nonconsecutive days) in adults and children with type 2 diabetes who have no contraindications to such exercise. The exercises should target all major muscle groups and progress to 3 sets of 8–10 repetitions. The amount of weight used should be that which cannot be lifted more than 8–10 times.

Exercise Precautions for Type 1 Diabetes with Hyperglycemia

Hyperglycemia and ketosis can worsen if a person with type 1 diabetes initiates exercise while blood glucose is greater than 250 mg/dL and ketones are present. These clients should be advised to avoid exercise until blood glucose improves and ketones are absent.

If a client with type 1 diabetes has blood glucose of 250–300 mg/dL following overconsumption of carbohydrate and ketones are negative, exercise is probably safe. The absence of ketones signals that the person is not insulin-deficient at that time and the risk for ketosis is small.

If a client with type 1 diabetes has blood glucose greater than 300 mg/dL, it is prudent to delay exercise even in the absence of ketones.

Sometimes a person with type 1 diabetes experiences an acute rise in blood glucose following intense exercise, such as engaging in competitive sports. In this case, additional insulin should not be administered because its action will coincide with the increased insulin sensitivity that follows exercise.

Exercise Precautions for Type 2 Diabetes with Hyperglycemia

While people with type 1 diabetes are usually advised to delay exercise when hyperglycemia and ketones are present, this is usually not necessary for people with type 2 diabetes because they do not have a risk for severe insulin deficiency.

If a person with type 2 diabetes has a blood glucose level greater than 300 mg/dL, it is not necessary to advise them to abstain from exercise at that time, especially if they are in a postprandial state. As long as the person is not severely insulin deficient, increasing physical activity is likely to decrease blood glucose levels. If ketones are negative, insulin deficiency is not present.

The client should be advised to remain well-hydrated during exercise, especially when blood glucose is high.

If ketones are present in the hyperglycemic client with type 2 diabetes, strenuous exercise should be avoided.

Precautions for Preventing Exercise-Induced Hypoglycemia

For individuals taking insulin or insulin secretagogues, blood glucose should be monitored before exercise and additional carbohydrate consumed if results are less than 90 mg/dL. Risk for hypoglycemia is especially high when injected insulin is at its peak action or exercise is prolonged.

For those not treated with insulin or secretagogues, exercise-induced hypoglycemia is rare. Updated American Diabetes Association (ADA) guidelines indicate that supplemental carbohydrate is not needed prior to exercise, even if blood glucose is less than 90 mg/dL when:

- Treating diabetes by lifestyle modification alone
- Using metformin, alpha-glucosidase inhibitors, or thiazolidinediones without insulin or secretagogues

The risk of exercise-induced hypoglycemia associated with the amylin analog pramlintide or the incretin mimetic exenatide has not been studied. The ADA suggests that neither drug has high potential for causing exercise-induced hypoglycemia when used alone or in combination with metformin or a thiazolidinedione. If these medications are taken with insulin or a secretagogue, supplemental carbohydrate would be needed prior to exercise when blood glucose is below 90 mg/dL.

Post-Exercise, Late-Onset Hypoglycemia

Post-exercise, late-onset hypoglycemia (PEL) is exercise-induced low blood glucose that occurs 4 or more hours after exercise. It happens most commonly to people with type 1 diabetes, but anyone using insulin or insulin secretagogues is at risk. The risk is increased after exercising at moderate to intense levels for more than 30 minutes.

Physiologically, PEL is the result of exercise-related increases in glucose utilization and insulin sensitivity and the replenishment of glycogen stores post-exercise.

Clients who use insulin or insulin secretagogues should be educated about the risk for PEL and be instructed to watch for signs of impending hypoglycemia beyond the immediate post-exercise period. Adjustments to insulin can be made to avoid having peak action occur during the post-exercise period. Another option to prevent PEL is to have the client increase carbohydrate consumption after exercise. Clients at risk for PEL should not exercise prior to bedtime to prevent nocturnal hypoglycemia.

Impact of Insulin Injection Technique on Absorption During Exercise

It is important to ensure that insulin is injected into the subcutaneous fat layer and to avoid intramuscular injection. Muscle contractions can hasten the absorption of insulin into the circulation and injecting into muscle increases the risk for exercise-induced hypoglycemia.

In the past, it was recommended to avoid injecting insulin into the part of the body involved in exercise. For example, injecting into the arm would have been recommended if the person was planning to jog or walk.

More recent research has indicated that this practice does not decrease the risk for exercise-induced hypoglycemia in the person taking insulin injections. Exercise increases insulin absorption no matter the site of injection, so exercise always increases the risk for hypoglycemia in these clients. To avoid hypoglycemia, they should decrease or adjust the insulin dose so that peak action does not coincide with the planned exercise period.

Carbohydrate Replacement During Exercise

If the person does not use insulin or an insulin secretagogue, carbohydrate replacement during exercise is usually not required since the risk for hypoglycemia is low. For those using insulin, the best strategy is to reduce the dose or make adjustments so that peak insulin action does not coincide with exercise. When exercise occurs during the postprandial period, 1 -3 hours after a meal, carbohydrate supplementation may not be needed.

Carbohydrate supplementation may be needed to prevent hypoglycemia when exercise is unplanned or insulin adjustments are not possible. Blood glucose monitoring before, during and after exercise helps determine the individual's glycemic response to exercise and the need for supplementation.

For moderate exercise of 30 -60 minutes duration, 15 extra grams of carbohydrate is often appropriate.

For high-intensity exercise or exercise lasting for more than an hour, 30 -50 grams of additional carbohydrate may be needed for each hour of activity.

Effect of Exercise on Weight Loss

Exercise has long been recognized as an integral part of successful **weight loss** programs. However, exercise alone, without modification of diet or behavior, tends to result in only modest weight loss of approximately 4–5 pounds on average. Higher volume exercise regimens, such as 1 hour daily of moderate intensity aerobic exercise, have the most beneficial effect on weight loss.

For people with diabetes, the health benefits of exercise are greatest with regard to improved glycemic control and cardiovascular health but less pronounced with regard to weight loss. The greatest effect of exercise on weight loss seems to be in maintaining the loss over time. It has been found that people who have been able to maintain larger loss of weight for a year or more typically engage in about 7 hours per week of moderate to vigorous exercise.

Optimizing Fitness Level and Glycemic Response

To optimize fitness level and glycemic response, at least 150 minutes of moderate to vigorous exercise per week is recommended. For optimal insulin sensitization, exercise should occur about every other day, or at least 3 days per week with no more than two days between exercise sessions.

For weight loss, more frequent exercise (e.g., 5–7 days per week) is needed.

For minimum health conditioning, 700 calories should be expended per week on exercise. Expending 2,000 calories per week yields maximum health and fitness benefits. There is little evidence to suggest that expending more than 2,000 calories per week on exercise substantially increases health and fitness benefits.

Intensity of exercise should be such that the client's heart rate is 50–85% of their maximum age-adjusted heart rate. A target heart rate in that range is selected based on the results of exercise stress testing or the individual's fitness level, age, duration of diabetes, and presence of complications and comorbidities. In the absence of stress testing, maximum age-adjusted heart rate can be estimated by subtracting the client's age from 220.

Modifying the Exercise Program of Those with Microvascular Complications

Modifications to the exercise plan based on microvascular complications include the following:

- **Proliferative or severe nonproliferative retinopathy:** Clients should be instructed to avoid vigorous aerobic or resistance exercises to prevent vitreous hemorrhage and retinal detachment.
- **Peripheral neuropathy:** Clients who have lost protective sensation in the lower extremities should be advised to avoid exercises that increase the risk for skin breakdown, joint injury, and Charcot fracture. At the very least, protective and well-fitting shoes and socks should be worn at all times. In cases of severe loss of protective sensation, non-weight-bearing activities such as cycling or swimming are recommended.
- **Autonomic neuropathy:** This poses risk for decreased cardiac response to exercise, postural hypotension, silent angina, and impaired thirst sensation. These clients should undergo thorough cardiac evaluation before being recommended an exercise program.

- **Microalbuminuria:** Exercise can increase urinary protein excretion but studies have not confirmed that exercise accelerates decline in kidney function. Therefore, the presence of microalbuminuria should not limit exercise. However, the cardiovascular status of microalbuminuric individuals should be considered since microalbuminuria and nephropathy are associated with increased cardiovascular risk.

Exercise Program for Clients with Peripheral Vascular Disease (PVD)

Intermittent claudication is PVD-related ischemic pain resulting from an inadequate oxygen supply to the muscles of the lower extremities. The pain is exacerbated by walking and alleviated by rest. Although it causes discomfort, a walking program is usually recommended to increase collateral circulation and improve condition. However, when the person has pain at rest or during the night, the degree of PVD is severe and a walking program is contraindicated.

The walking program is usually developed to provide intervals of activity and rest. The client is instructed to walk at a low intensity and to continue walking through low to moderate pain. Distraction techniques such as listening to music or talking to a partner can help. The client should rest when pain begins to elevate from moderate to intense.

Benefits from the interval exercise program are optimized when the client participates every day and engages in weight-bearing exercise.

Person-Centered Education on Self-Care Behaviors: Medication Management

Physiological Effects of Insulin on Body Tissues and Hormones

Insulin is a hormone secreted by the beta cells of the Islets of Langerhans in the pancreas.

Actions of insulin on body tissues include:

- Augments protein synthesis by promoting the entry of amino acids into the cells
- Promotes utilization of glucose for energy by stimulating its entry into the cells
- Enhances storage of unused glucose as glycogen in muscle and liver cells
- Enhances the storage of fat and prevents the use of fat breakdown for energy
- Impedes glycogenolysis, the making of glucose from glycogen stored in muscle and liver cells
- Impedes the formation of glucose from amino acids and other non-carbohydrate sources

Counter-regulatory hormones antagonize the hypoglycemic effects of insulin. These include glucagon, epinephrine, norepinephrine, growth hormone, and cortisol.

Classification of Insulin

Insulin type	Onset	Peak	Duration	Teaching
Rapid-acting	5–15 min	30–90 min	Less than 5 hours	Inject less than 15 minutes before eating. Injecting too early can cause profound hypoglycemia.

Insulin type	Onset	Peak	Duration	Teaching
Short-acting	30 min	2–4 hours	5–8 hours	Like rapid-acting, used as bolus insulin to provide postprandial glucose control.
Intermediate-acting	1–2 hours	4–10 hours	10–18 hours	Cloudy insulin; gently roll and rotate vial prior to filling syringe to resuspend particles.
Long-acting	1–2 hours	None	Up to 24 hours	Do not mix in same syringe with other insulins.

Rapid-Acting Insulins

Rapid-acting insulins are given as bolus doses to provide post-meal blood glucose control. They include lispro, aspart, and glulisine insulin. They are usually used in place of regular (short-acting) insulin and have shorter onset, peak, and duration times.

Rapid-acting insulin begins to work in 5–15 minutes after injection. Clients should be cautioned to avoid injecting this type of insulin too early because profound hypoglycemia can result, especially with lispro. However, when compared with regular insulin, both lispro and aspart have a lower overall risk for hypoglycemia.

Peak action for rapid-acting insulin is 1–2 hours. Duration is usually less than 5 hours. The injection of aspart insulin into the abdominal subcutaneous tissue has been shown to shorten the duration of its action time.

The rapid-acting insulins are suitable for multiple daily injections and for use with an insulin pump.

Long-Acting Insulins

Long-acting insulins include glargine, detemir, and degludec. They are options for basal insulin therapy and should provide about 50% of the daily insulin requirement continuously over 24 hours. Long-acting insulin is often used in combination with bolus insulin or oral agents that provide postprandial blood glucose control.

Long-acting insulin can be given once or twice daily. When administered once daily, the dose is usually given at bedtime. It should always be given at the same time each day.

Long-acting insulins have a "peakless" action and therefore pose a lower risk for hypoglycemia than insulins with shorter action times. The risks for nocturnal hypoglycemia and weight gain are lower in people with type 2 diabetes who use long-acting insulin as compared to those who use NPH.

Patients using long-acting insulin should be instructed that the insulin is not to be mixed in the same syringe with other types of insulin.

Routine Insulin Injections

Routine insulin injections should be made into subcutaneous tissue. Most people can accomplish this by grasping a fold of skin and injecting at a 90-degree angle. If a person is very thin, injecting at a 45-degree angle is advised. Shorter needles are also available.

Aspiration of the needle to check for blood is no longer considered necessary.

When using an insulin pen, the needle should remain embedded within the tissue and the plunger depressed for at least 5 seconds to ensure complete delivery of insulin from the device.

Air bubbles should be removed from the filled syringe to ensure proper insulin dose.

When clear fluid escapes the puncture site, pressure should be applied for 5–8 seconds. Rubbing the site is not advised. If it is suspected that a significant portion of the insulin has been lost due to leakage, blood glucose should be monitored within a few hours.

Injecting insulin at room temperature decreases the risk for a painful injection.

STARTING DOSES FOR INSULIN THERAPY

Starting doses for insulin therapy are as follows:

- **Type 1 diabetes:** Daily insulin requirements are usually 0.5–1.0 units per kilogram of body weight. Requirements can be much higher during periods of illness or metabolic instability. During the "honeymoon phase," when some endogenous insulin is still being produced, injected daily insulin requirements are usually 0.2–0.6 units/kg of body weight.
- **Type 2 diabetes:** There is more variability in the starting does of insulin for people with type 2 diabetes. The decision is based on body weight, degree of insulin deficiency, suspected insulin resistance, glycemic goals, and concurrent use of oral antidiabetic agents. Oral medications are often continued while insulin is added to the regimen.

For a single daily injection of basal insulin, 10 units per day is a common starting dose. Because of insulin resistance, initial starting dose relative to body weight is usually higher for type 2 diabetes, often 0.7–2.5 units/kg body weight daily.

BASAL BOLUS INSULIN THERAPY

Basal bolus insulin therapy is designed to mimic the normal patterns of insulin secretion, such as that observed in a person without diabetes.

Basal insulin refers to small amounts of insulin that are secreted continuously. This is sometimes referred to as "background insulin" because it is secreted in steady states and causes no peaks in action.

Bolus insulin refers to bursts of insulin secretion that occur in response to increased blood glucose.

With exogenous insulin therapy, it is possible to closely mimic the normal basal bolus insulin production of the non-diabetic pancreas. The choices for doing this include:

- **Continuous subcutaneous insulin infusion (CSII),** also known as an insulin pump. The pump is programmed to release basal insulin at selected rates. Bolus insulin is controlled by the user each time food is ingested to deliver the calculated insulin-to-carbohydrate ratio.
- **Multiple daily injections.** This choice involves injecting a long-acting insulin analog at least once or twice a day and possibly several times a day or more to provide basal insulin. The user injects a calculated dose of fast or rapid-acting insulin to cover meals.

Advantages and Disadvantages in Type 1 Diabetes

Basal bolus insulin therapy is the preferred choice for people with type 1 diabetes because they produce neither basal nor bolus insulin of their own. Using basal insulin reduces hepatic glucose production, while bolus insulin limits excursions in post-meal blood glucose. Basal bolus insulin therapy, which is delivered via insulin pump or by multiple daily injections, allows for a more flexible lifestyle and the best possible blood glucose control.

Basal bolus insulin therapy requires the client and provider to have a good understanding of the action times of different insulins. The client must also be able to understand the basal bolus concept and to consistently follow through with this type of regimen. A certain level of math literacy (numeracy) is also needed.

For some clients, premixed insulin such as 70/30 NPH/regular may be desirable. However, this does not allow for as much flexibility in the timing of eating or exercise. It also does not allow for the best possible control of blood glucose.

Insulin Regimens for Single Daily Injections and 2 Injections Per Day

Single and 2-dose daily insulin regimens can be utilized as monotherapy or in combination with oral antidiabetic agents in type 2 diabetes.

Single daily injection:

- Contraindicated for type 1 diabetes
- Used when dose requirement is less than 30 units/day
- Administered in the morning or at bedtime using intermediate or long-acting insulin
- Intermediate-acting insulin can be mixed with rapid or short-acting insulin
- Often administered at bedtime to improve fasting blood glucose or to suppress nocturnal glucose production by the liver

Two-injection regimen:

- Administered before breakfast and in the evening, either before dinner or at bedtime
- May include 2 doses of intermediate or long-acting insulin only, or mixed intermediate and rapid or short-acting insulin at either or both injection times
- Typically, two-thirds of the total daily dose is given at the morning injection and one-third in the evening.

Mixing Two Types of Insulin in the Same Syringe

Rapid-acting and regular insulin are drawn into the syringe before intermediate-acting insulin to avoid protamine contamination of the clear insulin. Glargine should never be mixed with another type of insulin.

Some mixtures come premixed by the manufacturer in predetermined ratios. An example is Humulin 70/30, which includes 70% NPH plus 30% regular insulin. While convenient, these mixtures have the disadvantage of decreasing the flexibility and fine-tuning of the regimen. They are most appropriately used with clients who need a simple regimen or who have cognitive or functional issues that impair their ability to mix insulin.

Prefilling syringes is acceptable if guidelines to protect the potency of the insulin are followed. Regular and NPH insulins can be mixed and stored in the refrigerator for 1 month. The syringes should be stored vertically with the needle pointing up to prevent the suspended insulin particles from clogging the needle.

Pros and Cons of Using Insulin to Treat Type 2 Diabetes

The decision to initiate insulin should be based on the need for glycemic control. If lifestyle interventions and oral medications do not achieve control, starting insulin improves the chances for a better outcome. Unfortunately, some patients perceive this as a sign of failure or punishment for not achieving control.

An advantage of insulin therapy is that, as beta cell function naturally declines, the insulin dosage can be adjusted up, with no ceiling, to achieve glycemic goals.

Weight gain when initiating insulin is a concern. Patients can count carbohydrates and increase exercise to offset this risk. Concurrent use of metformin can also help.

Hypoglycemia is a significant risk for patients using insulin. Patients must be taught to closely match the timing and content of meals with their insulin dosing and to be alert for signs of impending hypoglycemia.

Pain, inconvenience, and fear of needles are all reasons why patients resist starting insulin. Because of its effectiveness in gaining glycemic control and producing better outcomes, educators must communicate positively about the advantages of insulin.

Using Pattern Management to Adjust Insulin Doses

Normally, pattern management involves observing and recording blood glucose for 2–3 days and making insulin adjustments based on a pattern of high or low blood glucose at a given time of day. However, for very high blood glucose values, supplemental insulin can be taken immediately.

Changes in insulin doses are made according to the time of day being observed and the type of insulin being used. Although treatment regimens are always individualized, a rule of thumb is to adjust only after a pattern is observed for 2–3 days and changes are made in 10–20% increments until target blood glucose is achieved.

Examples of **insulin adjustments** in response to patterns include:

- Glucose high or low before breakfast → Adjust bedtime intermediate (NPH) or long-acting (glargine, detemir) insulin
- Glucose high after breakfast → Adjust pre-breakfast rapid-acting insulin
- Glucose high after lunch → Adjust pre-lunch rapid-acting insulin
- Glucose high after dinner → Adjust pre-dinner rapid-acting insulin

Interactions of Food, Exercise and Medications

Pattern management is a comprehensive approach to diabetes self-management that is often associated with intensive insulin therapy. However, it can also be useful for identifying any appropriate changes that could be made to improve glycemic control.

Pattern management involves analyzing 3–5 days' worth of blood glucose readings and identifying patterns of high or low blood glucose that occur at the same time each day. Adjustments can then be made based on a blood glucose trend, rather than responding to a single reading.

Pattern management allows choices in how to respond to these patterns. For example, the insulin or medication doses could be adjusted up or down based on a blood glucose pattern. Other choices would be to increase or decrease carbohydrate consumption or to change exercise frequency, timing, or intensity.

Intensive Insulin Therapy

Intensive insulin therapy includes 3 or more injections per day. Glycemic control is optimized when a basal bolus regimen mimics the physiologic profile of insulin secretion as closely as possible.

Basal insulin is intermediate or long-acting insulin that provides an ongoing low level of insulin to provide for basic metabolic needs. Bolus insulin is rapid or fast-acting insulin that is given to control post-meal blood glucose.

Examples of 3 and 4 daily-injection regimens include:

- Bolus insulin given before each meal
- Bolus insulin before each meal and basal insulin at bedtime
- Bolus insulin given before breakfast and lunch and basal insulin given at bedtime
- Bolus regimen with intermediate-acting insulin before breakfast + bolus insulin before the evening meal + intermediate-acting insulin at bedtime

When intermediate-acting insulin is given in the morning, bolus insulin should NOT be given at lunchtime, as the peak times for both insulins would coincide and could cause profound hypoglycemia.

Storage and Preparation Guidelines for Insulin

Insulin vials that are currently in use can be stored at room temperature for the number of days that the manufacturer specifies, as long as room temperature remains between 36° and 86° F. Vials of insulin not in current use should be stored in a refrigerator and used by the printed expiration date. The client should always have a spare bottle of each type of insulin that he or she is using.

Care should be taken to avoid vigorous agitation of the insulin vial, as this can cause loss of potency.

Prior to drawing an injection, the client should inspect the insulin for signs of degradation, such as clumping, frosting, precipitation, or change in clarity or color. Rapid and fast-acting insulins, as well as glargine, should remain clear. Intermediate-acting insulin should remain uniformly cloudy without clumping.

In situations where a client has otherwise unexplained loss of glycemic control, reduction in insulin potency should be considered.

Safety Precautions Related to Insulin Syringes

Clients using insulin should be carefully instructed that insulin syringes are manufactured in different sizes, according to the capacity of insulin they can hold. This can affect the value of the markings on the syringe used for measuring the insulin. For example, a 0.3 cc (30 unit) or 0.5 cc (50 unit) syringe has measurement marks in 1-unit increments, whereas a 1.0 cc (100 unit) syringe has measurement markings in 2-unit increments. When a client switches from one type of syringe to another, there is the risk that he or she will assume the measurement marks are the same for both syringes; this could lead to potentially dangerous dosing errors.

Insulin syringes should never be shared with another person.

Because bending or breaking needles increases the risk for needle-stick injury, these practices should be discouraged.

Educators should instruct clients on the appropriate disposal of medical sharps waste in compliance with their local ordinances.

Reusing Insulin Syringes and Needles

Manufacturers of disposable needles and syringes recommend single use only. The American Diabetes Association (ADA) neither encourages nor prohibits needle and **syringe reuse** but provides guidelines for those who choose to reuse for convenience or economic reasons.

Personal hygiene will help reduce risk for infection related to using unsterile needles. Insulin is manufactured with bacteriostatic additives that are active against common skin contaminants, but the used needle may carry bacteria. Those who are immunocompromised should not reuse needles.

Guidelines for needle reuse include:

- Discard needle when it is visibly dull or damaged.
- Discard needle if it comes into contact with any environmental surface.
- Cap the needle to be reused after each use.
- Store the syringe at room temperature.
- Do not clean the needle with alcohol or any other disinfectant. This will remove the silicone coating that makes the injection more comfortable.
- Inspect injection sites for signs of infection or lipodystrophy.

Amylin Analog as a Treatment for Insulin Deficiency

People with insulin deficiency are also amylin deficient. Amylin is a hormone that is normally secreted by the pancreatic beta cells along with insulin. It serves to reduce postprandial hyperglycemia and cause satiety, leading to weight loss.

Pramlintide is an amylin analog given as an injection.

Nausea is a common side effect of pramlintide, but it is usually dose-related and subsides over time.

The potential for insulin-induced hypoglycemia is a major concern with using pramlintide. The insulin dose must therefore be adjusted down when the amylin analog is started. Also, the client must be willing to test blood glucose numerous times a day to monitor and prevent hypoglycemia when using pramlintide.

Determining Appropriate Oral Medications for Type 2 Diabetes

While the American Diabetes Association (ADA) recommends starting with **metformin** (an oral medication) at the onset of type 2 diabetes, individual characteristics may alter the decision.

- Liver and kidney function must be tested before starting any oral diabetes medication.
- Metformin is not used when glomerular filtration rate (GFR) is less than 30 and/or serum creatinine is greater than 1.5 mg/dL in women or greater than 1.4 mg/dL in men.
- When renal function is decreased, the risk for hypoglycemia is greater with the use of insulin secretagogues.
- When the alanine aminotransferase (ALT) level is elevated above 2.5 times normal, the use of metformin and thiazolidinediones is contraindicated.
- Metformin is contraindicated in clients who drink alcohol excessively or engage in binge drinking.

- Thiazolidinediones are contraindicated in people with heart failure and severe cardiac disease. Metformin should be used with caution in these clients.
- Glucose toxicity usually requires insulin prior to initiation of oral medications. Signs of glucose toxicity include prolonged hyperglycemia, HbA1c >9%, and possibly ketones.

METFORMIN

Metformin prevents high blood glucose primarily by decreasing glucose dumping from the liver. A secondary effect is that it decreases insulin resistance. In patients on certain medications, such as high-dose glucocorticoids or PI3Kα inhibitors, metformin should be considered as a preventive measure for the known risk for hyperglycemia that is associated with these medications.

The dosage range is 500–2,550 mg/day.

The most common side effects are gastrointestinal. These include nausea, bloating, gas, diarrhea, and metallic taste in the mouth. They are more common with higher doses and in the first 2 weeks of therapy. Long-term metformin use is associated with deficiency of vitamin B12, so 2026 ADA guidelines suggest periodic assessment of B12 levels. Supplementation may be required in individuals with concomitant anemia or peripheral neuropathy.

Metformin is contraindicated in patients with decreased renal function. Metformin should not be prescribed in those with a glomerular filtration rate less than 30. Metformin should not be used in people who drink more than 2 alcoholic beverages a day or engage in binge drinking.

Caution is advised when there is concurrent heart failure, dehydration, acidosis, NPO status, or pending iodine radio contrast studies.

PATIENT EDUCATION

Patient education for metformin:

- Take the medication with food to reduce risk for gastrointestinal side effects.
- If gastrointestinal side effects are severe, call your healthcare provider.
- The medication takes up to 1 month to reach maximum effectiveness.
- Use caution when drinking alcohol. Drinking in excess can cause a serious and life-threatening condition called lactic acidosis. Consult with your healthcare provider to ascertain if moderate alcohol consumption (less than 2 drinks per day) is safe for you.
- Stop taking metformin if you are not eating and drinking or become dehydrated.
- Stop taking metformin on the day of surgery or when having studies using radio contrast dye.
- This medication increases chances for becoming pregnant in patients who have polycystic ovary syndrome. Discuss birth control options with your healthcare provider.
- Always carry medical identification stating that you have diabetes.

SULFONYLUREAS

Sulfonylureas include glipizide, glyburide, and glimepiride. They work by stimulating the pancreas to produce more insulin. They are only effective in people who maintain some beta cell function.

The most common side effect is hypoglycemia. The risk for this is greatest in the first few months of starting the medication. To prevent hypoglycemia, the patient should check blood glucose regularly, avoid delaying or missing meals, and avoid drinking alcohol. Other side effects include weight gain, sun sensitivity, headache, and nausea.

Liver and kidney function should be tested prior to starting a sulfonylurea. If either function is low, the risk for hypoglycemia is increased. Healthcare providers should exercise caution when prescribing to the elderly, who often have decreased liver and kidney function as well as a higher risk for hypoglycemic unawareness. Patients with adrenal or pituitary insufficiency are also at higher risk for hypoglycemia when taking sulfonylureas.

People with severe sulfa allergies may not be able to take sulfonylurea medications.

Thiazolidinedione Medications (TZDs)

TZDs include pioglitazone and rosiglitazone. They work by increasing the insulin sensitivity of liver and skeletal tissues and by suppressing glucose production by the liver. ADA guidelines recommend the use of pioglitazone for stroke and myocardial infarction risk reduction in individuals with a history of stroke with insulin resistance.

Side effects include weight gain, mild to moderate edema, bone fractures in women, and upper respiratory symptoms. When used alone, these agents do not cause hypoglycemia. However, when used with a sulfonylurea or insulin, risk may be increased.

TZDs have a black box warning that they may cause or exacerbate congestive heart failure (CHF) in some patients and are contraindicated in people with class III or IV heart failure. The manufacturer of rosiglitazone advises against prescribing this medication for any patient who uses nitrates or insulin, as these drug combinations have been associated with increased risk for cardiac problems.

TZDs are associated with rare cases of idiosyncratic hepatocellular damage. TZDs are used with caution in people with hepatic dysfunction. Serum transaminase should be checked every 2 months during the first year of therapy and periodically thereafter.

Patient Education

Patient education for thiazolidinediones (TZDs):

- Notify a healthcare provider immediately if edema, sudden weight gain, shortness of breath, or other signs of fluid retention develop.
- TZDs may induce ovulation in premenopausal women with insulin resistance. If applicable, discuss family planning and birth control with a healthcare provider.
- It may take several weeks of therapy to realize optimal effect.
- Drug effectiveness and risk for side effects are not altered by food. Take with or without food.
- If using with insulin or a sulfonylurea, there is an increased risk for hypoglycemia. Monitor blood glucose regularly and be prepared to treat hypoglycemia with a fast-acting carbohydrate.
- Do not take TZDs if you are pregnant or breastfeeding.
- Always carry medical identification stating that you have diabetes.

Dipeptidyl Peptidase-4 (DPP-4) Inhibitors

DPP-4 inhibitors include sitagliptin, saxagliptin, linagliptin, and alogliptin.

DPP-4 is an enzyme that rapidly inactivates the incretin hormones. Incretins are digestive hormones that are released from the small intestine after eating in response to the post-meal rise in blood glucose. They lower blood sugar by stimulating insulin release and by decreasing glucagon production in the pancreas. The DPP-4 inhibitors prolong active incretin levels, allowing for increased insulin action following the post-meal rise in blood glucose.

The most common side effects of DPP-4 inhibitors are upper respiratory infection, urinary tract infection, and headache. They are unlikely to cause hypoglycemia because they do not work well when blood glucose is low.

These medications may be used in patients with renal issues when guidelines for dosage adjustments are followed.

Alpha-Glucosidase Inhibitor (AGI) Medications

AGIs include acarbose and miglitol. They work by reducing the rate of starch digestion and slowing its absorption through the small intestine, thus lowering post-meal blood glucose levels.

The most common side effects of AGIs are abdominal pain, diarrhea, and flatulence. Side effects can be minimized by starting with a low dose and titrating upward.

When used alone, AGIs do not cause hypoglycemia. However, patients also using insulin or a sulfonylurea remain at risk for hypoglycemia. When taking these medications concurrently, patients require special instructions for treating hypoglycemia since the AGIs block the absorption of complex sugars. Only glucose and lactose are effective in treating hypoglycemia in patients who take AGIs.

AGIs are contraindicated in inflammatory bowel disease, cirrhosis, malabsorption disorders, pregnancy, and lactation. They are not recommended in patients with serum creatinine greater than 2.0 mg/dL or with creatinine clearance of less than 25 mL/min.

Patient Education

Patient education for AGIs should include the following points:

- To be effective, acarbose and miglitol must be taken with the first bite of food at the meal. Initially, the medication might be used only once a day to minimize gastrointestinal side effects. GI side effects should lessen over a few weeks. If the low initial dose is tolerated, it will be titrated upward until the desired therapeutic effect is reached. By that point, AGI therapy is usually being taken at all three meals each day.
- Patients using an AGI concurrently with a sulfonylurea or insulin are at risk for hypoglycemia from the latter two medications. If hypoglycemia occurs while using an AGI, most standard treatments will not be effective because the medication blocks the absorption of complex sugars through the small intestine. The only types of carbohydrate that will be effective are lactose (milk) and glucose (usually tablets).
- Carry medical identification that states you have diabetes.

Meglitinides

Meglitinides include repaglinide and nateglinide. They work by stimulating the pancreas to promptly release insulin in a glucose-dependent fashion with a shorter duration of action than sulfonylureas.

Hypoglycemia is a potential side effect of meglitinides. However, the risk is significantly lower as compared to sulfonylureas. Other side effects are not common but may include gastrointestinal complaints, upper respiratory symptoms, back pain, and arthralgia.

Meglitinides must be taken within 30 minutes of the meal. If a meal is skipped, the medication dose is to be withheld. For this reason, meglitinides may be a good choice for patients with erratic eating habits.

Meglitinides are normally started at a low dose and titrated upward until glycemic goals are met. These medications should be used cautiously in patients with impaired hepatic function. Cautious use is also recommended in any patient with increased risk for hypoglycemia, such as the elderly and those with impaired renal, adrenal, or pituitary function.

INCRETIN MIMETICS

Incretin mimetics (also referred to as GLP-1 receptor agonists) include exenatide, liraglutide, dulaglutide, and semaglutide. They mimic the action of the incretin hormones glucagon-like peptide-1 (GLP-1) and gastric inhibitory polypeptide (GIP), causing an increase in insulin secretion from the pancreas. They also delay gastric emptying, increasing satiety and promoting weight loss. GLP-1 receptor agonists should be considered in the management of type 2 diabetes along with metabolic dysfunction-associated steatohepatitis (MASH), metabolic dysfunction-associated steatotic liver disease (MASLD), overweight, and obesity. GLP-1 RAs also facilitate heart failure prevention benefits, and are recommended (with or without GIPs) for clients with type 2 diabetes and high risk for cardiovascular disease and/or mild to moderate heart failure. Additionally, new evidence has supported a decrease in risk for lower extremity amputation with GLP-1 RA therapy for peripheral artery disease.

Exenatide is given within 60 minutes prior to the morning and evening meals. Missed doses should not be administered after the meal. Exenatide is not labeled for use with insulin and is contraindicated in type 1 diabetes. Exenatide has been associated with pancreatitis and is contraindicated in patients with a history of this condition. The most common side effects are nausea, vomiting and diarrhea. Hypoglycemia can occur if exenatide is used in conjunction with a sulfonylurea.

Liraglutide is delivered as a once-daily subcutaneous injection. Dulaglutide is available in the subcutaneous form through the use of a pen injector, administered once weekly. Semaglutide is available in both oral (Rybelsus) and subcutaneous (Ozempic) forms. The oral form is administered 30–60 minutes prior to the first meal of the day, and the subcutaneous form is administered once weekly.

PRECAUTIONS AND CONTRAINDICATIONS

Liraglutide, dulaglutide, and semaglutide are not considered first-line treatments for those with type 2 diabetes. Rather, they are recommended in conjunction with diet and exercise for those for whom metformin has not proven effective. These medications may be recommended as an alternative first-line treatment for those with type 2 diabetes and concurrent atherosclerosis/cardiovascular disease due to their inhibitory effect on the buildup of atherosclerotic plaque.

Exenatide, liraglutide, dulaglutide, and semaglutide carry a black box warning cautioning that thyroid tumors were observed in rodent tests of this medication. For this reason, these medications are contraindicated in those with multiple endocrine neoplasia syndrome and/or a history/family history of medullary thyroid carcinoma.

PATIENT EDUCATION

Patient education for incretin mimetics:

- Exenatide and liraglutide are administered subcutaneously by injection into the abdomen, thigh, or upper arm.
- The injection should be given as directed, including number of doses, time of day, and whether they should be taken before or with a meal.

- Store the prefilled syringes in the refrigerator. Remove the needle from the pen after each use.
- Gastrointestinal side effects are common. These can sometimes be alleviated by injecting the medication closer to the mealtime. Nausea frequently subsides with continued use.
- The patient should report possible signs and symptoms of pancreatitis, such as persistent abdominal pain or vomiting.
- Oral antibiotics and contraceptives should be taken 1 hour apart from incretin mimetics.
- Always carry medical identification stating that you have diabetes.

Sodium-Glucose Cotransporter 2 Inhibitors

Sodium-glucose cotransporter 2 inhibitors (SGLC2 inhibitors) include ertugliflozin, dapagliflozin, empagliflozin, and canagliflozin. They work by inhibiting the reabsorption of glucose in the proximal tubule of the kidney by 50–90%. Excess glucose is therefore excreted by the kidneys. SGLC2 inhibitors share the cardiovascular benefits of GLP-1 receptor agonists and are similarly recommended by the ADA as a first-line or alternative treatment for patients with type 2 diabetes and concurrent cardiovascular disease, particularly in the context of heart failure. ADA guidelines recommend the initiation of SGLC2 inhibitors when the eGFR is less than 20 mL/min/1.73 m^2 and the urinary albumin-to-creatinine ratio is less than 200 mg/g. SGLC2 inhibitors should not be used in individuals with kidney failure.

SGLC2 inhibitors are administered orally, once daily in the morning regardless of mealtime. Maximum effect requires that SGLC2 inhibitors are used in conjunction with diet and exercise. They may be added to a regimen that includes metformin if metformin alone was not effective.

Using Combination Therapy in Individuals with Diabetes

As a naturally progressive disorder, diabetes usually requires increasingly intensive therapy over time. This is due to progressive loss of beta cell function and/or increasing insulin resistance.

Various classes of diabetes medications target the different physiological defects of type 2 diabetes. Often, combination therapy, or simultaneously using medications from different classes, is necessary to gain and maintain glycemic control.

In addition to glycemic control, ameliorating the high risk for cardiovascular disease is imperative for good diabetes management. As hypertension and dyslipidemia are often comorbidities with insulin resistance, these usually require their own pharmacological intervention in addition to the medications patients with diabetes may need to achieve and maintain glycemic control.

Due to the complexity of the type 2 diabetes disease process, coupled with the need for cardiovascular protection, polypharmacy is common in the treatment of type 2 diabetes.

Insulin Pump Therapy

Basal and Bolus Components

Although an insulin pump is designed to provide both basal and bolus insulin, the only type of insulin used with the pump is rapid-acting, such as lispro or aspart.

The basal dose is programmed to deliver a constant supply of insulin at a low level. The basal dose can be set to vary for particular time periods throughout the day. For example, a patient with elevated early morning blood glucose may set the pump to deliver more insulin in the pre-waking and early morning hours. Basal rates are highly individualized and depend on blood glucose patterns and usual activity level. Typically, 4–6 different basal rates are set for a 24-hour period.

Bolus rates are designed to correct for episodes of high blood glucose and to cover the anticipated carbohydrate load of a meal. The client pushes a button on the pump to deliver the bolus dose at the appropriate time.

Patient Education

Technical malfunction of the pump can cause interruptions in insulin delivery and may result in ketosis.

As with any insulin use, hypoglycemia is a risk.

The risk for inflammation and infection at the catheter insertion site can be reduced by following good personal hygiene, careful hand washing, and changing the site and tubing every 3 days. Changing the tubing at this interval also prevents clogging.

Tube and reservoir changes should be done early in the day to avoid undetected malfunctions during sleep.

Consistently rotating insertion sites reduces the risk for lipodystrophy and maintains good absorption of the insulin.

The insulin pump should be removed when the client is undergoing x-rays, CT scans, MRIs, or radiation therapy and the device should be kept out of these treatment areas.

1700 Rule for Bolus Doses

The 1700 Rule assumes that only rapid-acting insulin is being used as a bolus to correct high blood glucose. If correcting with regular insulin, the 1500 Rule is used. There is no standard formula for safely correcting hyperglycemia with intermediate or long-acting insulin.

The 1700 Rule determines by approximately how many mg/dL the blood glucose will be lowered by 1 unit of insulin.

1. Add up total daily insulin dose. This includes rapid, short, intermediate, and long-acting insulin.

Example: 10 units of aspart before each meal and 30 units of NPH at bedtime. Total daily dose = 60 units

2. Divide 1700 by the total daily dose.

Example: 1700 divided by 60 = 28

3. One unit of aspart will lower the blood glucose by approximately 28 mg/dL.

4. If blood glucose is 210 mg/dL and the target is 100 mg/dL, the correction dose would be approximately 4 units of aspart.

Example: 210 – 100 = 110

110 divided by 28 = 3.93 (round to 4.0)

Initial Dosing and Adjustment for Oral Diabetes Medications

Initial dosing and adjustment of oral medications:

- Sulfonylureas are initiated at the lowest dose and titrated upward until glycemic goals are attained or maximum dose is reached.
- Meglitinide doses do not need titration. The initial and maintenance dose is normally 120 mg taken before each meal.
- The biguanide dose usually starts at 500 mg per day for adults and 250 mg daily for children. Although normally subtherapeutic, the starting dose is low to minimize gastrointestinal side effects. Gradual increases are made about every 2 weeks.
- Thiazolidinediones are typically started at a low dose and gradually titrated upward to achieve glycemic targets. Adjustments should be made every 8–12 weeks, as this much time is needed for the optimal benefit to be realized.
- Alpha-glucosidase inhibitors are initiated at lower doses to minimize gastrointestinal effects. The initial dose is usually 25 mg with meals, starting with one meal per day, and increased to patient tolerance.
- Dipeptidyl peptidase-4 (DPP-4) inhibitors have once-daily dosing that does not require titration. Dosage adjustments are made for patients with renal issues.

Medications that Interact with Diabetes Treatment

Medications that can raise blood glucose levels:

- Glucocorticoids, such as prednisone
- Thiazide diuretics, such as HCTZ
- Phenytoin
- Estrogen compounds
- Antipsychotics, such as clozapine, olanzapine, and risperidone
- Anticancer medications, such as immune checkpoint inhibitors, phosphoinositidylinositol 3-kinase α (PI3Kα) inhibitors, and mTOR inhibitors

Clients on any of these medications should have routine plasma glucose monitoring for hyperglycemia.

Non-diabetes medications that can lower blood glucose:

- Some antibiotics, such as clarithromycin and levofloxacin
- Salicylates in large doses
- Ethanol (alcohol), especially if consumed without food

Medications that can raise blood pressure or interfere with effectiveness of blood pressure medications:

- Anti-inflammatory agents, such as ibuprofen
- Glucocorticoids
- Over-the-counter nasal decongestants and cold remedies
- Oral contraceptives
- Tricyclic antidepressants, such as nortriptyline

Medications that mask hypoglycemia:

- Beta blockers, such as propranolol

Clients should be encouraged to keep an updated list of all of their medications and to bring it to each appointment so that possible drug interactions can be detected.

Safety Issues Related to the Use of Herbs

An evaluation of the use of herbs should be included in the medication assessment. Although these are sold over-the-counter, there are potential safety issues with their use. These issues include:

- Gastrointestinal side effects such as diarrhea (dandelion), or fecal impaction (guar gum).
- Dosages are not well-established, increasing the risk for toxicity.
- Some have potential to raise blood glucose (ma huang, rosemary).
- Some have potential to lower blood glucose, thereby increasing risk for hypoglycemia in clients using insulin or secretagogues (fenugreek, ginseng, prickly pear/cactus).
- Some have the potential to raise blood pressure (ma huang, licorice).
- Some have potential for liver damage (chaparral, sassafras, comfrey).
- All have potential for interaction with other medications.
- Most herbs have not been adequately studied for safety and efficacy.
- They are not standardized for purity and strength.

Assessment of liver and kidney function is important for the client who uses herbs. Many herbs are deemed unsafe for use during pregnancy.

ADA's Position on Alternative Therapy

ADA criteria for deeming an alternative therapy to be safe and effective are that they must be approved by Food and Drug Administration (FDA) and be supported by at least 2 studies published in a scientific, peer-reviewed journal.

When clients are interested in using alternative therapies, the educator should help them evaluate the claims made by the product and identify the symptoms being targeted by the therapy. Clients should keep a journal of symptoms and their response following implementation of the therapy. Professional complementary care providers are available through the American Holistic Nurses Association and Healing Touch International.

Although not endorsed by the ADA, some alternative modalities that are potentially useful for diabetes are:

- Omega-3 and omega-6 fatty acids to improve lipid profile
- Alpha lipoic acid and capsaicin for symptoms of neuropathy
- Fenugreek seeds, chromium picolinate, and psyllium to lower blood glucose

At one time, cinnamon was believed to lower blood glucose, but several follow-up studies did not support this.

Person-Centered Education on Self-Care Behaviors: Monitoring and Interpretation

Interpretation of Blood Glucose Results

Interpretation of food records, medication practices, and exercise logs are valuable in interpreting blood glucose values and directing changes in therapy. Medication changes should be made based on blood glucose trends rather than a single reading.

When blood glucose is high after meals, possible causes are:

- Too much carbohydrate at the meal
- Not enough pre-meal insulin
- Inadequate dose of oral agent (except metformin)
- Not enough exercise in preceding hours or days

When fasting blood glucose is high, possible causes are:

- Not enough basal insulin
- Inadequate oral medication in the evening or at bedtime

When blood glucose is high most of the time, possible reasons are:

- Insufficient medication dose
- Patient requires combination therapy
- Medication has not been taken for long enough time
- Not enough exercise
- Too much carbohydrate overall
- Excessive stress

When blood glucose values are erratic, possible causes are:

- Inconsistent timing of meals or quantity of carbohydrate intake
- Irregular insulin injection technique, such as changing injection site from the abdomen to the arm
- Insulin has lost potency
- Excessive stress

Assessing Blood Sampling Technique for Self-Monitoring

The most common source of user error in blood glucose monitoring at home is failure to obtain an adequate blood sample. Take every opportunity to assess clients' ability to obtain an adequate sample and always ensure proper placement on the test strip. Educators should be familiar with the type of meter and strip system that the client is using, as different systems require different amounts of blood and different blood drop placement techniques.

Assess client's procedure for collecting an adequate blood sample. This should include:

- Using warm water to wash hands
- Dangling or shaking hand below the waist for approximately 30 seconds
- Setting the adjustable end cap on the lancing device to an appropriate puncture depth
- Using the "milking" technique to push blood to the fingertip (This involves pushing the blood from the base of the finger to the tip, which is more effective than just squeezing the fingertip.)

Equipment/Meter-Related Errors in Self-Monitoring

Additional causes of inaccurate blood glucose readings can be equipment/meter-related, including:

- **Defective test strips** can lead to inaccurate results. The client should check the expiration date before each use, keep the reagent vial tightly capped between uses, and perform periodic control tests of strips. Strips should also be stored away from extreme heat, cold, or humidity.
- Clients using certain types of meters should know how to properly **calibrate the meter** using an inserted strip or setting a code number.
- Some older meters use a reflective technology to read blood glucose. These types of meters need to be **cleaned** if the optic window becomes soiled. Assess the client's ability to properly clean this type of meter according to manufacturer instructions.

Glycated Hemoglobin A1c (HbA1c) Test

The glycated hemoglobin A1c (HbA1c) test is the gold standard test for measuring glycemic control in people with diabetes. Results of the landmark Diabetes Control and Complications Trial (DCCT) and other major studies have shown that elevated HbA1c levels are directly related to long-term complications of diabetes.

The HbA1c provides a depiction of the average blood glucose over the previous 2–3-month period. Glucose in the blood attaches to the hemoglobin molecule, which is measured by the HbA1c test. While recommendations for glycemic control are always individualized, the target HbA1c for most people is 7% or less. According to the ADA, an HbA1c test should be performed at least twice a year in patients that are meeting their treatment goals, and quarterly for patients with a change to their treatment plan and patients that are not meeting their glycemic goals. Point-of-care testing for HbA1c provides a timelier opportunity for treatment changes.

In 2010, its use a tool for diagnosing diabetes was established by the American Diabetes Association (ADA). An HbA1c ≥6.5% is now an accepted diagnostic criterion for diabetes. The ADA states that in order to be valid, the HbA1c test must be done by a standardized and certified laboratory method.

ADA Goals for Self-Monitoring Blood Glucose and HbA1c

Adults

Recommended target ranges for self-monitoring of blood glucose should be individualized and can vary according to age group. While the gold standard test of glycemic control is the HbA1c, daily blood glucose values from self-monitoring should correlate with HbA1c results.

According to the ADA, general **target blood glucose** goals from self-monitoring for most adults are:

- Fasting: 80–130 mg/dL
- Postprandial: <180 mg/dL

Like target ranges for self-monitoring of blood glucose, HbA1c targets should be individualized. Age, pregnancy status, hypoglycemic awareness, and comorbidities are factors to consider when recommending a goal for glycemic control.

In general, the 2026 ADA guidelines recommend a **target HbA1c** of 7% or less for most people. The goal may be less stringent for someone with limited life expectancy or with hypoglycemic unawareness. A more stringent goal may be recommended for a younger person if this can be achieved without significantly increasing the risk for hypoglycemia.

Children

Blood glucose target ranges should be individualized based on assessment of risk and benefit for each patient. As a general guideline, the ADA recommends the following for infants through age 19 with type 1 diabetes, but acknowledges that these goals should be individualized to the risks of each child:

- Ages 0–6
  - 100–180 mg/dL before meals
  - 110–200 mg/dL at bedtime
  - HbA1c <7.5%
- Ages 6–12
  - 90–180 mg/dL before meals
  - 100–180 mg/dL at bedtime
  - HbA1c <7.0% (<7.5% for children that cannot communicate symptoms of hypoglycemia or with higher risk of hypoglycemia)
- Ages 13–19
  - 90–130 mg/dL before meals
  - 90–150 mg/dL at bedtime
  - HbA1c <7.0% (<7.5% for children that cannot communicate symptoms of hypoglycemia or with higher risk of hypoglycemia)

Infants and very young children have more liberal goals to prevent undetected hypoglycemia and protect the developing central nervous system. Goals for all age groups should be adjusted if the child experiences frequent hypoglycemia. The 2026 ADA Standards recommend the use of real-time continuous glucose monitoring (CGM) with insulin therapy to meet glycemic control targets.

Considerations When Recommending Glycemic Targets in Older Adults

Goals for glycemic control should not automatically be raised for elderly clients, as a target HbA1c of 7.0–7.5% may be appropriate for some people over the age of 65.

However, certain factors related to the aging process do require special consideration when recommending glycemic targets for this population. Reasons to consider more lenient targets for older people may include:

- Impaired functional status
- Poor social support or isolated living situation
- Decline in cognitive function
- Hypoglycemic unawareness
- Decreased life expectancy

The ADA recommends an HbA1c goal of less than 7.0–7.5% for the elderly without comorbidities or cognitive decline. Hypoglycemic unawareness is a common change with aging, so choice of medication should take this into account. Selection of medication for elderly clients should also take into account declining kidney and liver function.

Using the Estimated Average Glucose to Correlate HbA1c with Blood Glucose

The HbA1c test is the gold standard for monitoring blood glucose control. By measuring the degree of glycation of the red blood cells, it provides a picture of blood glucose control over the previous 2–

3 months. There is a linear relationship between HbA1c and blood glucose, so as one goes up or down, so does the other.

Recent research has refined a formula for correlating blood glucose and HbA1c values (see table below for the correlations). This is called **estimated average glucose (eAG).** Its purpose is to help patients better interpret their HbA1c in relation to their self-monitoring.

The American Diabetes Association advocates using the eAG to enhance communication with patients about the results of their laboratory values. Using mg/dL as the unit of measure for reporting results is thought to be more understandable to patients, as this is what they are accustomed to seeing on their home testing equipment.

HbA1c	eAG
6%	126 mg/dL
6.5%	140 mg/dL
7%	154 mg/dL
7.5%	169 mg/dL
8%	183 mg/dL

Selecting and Preparing the Fingertip for Self-Monitoring

Capillary blood, usually from the fingertip, is used for self-monitoring of blood glucose. Fingertip testing is more comfortable when the prick is situated along the sides of the fingertip, rather than the tip or the pad where more nerve endings are clustered. The client should also select a site that does not have callus formation and rotate testing sites.

Inadequate blood sample is one of the most common user errors in blood glucose monitoring. Tips for helping a client get an adequate sample from the fingertip include:

- Wash hands vigorously with warm water prior to testing.
- Dangle hand below the waist and shake it for 30–60 seconds to increase blood flow.
- Gently "milk" the finger after the puncture rather than squeezing it.
- Adjust the depth of puncture on the lancing device if necessary.

Using Alternate Sites

Obtaining capillary blood from the fingertip is the most common method for self-monitoring of blood glucose. Some clients prefer alternate-site testing to avoid repeated pricks to the sensitive areas of the fingertips. Alternate sites include the fleshy parts of the palm of the hand, such as the thenar aspect, as well as the forearm, abdomen, or thigh. Clients should only perform alternate-site testing if approved by the manufacturer of their equipment and the proper device for pricking is used. Often a special end cap to the lancing device is required.

Obtaining a blood drop from alternate sites can be more challenging than getting blood from the fingertip. It takes more time for the blood drop to form from these other sites. The lancing device usually needs to be held firmly on the site for several seconds before and after the puncture to produce the drop. Gently rubbing the site for 30–60 seconds before testing may improve blood flow. Instruct the client to follow the manufacturer's instructions for how to place and hold the lancing device on the site.

CONTINUOUS GLUCOSE MONITORING

Continuous glucose monitoring (CGM), is a technology that is gaining more widespread use. The device uses a sensor to measure the glucose of interstitial tissue on a continuous basis. This type of monitoring was initially created for those on intensive insulin regimens (frequent injections or continuous infusions) as the close, real-time monitoring allows for on-the-spot insulin adjustments, but CGM is now more broadly recommended for early initiation at the time of diagnosis with diabetes, to include the diagnosis of type 1 diabetes in children. Because there is a 2- to 3-minute lag between interstitial glucose and capillary blood glucose, alarms for hypoglycemia should be set to go off at a higher-than-usual target to allow for prompt detection of hypoglycemia.

Careful client selection for CGM is important and education/training should be provided on an ongoing basis. Insurance reimbursement for CGM is minimal, so many clients cannot afford the device. Clients selected for CGM should have the cognitive skills and desire to work with technology and be able to use a software system to analyze blood glucose data.

FACTORS TO CONSIDER WHEN SELECTING A BLOOD GLUCOSE METER

When selecting a meter for the client, the insurance formulary often dictates the choices available. In general, all meters meet similar criteria for accuracy as long as the manufacturer's instructions are followed. Test strips for the various meters are comparatively priced.

A plasma-referenced meter may be preferred over a meter that reports results as whole blood. While all meters use a whole blood sample, laboratory glucose values are reported from plasma. Meters that self-calibrate to report results as a plasma value allow better comparison between home and laboratory results.

Some clients may need a meter that helps them adapt to functional limitations in vision, manual dexterity, or cognition. Some meters have strips that come in a cassette that helps reduce the need for inserting a strip into the meter each time. Other meters require fewer steps in the procedure and some have larger screens.

Some clients' lifestyles, occupations, or preferences may indicate that a meter allowing for alternate-site testing is the best choice.

Clients who like technology may prefer a meter with advanced electronic features and data management capabilities.

ASSESSING THE ACCURACY OF A BLOOD GLUCOSE MONITOR

According to the American Diabetes Association, at home blood glucose meters should have at least 95% accuracy (*accurate* is defined as the reading being within 15% of the actual value) for all blood glucose levels that are within "usable range," and in-hospital meters should have at least 98% accuracy for all levels of 75 mg/dL or greater.

When the accuracy of the meter is in question, assessment can be done by comparing meter results with laboratory values using the following procedure:

- Meter accuracy should be checked against laboratory values, not against another meter.
- The laboratory test used for comparison should be a fasting plasma glucose test.
- The laboratory test and the meter test should be performed at the same time.

- The test done using the meter should use capillary blood collected from the fingertip or alternate puncture site. A drop of blood from the venous sample should not be placed on the meter strip.
- The venous blood collected in the laboratory should be spun in the centrifuge within 30 minutes of collection.

It should be noted that meters reporting whole blood results will give a reading 11–15% lower than the plasma levels measured in the laboratory.

Self-Monitoring for Ketones

Ketones, byproducts of fat metabolism, can cause acidosis when present in excessive amounts. They can be measured with a home monitoring system that detects ketones in the blood or with dipsticks that test for ketones in the urine.

People with type 1 diabetes are more prone to ketosis than those with type 2 diabetes. These clients should test for ketones whenever blood glucose is persistently elevated over 300 mg/dL. They should also monitor for ketones when they are on a weight reduction diet or when ill, especially with febrile illness of infectious process.

Clients with type 2 diabetes should monitor for ketones during illness or when an infection is present. It is also recommended that they monitor regularly when they are on hypocaloric weight loss diets.

Some pregnant clients with diabetes should monitor for ketones daily, especially if inappropriate calorie restriction is suspected. Pregnant clients should also check for ketones when ill, undergoing severe stress, or significantly increasing physical activity.

Blood Pressure Monitoring

Control of blood pressure is considered paramount for the reduction of cardiovascular risk in people with diabetes.

For the fifth straight year, the American College of Cardiology has endorsed the American Diabetes Association (ADA) Standards regarding cardiovascular disease and risk management. The 2026 ADA Standards recommend a blood pressure goal of less than 130/80 mmHg for most people with diabetes. In pregnant patients with diabetes and preexisting hypertension, blood pressure goals should be maintained between 110/85 and 135/85 mmHg, while pregnant individuals without preexisting hypertension should have a threshold of 140/90 mmHg for initiating or titrating antihypertensive therapy. In individuals with high cardiovascular or kidney risk, a systolic blood pressure goal of <120 mmHg is recommended. Older adults with poor health or high risk for complications secondary to hypertensive medications can have a more relaxed blood pressure goal of less than 140/90 mmHg.

When the patient's blood pressure is greater than 130/80 mmHg (or the targeted goal for special populations), antihypertensive medication is usually added to therapeutic lifestyle interventions, even when only either the diastolic or systolic value is elevated. One agent is recommended if the blood pressure is between 130/80 and 160/100 mmHg; if greater than 160/100 mmHg, two agents should be utilized.

Angiotensin-converting enzyme (ACE) inhibitors or angiotensin receptor blockers are considered first-line pharmacologic therapy for hypertension in people with diabetes, and calcium channel blockers and diuretics are considered second-line.

Lipid Monitoring

Dyslipidemia associated with type 2 diabetes includes reduced HDL cholesterol and elevated triglyceride levels. These abnormalities, along with hypertension, are known as metabolic syndrome and are associated with increased risk for cardiovascular disease. **Elevated LDL cholesterol** is not specifically associated with type 2 diabetes. However, since LDL cholesterol particles are atherogenic and their presence increases cardiovascular risk, this type of cholesterol is also targeted for control in people with diabetes. The American Diabetes Association (ADA) recommends an LDL cholesterol of less than 100 mg/dL. Further reduction to less than 70 mg/dL is recommended for people with high risk, and less than 55 mg/dL for people with very high risk.

Goals for HDL cholesterol and triglycerides vary among the authoritative bodies, but it is agreed that lipid testing and treatment is paramount in diabetic care. Fasting lipids should be tested at least annually, or every two years if the patient is at low risk. Because the dyslipidemia associated with diabetes includes reduced HDL cholesterol and increased triglycerides, a complete lipid panel is usually warranted. Lifestyle modifications, such as increased physical activity and a diet low in saturated fat, are recommended for dyslipidemia. Statin medication is recommended when LDL cholesterol is greater than 135 mg/dL if the person has no other cardiovascular risk factors. Statin medication should be started in all patients with diabetes who have increased cardiovascular risk, regardless of baseline lipid levels. Because statins have a moderate risk of contributing to type 2 diabetes, these individuals should be closely monitored for hyperglycemia. Despite this, since the benefits of the statins outweigh these risks, it is not recommended that statins be discontinued.

Additionally, 2026 ADA guidelines recommend bempedoic acid treatment as an option for treating individuals with diabetes (without cardiovascular disease) for whom statin therapy is ineffective at lowering cholesterol.

Metabolic Monitoring for Prevention of Cardiovascular Disease

Because cardiovascular disease is the leading cause of death among people with diabetes, measures to prevent heart attack and stroke in these patients are paramount. Studies show that reducing risk factors saves lives.

- While monitoring blood pressure and lipids are essential to risk management, it should be noted that **microalbuminuria** is another important marker of cardiovascular risk. **Urine microalbumin** should be measured annually, starting at 5 years after diagnosis in type 1 diabetes and upon diagnosis in type 2 diabetes. The normal value for spot urine collection is <30 µg/mg.
- **Blood pressure** should be monitored at every visit. The target blood pressure goal for people with diabetes and average cardiovascular risk is less than 130/80 mmHg. For those with high cardiovascular or kidney risk, the systolic goal is less than 120 mmHg. If the patient is pregnant, the goal is less than 135/85 mmHg, to reduce the risk for accelerated hypertension, which may impair the growth of the fetus.
- **Fasting lipid levels** should be measured at least annually. Target goals, according to the American Diabetes Association, are:
    - LDL-C <100 mg/dL
    - HDL-C >40 mg/dL (men)
    - HDL-C >50 mg/dL (women)
    - Triglycerides <150 mg/dL

Additionally, ADA guidelines stress the importance of monitoring for risk of bone fracture in high-risk populations, most effectively using dual-energy x-ray absorptiometry (DEXA scan), as some pharmacological treatment plans enhance the risk for fracture.

Monitoring Renal Function

Tests for measuring renal function include the following:

Microalbuminuria measured by any of three methods:

- Spot urine collection to measure albumin-to-creatinine ratio:
  - Most commonly used of the three options
  - Normal value is less than 30 μg/mL
- 24-hour urine collection to compare simultaneous urine and serum creatinine clearance
- Timed urine collection, such as overnight or for 4 hours

Creatinine clearance to estimate glomerular filtration rate (GFR):

- Depends on carefully timed urine sample, usually over 24 hours
- Inaccuracy in timing or an incomplete sample can lead to erroneous results
- Provides a direct method of estimating GFR

Serum creatinine (SCr) to estimate GFR indirectly:

- Can be calculated based on patient age and weight
- Subtle changes in SCr can herald major loss of renal function

Blood Urea Nitrogen (BUN) also to indirectly measure GFR:

- Less-sensitive marker of early diabetic nephropathy
- Used with SCr to monitor renal function on a day-to-day basis
- Inexpensive and relatively easy test to perform

Microalbuminuria

Microalbumin is a protein that is normally absent from the urine or found in very small amounts when kidney function is normal. The purpose of the microalbumin urine (MAU) test is to detect early microalbuminuria so that further decline in kidney function can be prevented or delayed. The ADA recommends annual screening for microalbuminuria for patients with type 1 diabetes for more than 5 years, all patients with type 2 diabetes, and diabetic patients with comorbid hypertension.

The most commonly used test for albuminuria is the random spot urine sample to evaluate microalbumin-to-creatinine ratio. Results are interpreted as follows:

- Normal is less than 30 μg/mg.
- Microalbuminuria is defined as 30–299 μg/mg.
- Clinical albuminuria is ≥300 μg/mg.

Repeat MAU testing is usually required to confirm findings, as several factors can influence the results. These factors include exercise within 24 hours of the test, infection, fever, inflammatory processes, hyperglycemia, and hypertension. It is recommended that at least two of three tests

Care and Education Interventions

performed within a 6-month period be elevated before confirming that the patient has microalbuminuria.

When clinical albuminuria is present, further testing of glomerular filtration rate (GFR) is indicated.

Liver Function Testing

Although diabetes is not known to directly affect liver function, most people with diabetes undergo routine liver function testing. Because polypharmacy is part of standard diabetes treatment, liver function tests are necessary to evaluate the safety of initiating medications and to monitor the effects of ongoing medication therapy on liver function. Guidelines recommend the use of the Fibrosis-4 (FIB-4) index to identify individuals with risk factors for liver fibrosis by estimating liver scarring.

Use of multiple medications increases the risk for drug interactions that cause inadequate clearance of byproducts from the liver. Elderly patients and patients who abuse alcohol are especially prone to impaired liver function. Caution should be used when prescribing medications that are metabolized by the liver.

The alanine aminotransferase (ALT) test is a common liver function test for medication hepatotoxicity. The reference range for this test is 8–20 U/L.

Handwritten vs. Downloaded Blood Glucose Records

Handwritten records offer greater opportunity to keep a journal of factors that affect blood glucose and may provide more opportunity for problem-solving than downloaded records. With written records, the person with diabetes may be able to more clearly associate such things as food, activity, stress, emotions, and medications to blood glucose results.

Cables and software for downloading meter results are available from most meter manufacturers. Downloading blood glucose records may be more convenient for some people and make testing and recordkeeping more portable. Many providers prefer downloaded records from their patients. When patients use downloaded records exclusively, they may miss opportunities to make important adjustments to the meal or exercise plans or the medication regimen.

Person-Centered Education on Self-Care Behaviors: Acute Complications

Hypoglycemia

Mild to Moderate Hypoglycemia

Hypoglycemia is usually defined as plasma glucose less than 70 mg/dL. Risk for and occurrences of hypoglycemia should be assessed at each encounter, according to the 2026 ADA Standards.

Clients should check blood glucose as soon as symptoms appear to verify hypoglycemia.

When testing for hypoglycemia, the blood sample should be taken from the fingertip. Blood samples from alternate sites, such as the forearm, are not appropriate for detecting hypoglycemia.

Treatment for **mild to moderate hypoglycemia** (plasma glucose 51–70 mg/dL) is 15–20 grams of oral carbohydrate. For glucose of 50 mg/dL or less, 20–30 grams of oral carbohydrate should be consumed.

Blood glucose should be rechecked 15 minutes after taking the carbohydrate. The treatment is repeated if blood glucose remains below 70 mg/dL.

The treatment should be followed with a planned meal or with an additional snack if the meal is more than 1 hour away.

Severe Hypoglycemia

Risk Factors

Severe hypoglycemia is defined as the level at which the patient requires the assistance of another person to treat the symptoms.

Risk factors for severe hypoglycemia include:

- Type 1 diabetes. About 2–4% of deaths in people with type 1 diabetes are due to hypoglycemia. In type 1 disease, the normal glucagon response to low blood glucose diminishes, leading to an increased risk for hypoglycemic unawareness.
- History of recurrent hypoglycemic episodes. The brain adapts to previous hypoglycemia by shifting the sympathetic nervous system response to a lower plasma glucose concentration. The result is an increased risk for severe hypoglycemia.
- Insulin excess. Inappropriate insulin dosing or increased insulin sensitivity can create insulin excess. People with type 2 diabetes using insulin may experience insulin excess if they also use insulin sensitizing medication at the wrong time or take the wrong dose.
- Alcohol consumption. Alcohol can inhibit gluconeogenesis and can lead to hypoglycemia, especially if the person is in a starved state.

Treatment

For people who are alert enough to follow instructions and can swallow, ingestion of 15–20 grams of oral carbohydrate is appropriate to treat severe hypoglycemia. This step can be repeated after 15–20 minutes if hypoglycemic symptoms persist or blood glucose remains below 70 mg/dL.

For people who are unconscious or cannot swallow, intravenous glucose or glucagon, delivered subcutaneously or intramuscularly, are the classic treatment choices. Intranasal glucagon and a solution-based glucagon for subcutaneous injection were recently approved by the FDA for use in treating hypoglycemia in these patients. No oral treatment should be administered to or placed buccally in people who are not alert enough to swallow.

Family members can be taught to administer glucagon to high-risk clients. It is most helpful with type 1 diabetes. Side effects, such as nausea, vomiting, and headache, are common following glucagon injection. Intravenous treatment for hypoglycemia is usually 10–25 grams of 50% dextrose administered over 1–3 minutes. People treated with either glucagon or intravenous glucose should consume oral carbohydrate as soon as they are able to eat.

Patient Education

Teaching points for clients at risk for hypoglycemia include the following:

- Clients using insulin and/or oral blood glucose-lowering medications need to be aware of the peak action times for these medications. Other measures to prevent hypoglycemia include taking care to administer the proper dose of medication at the right time and to avoid delaying or missing meals.

- Clients on insulin should have a glucagon kit available and have significant others who know where it is located and how to administer it. This kit should also contain oral glucose for mild hypoglycemia.
- Medical identification stating that the person has diabetes and is on insulin is critical, as this may prevent treatment delay in an emergency.
- Clients should be instructed to initially treat symptoms of hypoglycemia with 15–20 grams of oral carbohydrate. Over-treatment with too much carbohydrate is to be avoided so that hyperglycemia does not occur later. If the initial treatment does not raise the blood glucose to more than 70 mg/dL after 15 minutes has passed, an additional 15 grams of carbohydrate should be consumed.

Glycemic Goals for Hospitalized Patients with Diabetes

Research supports the goal of optimal glycemic control for hospitalized patients with diabetes, showing that this reduces morbidity, mortality, length of stay, and hospital cost.

However, other recent studies indicate that tight glycemic control in critically ill patients can increase the risk for severe hypoglycemia and mortality.

The American Diabetes Association (ADA) provides the following guidelines for glycemic control in hospitalized patients:

- Critically ill patients: A plasma glucose range of 140–180 mg/dL is recommended for most critically ill patients. Insulin should be started at a threshold of no greater than 180 mg/dL. In patient-specific cases, the goal may be lowered to 110–140 mg/dL, but only if hypoglycemia is not a high risk.
- Non-critically ill patients: Pre-meal plasma glucose should be 100–180 mg/dL if this can be achieved safely. Less-strict goals may be appropriate for patients with severe comorbidities.

Diabetic Ketoacidosis

Diabetic ketoacidosis (DKA) is a syndrome of hyperglycemia, ketosis, dehydration, and electrolyte imbalance caused by insulin deficiency. It is most commonly associated with type 1 diabetes.

Many cases of DKA are precipitated by illness, infection, or trauma. Omission of insulin doses is the second leading cause of DKA. Cardiovascular events, such as myocardial infarction, can also precipitate DKA.

Profound insulin deficiency results in:

- Decreased glucose uptake, leading to hyperglycemia
- Excessive protein degradation, leading to increased hepatic glucose production, which in turn exacerbates hyperglycemia
- Increased action of counter-regulatory hormones, leading to:
  - Production of free fatty acids that change into ketone bodies, which precipitate acidosis when unbuffered
  - Decrease in the effectiveness of insulin

Hyperglycemia leads to:

- Osmotic diuresis, causing fluid loss and electrolyte depletion
- Excretion of ketone bodies, leading to depletion of sodium, potassium, chloride, and fluid

Laboratory Values and Precipitating Factors

Laboratory values for DKA include:

- Elevated plasma glucose (often to greater than 300 mg/dL but lower values do not preclude diagnosis)
- Arterial pH less than 7.2
- Bicarbonate value less than 15 mEq/L
- Positive ketones

Infection precipitates about 40% of DKA cases. Another common cause is the omission of insulin on sick days. Many patients are unaware that they should continue taking insulin even if they are not eating due to illness.

Less-common precipitating factors include myocardial infarction, trauma, stress, and surgery. Certain medications, such as corticosteroids and thiazide diuretics, can precipitate DKA.

Use of an insulin pump can increase the risk for DKA. This is because the insulin pump infuses only rapid-acting insulin, which has a very short duration of action. In the event of pump malfunction, there is no longer-acting insulin on board, resulting in insulin deficiency.

Signs, Symptoms, and Clinical Presentation

The classic symptoms of DKA are the "three polys": polydipsia, polyuria, and polyphagia. Polyphagia occurs after more-prolonged periods of insulin deficiency, such as days to weeks.

Other symptoms of severe hyperglycemia are blurred vision, weakness, lethargy, headache, malaise, and nausea.

The clinical presentation of DKA includes:

- Signs of dehydration. These signs may include orthostatic hypotension, which is a drop in systolic blood pressure of 20 mmHg after 1 minute of standing compared to a baseline measurement with the patient supine.
- Abdominal symptoms, such as vomiting or abdominal pain
- Hyperventilation manifested as deep, rapid Kussmaul respirations
- Acetone breath with a fruity odor
- Hypothermia, although patient may have a fever if illness precipitated DKA
- Abdominal pain characterized by tenderness and guarding
- Depressed mental status, such as stupor and eventually coma in severe cases

DKA may progress slowly over days if caused by mild insulin insufficiency. It can progress rapidly in acute illness or from other causes of severe insulin deficiency.

Treatment and Management

In mild cases of DKA, assuming the patient is able to ingest fluids, oral rehydration on an outpatient basis may be appropriate. The patient should be able to ingest and retain 3–5 ounces of fluid per hour. Insulin supplementation is also required.

For moderate to severe DKA, immediate intravenous fluid replacement and correction of electrolyte imbalance is critical. Insulin replacement with fast or short-acting insulin is also required.

In the absence of cardiac or respiratory arrest, hypovolemia is the most critical concern. Fluid replacement not only corrects hypovolemia, but also decreases hyperglycemia. Hyperglycemia will persist as long as acidosis is present and if fluid replacement is inadequate.

Replacement of potassium is crucial due to the profound potassium depletion associated with DKA.

If infection is the precipitating cause of DKA, it must also be treated.

Patients with prior DKA require education on the causes and prevention, with emphasis on sick day management to prevent future episodes.

Hyperosmolar Hyperglycemic State (HHS)

HHS is a syndrome of severe hyperglycemia and profound dehydration that can occur in people with type 2 diabetes.

Ketosis is absent in HHS because there is usually enough insulin present to prevent the excessive fat metabolism that produces ketone bodies. In the absence of acidosis, a patient with developing HHS does not usually experience the acute abdominal symptoms found in diabetic ketoacidosis (DKA). Because the patient is less likely to seek medical attention, extremely high blood glucose levels can result.

As glucose builds in the blood, it produces a hyperosmolar state. This causes water to be pulled from body cells, including the brain cells, accounting for the appearance of neurological/cognitive signs and symptoms such as decreased mental status and seizures.

Because of the profound dehydration of HHS, rehydration is the first priority of emergency treatment, followed by the correction of electrolyte deficits.

DKA vs. HHS

DKA and HHS are acute complications of hyperglycemia. Either can occur in patients with previously undiagnosed diabetes and evolve into a medical crisis. Illness and infections are precipitating factors for both conditions. Both conditions involve insufficiency of available insulin coupled with a substantial increase in the counter-regulatory hormones. The fundamental differentiating factor is ketosis, which is absent in HHS.

The degree of hyperglycemia varies between the two conditions. DKA occurs at plasma glucose levels as low as 250 mg/dL, while the blood glucose is usually greater than 600 mg/dL in HHS.

Both can potentially produce life-threatening hypovolemia.

HHS occurs in type 2 diabetes, most commonly in the elderly. It has a slower onset and longer duration of symptoms. HHS causes a slow decline in mental status over days or weeks and has a higher mortality rate.

DKA occurs in younger patients with type 1 diabetes, with a more rapid onset. Symptoms are more acute and include Kussmaul respirations and severe abdominal pain.

Characteristics and Presentation

HHS manifestations are characterized by the following:

- Profound dehydration
- Neurological manifestations
- The absence of ketosis

Characteristics of HHS include:

- Most commonly seen in elderly people with type 2 diabetes. Living alone or in a situation of inadequate monitoring increases the risk. Decreased thirst sensation contributes to the risk.
- Has a slow, insidious onset, causing it to be overlooked in many cases
- Can be confused with other conditions, such as stroke
- Condition is often precipitated by illness

Signs and symptoms include:

- Signs of dehydration, such as orthostatic hypotension and dry membranes
- Evidence of decreased mental function, such as lethargy and confusion
- Neurological signs that mimic cerebral vascular accident, such as hemiparesis and aphasia
- Hyperglycemia, usually with a blood glucose level greater than 600 mg/dL
- Abdominal pain that is mild and less marked than in diabetic ketoacidosis (DKA)
- No ketone bodies in blood or urine, except in small amounts in some cases

Treatment

Treatment for HHS includes:

- Emergency treatment and inpatient admission are required to treat HHS.
- Fluid replacement is the first priority. Initially, 0.9% normal saline is usually administered as rapidly as possible over the first hour followed by a less-concentrated saline solution at slower rates over the ensuing hours. As blood glucose declines, 5% dextrose may be used. Fluid replacement is individualized based on the patient's hydration and cardiovascular status. Care is taken to avoid fluid overload.
- Insulin therapy is required, although correction of dehydration alone improves glucose levels. Insulin dosing is conservative because rapid reduction of blood glucose can cause cerebral edema.
- Monitoring and correcting potassium is crucial due to the profound potassium depletion that results from treating a hyperglycemic emergency.
- If infection is the precipitating cause of HHS, it must be treated.
- Patients with prior HHS require education on the causes and prevention, with emphasis on sick day management to prevent future episodes. The importance of maintaining adequate hydration should also be emphasized.

Person-Centered Education on Self-Care Behaviors: Chronic Complications

ADA Clinical Practice Screening Recommendations

ADA screening standards for chronic complications from diabetes:

- **HbA1c:** Check at least twice a year in clients with stable glycemic control. Perform the test quarterly if not meeting glycemic goals or if changing therapy.
- **Hypertension:** Blood pressure should be measured at each routine medical visit. If blood pressure is greater than 130/80 mmHg, measure again on another day.
- **Dyslipidemia:** Fasting lipid profile should be measured at least annually.
- **Smoking/e-cigarette/vaping use:** Ask clients at each routine visit if they smoke or use e-cigarettes/vape and advise quitting if necessary.
- **Diabetes distress and anxiety:** Screen caregivers and clients annually and refer to a qualified mental health professional as needed
- **Cannabis use:** Ask clients at each routine visit if they use cannabis recreationally, and advise to quit if recreational use is noted.
- **Nephropathy:** Test for microalbuminuria annually. Perform serum creatinine measurement at least once a year.
- **Retinopathy:** An annual dilated eye exam is recommended for all people with diabetes, but it can be less frequent if client has had one or more normal exams. All screening exams for retinopathy should be performed by an ophthalmologist or optometrist.
- **Foot:** Perform comprehensive foot exam annually, including testing for loss of protective sensation.

The most recent ADA recommendations for chronic complication screening include following the Chronic Care Model, which has 6 core elements: Delivery System Design (moving from reactive to proactive care), Self-Management Support, Decision Support (based on evidence-based care guidelines), Clinical Information Systems (using registries that can provide patient-specific and population based support to care team), Community Resources and Policies, and Health Systems (to create a quality-oriented culture).

Eye Disease

Diabetic Retinopathy

Retinopathy results from damage to the microvasculature supplying the part of the eye responsible for focusing images and light.

Hyperglycemic damage causes small hemorrhages and blood leakage through the vessel walls. To compensate for the loss of normal blood flow from damaged vessels, new blood vessels develop (neovascularization). These new vessels are so fragile that they leak and bleed easily, causing adhesions between the retina and the vitreous. This leads to retinal traction and detachment followed by vitreous bleeding that causes blindness. Macular edema is an additional serious consequence of retinal vessel leakage.

- In **nonproliferative retinopathy**, microaneurysms and other evidence of vessel leakage are seen on fundus exam. The client does not experience any changes in vision at this time. Nonproliferative retinopathy is staged from mild to very severe.
- **Proliferative retinopathy** indicates that neovascularization has started and there is resulting impairment in vision. This can range to mild blurring to large blind spots in the field of vision.

Risk Factors for Development and Progression

Diabetic retinopathy can often be detected within 5 years of diagnosis of either type 1 or type 2 diabetes. Since type 2 diabetes can be present or undetected for years prior to diagnosis, a significant number of patients already have retinopathy at the time of diagnosis.

The development and progression of retinopathy is highly correlated with the duration of diabetes and the degree of glycemic control. Optimization of glucose control is imperative for lowering risk. Blood pressure control can significantly contribute to the prevention of retinopathy and in slowing its progression. Other **risk factors for retinopathy** include:

- Hypertension
- Pregnancy*
- Smoking/e-cigarette use/vaping
- Genetic predisposition
- Hyperlipidemia
- Puberty
- Renal failure

*Women with diabetes who plan to become pregnant should be counseled on the increased risk for the development or progression of retinopathy related to pregnancy. A comprehensive eye exam by an optometrist or ophthalmologist should take place before pregnancy and in the first trimester, with close follow-up throughout pregnancy and postpartum.

Treatment

Treatment of diabetic retinopathy includes:

- Glycemic control is paramount in preventing retinopathy and for minimizing its progression. Smoking/e-cigarette/vaping cessation and managing hypertension and dyslipidemia are also fundamental treatment measures.
- Patients with any evidence of retinopathy should be promptly referred to an ophthalmologist.
- Mild to moderate nonproliferative retinopathy requires only observation and optimization of glycemic, blood pressure and lipid control.
- For proliferative retinopathy, laser photocoagulation therapy is indicated. This may also be indicated for some cases of severe to very severe nonproliferative retinopathy. Multiple outpatient treatment sessions are usually necessary. Most patients require anesthetic eye drops, although a local anesthetic injection may be available if needed.
- Studies show that laser photocoagulation surgery is effective in preventing further vision loss, but not in restoring acuity that has already been lost. Some patients experience a small decline in acuity and peripheral vision following photocoagulation therapy, but this is generally offset by the preservation of central vision.
- Surgical vitrectomy may be required in cases of retinal detachment or when hemorrhages do not resolve after laser surgery.

Additional Ocular Complications

Blurred vision is a common symptom of hyperglycemia and is also common during periods of fluctuating glycemic control. It is a transient condition caused by osmotic changes in the eyeball. When this condition occurs, clients should postpone changes in eyeglass prescriptions until blood glucose has stabilized for 6–8 weeks.

Cataracts are more common in people with diabetes. They occur at a younger age and progress more aggressively than in people who do not have diabetes. They are easily detected on eye exam. They can be corrected with a minor outpatient surgery that replaces the clouded lens with an artificial one.

Open-angled glaucoma may not occur more frequently in diabetes. However, the risk for vision loss is greater when blood glucose control is suboptimal due to compromised circulation.

Ischemic optic neuropathy is optic nerve damage caused by microvascular impairment. It can cause irreversible loss of vision.

Adaptive Equipment

For measuring insulin, syringe magnifiers may be adequate for many clients with poor vision. Others may benefit from using preset dose gauges that assist with measuring insulin. Other devices measure insulin units by a series of audible or tactile clicks. Some devices require set-up assistance by a person with unimpaired vision.

Insulin pens are prefilled and can be operated nonvisually by many people. Although this is not specifically endorsed by the pen manufacturers, many people feel it is a safe practice for appropriate clients.

Some types of insulin pumps have auditory cues and are sometimes appropriate for a visually impaired person. Proper assessment should determine the safety of this for the individual.

For monitoring blood glucose, talking meters are available and regular meters can often be adapted to provide this feature. Some meters have test strips with distinctive tactile features that can assist the user. Blood drop guides are also available to help with placing the blood drop on the test strip.

Sexual Dysfunction

Sexual dysfunction in diabetes is related to autonomic neuropathy. Up to 75% of men and 35% of women with diabetes experience difficulty with sexual functioning.

Erectile dysfunction is a common problem in men with diabetes. This is usually accompanied by loss of testicular pain sensation with pressure and loss of perineal sensation. Assessment includes ruling out other causes such as antihypertensive medications or psychological reasons. The patient and partner can be referred to a urologist or an impotence clinic. Treatments include surgical penile implants, suction devices that produce erection, prostaglandin injections, and oral medications such as sildenafil.

Manifestations of female sexual dysfunction in diabetes include decreased lubrication; delayed, blunted, or absent arousal; and absent orgasmic response. Referral to a gynecologist may be appropriate. Treatment includes application of vaginal lubricant and use of estrogen. Causes of female sexual dysfunction other than autonomic neuropathy could be depression or vaginal infection.

Neuropathies

Sensory Neuropathy

Sensory neuropathy causes sensory deficits that usually begin in the distal portion of the lower extremities. The deficits sometimes progress to the distal upper extremities, in what is known as a "stocking-glove" distribution.

Identifying sensory neuropathy is a diagnosis of exclusion, although extensive testing to rule out other causes is not often necessary.

Assessment includes:

- Monofilament testing for loss of tactile sensation
- Testing for loss of vibratory sensation by applying a tuning fork at the distal first metatarsal head
- Checking temperature sensation by using the cool metal part of a reflex hammer or tuning fork on the skin and asking the patient to describe the temperature
- Testing position sensation by flexing and extending the big toes and asking the patient to describe the position

There are no treatments to reverse neuronal loss. Improved glycemic control and smoking/e-cigarette/vaping cessation can slow or halt further progression of nerve damage. Medications such as gabapentinoids, SSRIs, sodium channel blockers, and tricyclic antidepressants are ADA-recommended as first-line pharmacologic treatments for neuropathic pain. Anticonvulsants and capsaicin cream may also provide palliation.

Autonomic Neuropathy

Autonomic neuropathy has the potential to affect every system in the body. About 50% of people with diabetic peripheral neuropathy also have autonomic neuropathy.

The autonomic neuropathies and manifestations of each include:

- Neurogenic bladder: difficulty emptying bladder, dribbling, frequent bladder infections
- Sexual dysfunction: erectile dysfunction, decreased vaginal lubrication, absent orgasmic response
- Gastroparesis: early satiety, heartburn, anorexia, postprandial hypoglycemia
- Intestinal impairment: fecal incontinence, nocturnal diarrhea, constipation
- Orthostatic hypotension (drop in blood pressure from sitting position to standing): dizziness, lightheadedness, syncope
- Cardiac denervation*: fixed heart rate, silent myocardial infarction, abnormal cardiovascular response to exercise
- Hypoglycemic unawareness: lack of normal symptoms with low blood glucose
- Impaired insulin counter-regulation: "brittle diabetes" in type 1 diabetes
- Anhidrosis (failure to sweat): cracked, fissured heels
- Abnormal pupillary response to light: slow dilation of pupils

*Cardiovascular autonomic neuropathy is associated with significant morbidity and mortality.

Impact of Autonomic Neuropathy on the Gastrointestinal Tract

Because the entire gastrointestinal (GI) system has autonomic innervation, neuropathy may affect any part of it from the esophagus to the rectum.

Gastroparesis results in delayed emptying of stomach contents. It can interfere with the absorption of glucose and oral medications, leading to suboptimal glycemic control and unpredictable postprandial glycemic response.

Symptoms of gastroparesis include reflux, heartburn, anorexia, early satiety, nausea, vomiting, and erratic blood glucose levels.

Referral to a gastroenterologist and dietitian are indicated for gastroparesis. Dietary measures include a low-fat/low-fiber diet with multiple small meals. Medications that increase stomach motility, such as metoclopramide, are useful.

The most common lower-intestinal autonomic disorder is **constipation**. Adequate fiber in the diet along with good hydration and regular physical activity are recommended to treat and prevent constipation. Stool softeners, bulk laxatives (e.g., psyllium), and medications to increase intestinal motility are also used.

As with all complications of diabetes, optimal glucose control and smoking cessation are indicated for autonomic neuropathies affecting the GI system.

Impact of Autonomic Neuropathies on Cardiovascular Function

Both sympathetic and parasympathetic nerves innervate the cardiovascular system and can be affected by neuropathy. This can affect heart rate, heart rhythm, and blood pressure maintenance. Mortality associated with cardiovascular autonomic neuropathy is estimated to be as high as 56% within 5–10 years of onset. Sudden death is associated with silent ischemia and cardiac arrhythmias.

Manifestations of autonomic neuropathy affecting the cardiovascular system include:

- Fixed heart rate
- Orthostatic hypotension
- Decreased cardiac response to exercise
- Absence or altered perception of cardiac ischemia
- Insufficient hemodynamic response to cardiovascular stressors such as surgery and infection
- Predisposition to cardiac arrhythmias

Interventions for **orthostatic hypotension** include:

- Prevention of falls
- Making position changes slowly
- Use of elastic body stockings
- Sleeping with head elevated
- Increasing salt intake
- Fludrocortisone to expand fluid volume

Interventions for cardiac denervation and abnormal cardiovascular response to exercise include:

- Avoiding strenuous exercise and straining
- Stress testing prior to initiating a new activity program
- Avoiding hypoglycemia, which can cause arrhythmias

Nephropathy

Micro- and Macroalbuminuria

Microalbuminuria is defined as the persistent presence of albumin in the urine in the range of 30–299 mg/24 hr. It is considered to be the first stage of nephropathy in type 1 diabetes and a marker for nephropathy in type 2 diabetes. Microalbuminuria is also a marker of increased cardiovascular risk and is associated with retinopathy in diabetes.

Macroalbuminuria is defined as albuminuria greater than or equal to 300 mg/24 hr. This greatly increases the risk for progression to end stage renal disease.

Interventions to delay progression of renal disease include:

- Achievement of normal or near-normal glycemia
- Blood pressure control: systolic pressure ≤120 mmHg
- Use of ACE inhibitors* (or substitute with ARBs)
- Stage-based reduction in dietary protein intake
- Additional therapy to lower blood pressure, which may include calcium channel blockers, diuretics, and beta blockers

*ACE inhibitors also prevent major cardiovascular events and related mortality in people with diabetes.

Implications of Hypertension and Diabetic Nephropathy

Hypertension is considered the most significant factor in accelerating the progression of established renal disease. This is true for both systolic and diastolic pressures.

The American Diabetes Association (ADA) recommends blood pressure <130/80 mmHg for the prevention of renal complications in patients with diabetes.

Lifestyle modifications to reduce blood pressure include weight loss (if needed), exercise, tobacco cessation, and reduced salt and alcohol intake. If lifestyle modifications do not result in reaching the blood pressure goal, angiotensin-converting enzyme (ACE) inhibitors are considered the first-line pharmacologic intervention. If these medications produce side effects, angiotensin II receptor blockers (ARBs) are substituted. The most common side effect of ACE inhibitors is cough. Angioedema is a less common but more serious adverse effect.

Studies indicate that reduction of blood pressure may reduce the risk for microvascular complications.

Clients with diabetes should self-monitor their blood pressure as a part of comprehensive self-management. Educators should evaluate the client's technique to ensure accurate readings.

Management of Hypertension

Management of hypertension in diabetes is aggressive. It often involves initiating antihypertensive medications even if there is only a modest elevation of blood pressure. An angiotensin-converting enzyme (ACE) inhibitor is usually the first drug of choice.

Smoking cessation is of utmost importance due to the adverse effects of smoking on the vascular system. Routine assessment of smoking status and advice to quit when applicable are important.

Dyslipidemia is managed first with lifestyle interventions, such as low-fat diet, exercise, and weight loss, if necessary. Statins or other medications to treat dyslipidemia are recommended for most patients with diabetes.

Aspirin therapy helps overcome the hypercoagulability associated with insulin resistance syndrome. Aspirin is recommended for people with risk factors such as age over 40, smoking, hypertension, albuminuria, and dyslipidemia. The usual dose is 81 mg per day, though higher doses are used in cases of higher risk. Clopidogrel may be used as an alternative to aspirin.

Vascular Disease

Macrovascular Disease

Macrovascular disease comprises both arteriosclerosis and atherosclerosis. It accounts for more morbidity, mortality, and cost than any other complication of diabetes.

- **Arteriosclerosis** is a condition in which the walls of arteries and veins become thicker and lose elasticity.
- **Atherosclerosis** describes the process of plaque formation within blood vessel walls, especially the arteries.

Macrovascular disease affects the cerebral, coronary, and peripheral vessels, causing 3 types of macrovascular disease in people with diabetes. They are:

- Coronary artery disease
  - This develops at an earlier age and has a more aggressive course in people with diabetes.
  - Women with diabetes lose their gender protection from atherosclerosis.
  - People with diabetes are more likely to have an adverse outcome from acute coronary events.
- Cerebral vascular disease in people with diabetes results in 3–5 times greater risk for death from stroke than in the population without diabetes.
- Peripheral vascular disease in people with diabetes, along with peripheral neuropathy, accounts for approximately 50% of all nontraumatic lower limb amputations in the United States.

Coronary Artery Disease

People with diabetes who do not have coronary heart disease (CHD) are at similar risk for a coronary event as people without diabetes who have CHD.

Coronary artery disease is responsible for 50–60% of all deaths in people with diabetes.

Although female gender normally provides a degree of cardiovascular protection, women with diabetes lose this natural safeguard. Therefore, efforts to reduce macrovascular risk in women with diabetes should be as aggressive as efforts to decrease the risk in men.

Common symptoms of acute coronary insufficiency include:

- Angina
- Anxiety
- Diaphoresis
- Shortness of breath

It is important to remember that a significant number of people with diabetes have atypical myocardial infarction, also known as "silent MI," in which they do not display the normal MI symptoms.

Peripheral Artery Disease

Peripheral artery disease (PAD) is a vascular disorder involving obstruction of arterial blood flow to vessels outside the coronary and cerebral systems. Up to one-third of people with diabetes over the age of 50 suffer from this condition. Elevated levels of C-reactive protein in diabetes are responsible for the inflammation and cellular derangements that lead to PAD.

The presence of PAD serves as a marker for concomitant coronary and cerebral vascular disease. In diabetes, additional risk factors are:

- Duration of diabetes
- African American or Hispanic ethnicity
- Hyperglycemia
- Peripheral neuropathy
- Smoking
- Older age
- Dyslipidemia
- Hyperhomocysteinemia

The most common symptom of PAD is intermittent claudication. This produces cramping in the calves, thighs, and buttocks that occurs with activity and is alleviated with rest. The pain is described as a fullness, aching, or itching sensation. Clients with these symptoms should be referred for medical examination. ADA recommendations advise to screen the following individuals for peripheral artery disease using the ankle-brachial index:

- Individuals with diabetes who are over 65 years of age
- Individuals with a history of microvascular disease
- Individuals with foot complications or any end-organ damage secondary to diabetes
- Individuals who have been diagnosed with diabetes for more than 10 years

INTERVENTIONS

Interventions for PAD include the same lifestyle modifications recommended for cardiovascular disease. These include smoking cessation, hypertension and lipid management, healthy diet, aspirin therapy, and glycemic control. Tobacco cessation is especially important as it is associated with increased risk for amputation.

Although intermittent claudication causes pain with walking, clients should be instructed to continue exercising. Walking programs improve intermittent claudication by increasing blood flow to lower extremities and initiating development of collateral circulation.

Clients with PAD need education on prevention of injury to the feet and prompt care of problems since decreased blood flow impedes the healing process. Footwear that fits properly and provides adequate protection is crucial. Clients should learn to perform daily foot inspections and be taught the signs and symptoms of infection or inadequate healing. For those unable to do their own foot inspection, family members or other caregivers should be identified. The ADA recommends the use of technology for self-monitoring, including temperature-sensitive socks, mats, and insoles that can be used to identify insufficient perfusion early.

LOWER EXTREMITY PROBLEMS

FOOT SCREENING

Foot screening identifies the likelihood of lower extremity complications related to diabetes, such as ulceration and amputation.

History of lower extremity ulceration, use of insulin, and duration of diabetes greater than 10 years are risk factors. Having previous ulceration or amputation automatically places the person at high risk, with no further screening or examination necessary. Deformities such as Charcot foot, hammer toes, or claw toes also predict amputation.

Sensory neuropathy is an important risk factor for foot complications. To determine loss of protective sensation, a 5.07/10-gram monofilament is applied to several spots on the bottom of the foot. Clients should have their eyes closed during this exam. If the monofilament cannot be detected, the client has lost protective sensation and is at risk for undetected injury and subsequent complications.

Loss of vibratory sensation is a predictor of foot ulceration. This is tested using a 128-cycle tuning fork or a biothesiometer at the big toe.

Charcot Foot

Charcot foot is a complication of diabetes related to peripheral and autonomic neuropathy. Repeated trauma to insensitive, neuropathic joints leads to joint destruction and severe deformities of foot structure.

Acute Charcot foot appears unilaterally as a swollen and warm foot, often appearing like an infection without any outward signs of skin breakdown. Inspection may reveal loss of the arch, producing a "rocker bottom" shape to the sole.

In spite of the severe injury, many patients do not feel pain due to neuropathic loss of sensation. They may continue to walk on the injured foot, causing further joint destruction.

Immediate referral for orthopedic evaluation is crucial when Charcot foot is detected. Primary treatment involves non-weight-bearing status on the affected foot. Non-weight-bearing casts are often used to stabilize the foot while the healing process is monitored radiologically. Following healing, corrective shoes are needed to accommodate the change in foot shape.

Tailoring Foot Care Education

Education about foot care should be individualized to the client's current level of knowledge, risk level and foot care practices. Foot care practices should be discussed with high-risk clients at every visit.

The educator should begin by asking what the client already knows about foot care and what he or she is currently doing for foot care. Open-ended questions are best.

Special situations that may alter one's ability to perform good foot care may include homelessness, blindness, and obesity.

Instruction should be presented in a positive way with rationales.

Carefully selected handouts and written guidelines can be helpful. Handouts should be screened for literacy level and cultural appropriateness. Graphic presentations are often desirable. Handouts should be provided in the client's preferred language.

Teaching Points for Performing a Self-Foot Exam

Patients with neuropathy and loss of protective sensation should perform a self-foot exam every day. While those who maintain good sensation are at lower risk for serious foot problems, checking the feet every day is a good practice for all people with diabetes. The use of technology that measures foot temperature using socks, mats, and insoles should be discussed with the client as helpful options in their self-monitoring plan.

To check the feet, instruct the client to:

- Carefully inspect all surfaces of the feet, including top, bottom, and between toes.
- Note any areas of skin breakdown or irritation. Report infection or slow healing to a healthcare provider promptly.
- Note areas that indicate poorly fitting shoes, such as callus formation or red pressure areas upon removing shoes.
- Use a mirror if needed to visually access all areas of the feet. Enlist the help of a support person if necessary.

It is helpful to have the client provide a return demonstration of the foot inspection instruction that has been given.

Foot Care Guidelines

Foot care guidelines:

- Inspect feet daily.
- Inspect shoes for irregularities that may cause pressure or irritate skin. Shake out shoes before putting them on.
- Always wear well-fitting, protective shoes and socks.
- Wash feet daily with mild soap and warm water as part of the bath or shower. Foot soaks are not recommended. Dry the feet after the bath or shower, especially between the toes.
- Use moisturizer for dry skin. Avoid getting it between the toes. Avoid highly scented moisturizers and those containing alcohol, which may irritate or dry the skin.
- For calluses, gently rub with a pumice stone after the bath or shower, followed by application of moisturizing cream or lotion. Do not use sharp instruments to cut a callus and do not use over-the-counter treatments containing harsh chemicals that may burn the skin.
- Cut toenails straight across.
- Do not use heating pads or hot water bottles to warm the feet.
- Promptly report any problems, such as cuts, scrapes, or blisters that do not heal or appear to be infected.
- Assess toe pressures as a screening measure for peripheral artery disease.

Selection of Footwear

People with diabetes should wear protective footwear at all times, even in their own homes, at the beach, and at swimming pools.

Those who have lost protective sensation should have their shoes fitted by a professional. Sensory loss can impair the ability to recognize that shoes are not fitting properly.

Characteristics of a safe, protective shoe include:

- Oxford style or with a wide Velcro strap so that fit can be modified as feet swell later in the day
- Plenty of room for the toes. The toe box should allow "wiggle room" and be wide enough to accommodate conditions such as wide feet or bunions
- Made of leather or other breathable material. Avoid plastic or shoes made of "man-made" materials
- Adequate cushioning and support for the soles of the feet

Other safety tips include:

- Check inside shoes for rocks, other sharp objects, or anything else that may irritate the skin before putting them on.
- Change shoes and socks during the day if they become moist from sweating or water.
- Wear socks with shoes. Socks should be made from materials that wick moisture away from skin.

Potential for a Foot Injury to Progress from Trauma to Systemic Infection

The most common cause of foot ulcers is minor repetitive trauma, such as walking on a bony prominence or repeated pressure from shoes that are too tight.

Many minor traumas are preventable and come from poorly fitting shoes, walking barefoot, foreign objects in the shoes or inappropriate treatment of corns, calluses, or blisters. Most amputations are preventable with client education about footwear, foot inspection and proper care of common problems.

Ulceration involves full-thickness skin trauma that infiltrates the subcutaneous tissue. Proper wound management is essential to prevent infection and amputation. Management of foot ulceration includes optimization of glycemic control, debridement as needed, applying dressings and protection from further trauma to allow healing.

Signs of **infection** include redness, swelling, warmth, continuous drainage, and failure to heal. Localized infection of 30 days duration or less can usually be effectively treated with oral antibiotics. Clients with signs of systemic infection, such as severe hyperglycemia or fever, require prompt emergency referral.

Treating Diabetic Foot Ulcers

Diabetic foot wounds are often treated inadequately because patients and healthcare providers do not appreciate the seriousness of a non-healing ulcer. Because underlying osteomyelitis can occur with little evidence of inflammation, treatment may be deferred. Prompt and appropriate treatment of foot ulcers can lead to significant decrease in amputations. New evidence supports that GLP-1 RA therapy may help reduce lower-extremity amputation in this population, so this option should be discussed with a provider.

Wound debridement is essential to the treatment of a foot ulcer because it helps move the wound past the inflammatory phase, allowing healing to commence. Debridement involves chemically or mechanically removing necrotic, callused and any other physiologically impaired tissue.

Offloading is an ulcer management strategy that requires the patient not to place any weight on the affected foot. Noncompliance rates with this recommendation are high and present a significant barrier to healing. Some healthcare providers have the patient wear a non-removable cast to enforce offloading of the wound.

Meticulous documentation is needed to track the progression of wound healing. This includes objective measurements of wound size and measures of glycemic control.

DERMATOLOGICAL

COMMON SKIN PROBLEMS

Common skin problems include:

- **Anhidrosis:** An autonomic neuropathic condition that leads to little or no production of perspiration in the feet and lower legs, resulting in severely dry and cracked skin
- **Diabetic dermopathy:** Pigmented spots on the shins, usually asymptomatic but can be painful if they ulcerate. Most likely due to poor skin perfusion associated with diabetes.
- **Acanthosis nigricans:** Velvety brown or black lesions found in the folds of the skin, most commonly the folds of the neck and axillae. The condition is associated with obesity and insulin resistance. In the young, it is a marker of glucose intolerance and when present should prompt providers to screen for type 2 diabetes.
- **Skin infections:** High risk for skin infections is associated with poor glycemic control, as well as neuropathy and peripheral vascular disease. Common skin infections in diabetes include staph, fungal, and *Candida* infections.

YEAST AND FUNGAL INFECTIONS

Poor glycemic control increases the risk for developing **yeast and fungal infection** of the skin and nails.

Tinea pedis, also known as athlete's foot, is a common problem in people with diabetes. Avoiding prolonged exposure of the feet to moisture is an important preventive measure. Instruct the client to dry well between the toes after bathing and to avoid wearing moist shoes and socks. Antifungal foot powder can be applied sparingly in the shoes. It is a good idea to alternate shoes from day to day to allow thorough drying in between wearing.

Yeast infections commonly occur in the folds of the skin where moisture can accumulate. Vaginal yeast infections can also occur. Over-the-counter (OTC) products for treating vaginal yeast infections are available. However, a client should only use one if she is having symptoms similar to an episode previously diagnosed by a healthcare professional. These OTC products should not be used more than 4 times per year without medical supervision.

PATIENT EDUCATION

Elevated glucose can cause dry skin and increase the risk for skin infections. Common skin infections in people with diabetes include staph, beta-hemolytic strep, fungal, and yeast infections. Furthermore, comorbidities such as neuropathy and peripheral vascular disease can complicate infections and slow healing.

Teaching points for skin care include:

- Maintain glycemic control.
- Maintain healthy eating habits and adequate hydration status.
- Inspect skin daily and report infections promptly to a healthcare provider.
- Pay attention to skinfold areas where fungus and yeast tend to grow. Dry well in all skinfolds, including between the toes, after each bath or shower. Antifungal powders may be used in skinfolds and shoes.
- Avoid trauma to the skin.
- Wear protective footwear.

- Avoid overexposure to the sun, especially if taking sulfonylurea medication.
- Use mild soap to bathe and avoid harsh or drying skin care products, such as those that contain alcohol.

Dental and Gum Disease

Impact on Individuals with Diabetes

People with diabetes have a three-fold risk for **dental problems** such as caries, periodontal disease, and tooth loss. Studies have indicated that people with diabetes underestimate the importance of good dental care and do not appreciate the relationship of good oral health with general health.

Dental problems can negatively affect glycemic control, while poor glycemic control can complicate dental visits and procedures. Common issues related to diabetes that complicate dental care include poor wound healing, susceptibility for infection, vascular changes, and neuropathy.

Tooth loss or dental pain can affect what a person is able to eat and can lead to insufficient intake of healthy foods such as vegetables, fruits, and whole grains. Softer foods tend to cause a sharper rise in blood glucose.

Dental treatments, such as root canals or oral surgery, can require changes in food intake and adjustment in oral medications and insulin.

Patient Education for Promoting Good Dental Health

Educators should consider teaching about dental care as a standard component of the diabetes education program. The following **teaching points** should be included:

- There is an interrelationship between dental health and glycemic control. A decline in one can lead to a decline in the other.
- Maintain glycemic control and healthy eating habits.
- Maintain good routine brushing and flossing habits.
- See the dentist every 6 months—more often if there is periodontal disease.
- Notify the dentist that you have diabetes and know your most recent HbA1c value.
- Don't smoke, as it increases the risk for periodontal disease.
- Dry mouth, common in diabetes, promotes the formation of dental caries. Maintain good hydration and use fluoride mouth rinses and salivary substitutes as needed.
- Be prepared to make adjustments in food, oral medication, and insulin for dental procedures.

Presentation of Clients with Periodontal Disease

People with diabetes have a higher risk for periodontal disease; the risk is even greater in those who smoke. Increased age and longer duration of diabetes are also risk factors for periodontal disease.

Periodontal disease should be suspected with the following presentation:

- History of poor glycemic control
- Current and persistent poor glycemic control with no obvious reason
- Red, inflamed, tender gums
- Bleeding gums

- Foul breath odor
- Change in eating habits to soft foods

When periodontal disease is suspected, interventions include:

- Educating the client that gum disease can negatively affect control of blood glucose
- Referring to a dental health professional
- Continuing to work with the client to lower blood glucose levels
- Anticipating dietary changes, such as consuming more soft foods, that can have an influence on blood glucose control

Safety Factors Related to Dental Visits

People with diabetes have a greater risk for dental caries, periodontal disease, and other dental problems. Poor glycemic control is associated with impaired wound healing and increased susceptibility for infection. Dental procedures with sedation may require fasting prior to the procedure while post-procedural pain may affect what the person is able to eat afterward.

Teaching points for **safety related to dental care** and procedures includes:

- Notify your dentist that you have diabetes and know your most recent HbA1c result.
- Prevent hypoglycemia during examinations and procedures by having appropriate food intake before the dental visit.
- If fasting is required before a procedure, be aware that a reduction in medication or insulin may be necessary.
- Avoid scheduling a dental appointment during the hours when insulin action will be peaking.
- If at risk for hypoglycemia, have at least 15 grams of fasting-acting carbohydrate readily available.
- Avoid dental surgeries during periods of severe hyperglycemia, as this will affect healing and increase the risk for infection.

Impact of Socioeconomic Status on Utilization of Dental Care

Because diabetes increases the risk for dental problems and because dental problems can affect glycemic control, regular dental care is an important part of diabetes management.

There is a strong relationship between socioeconomic status and utilization of dental services. Dental care is often not covered by insurance to the same extent that medical insurance covers healthcare, so it represents a much greater out-of-pocket expense to patients. Furthermore, Medicare does not provide for dental care and Medicaid provides only limited coverage for dental care in some states.

A recent study has shown that, among people with diabetes, there is a greater disparity in utilization of professional dental care based on racial, ethnic, and socioeconomic status than for any other type of healthcare. Those with an income of less than $10,000 saw a dentist at roughly half the rate of those with income over $50,000. These disparities did not exist for physician visits or foot exams among the same groups.

Other Comorbidities

Celiac Disease in Type 1 Diabetes

Celiac disease associated with type 1 diabetes is often overlooked. Its prevalence rate is approximately 4–6% among people with type 1 diabetes.

- Celiac disease is an autoimmune disorder of the small intestine most commonly seen in people of European descent. It is thought to be triggered by a viral immune response in people with a genetic predisposition.
- Celiac disease causes an inability to digest certain nutrients and results in chronic diarrhea, failure to thrive, and loss of energy. A gluten-free diet relieves symptoms and improves general health. This diet must be maintained for life.
- 2026 ADA Standards recommend that adult clients with type 1 diabetes be screened for celiac disease when they present with gastrointestinal symptoms or laboratory manifestations of celiac disease.
- People with type 1 diabetes and celiac disease must avoid all wheat-based foods. This can be challenging because gluten is used as an additive in many food products and is found in processed cheese, ground spices, cosmetics, lip balms, and even postage stamps.
- Examples of grain products appropriate for a gluten-free diet are corn, rice, potatoes, and soy.
- Clients with celiac disease should be referred to a registered dietitian who can provide education and emotional support for making these complicated dietary adaptations.

Thyroid Disorders

Thyroid disorders are more common in people with diabetes than in the general population.

Since type 1 diabetes is an autoimmune disorder affecting the pancreas, other organs can be affected by the destructive process, including the thyroid. Thyroid dysfunction appears to be more common in people with type 2 diabetes as well.

The most common type of thyroid dysfunction is hypothyroidism. In the person with diabetes, this can affect glucose control and can affect response to medication. When the thyroid level is low, metabolism slows and the action of medications may be prolonged. This can increase the risk for hypoglycemia in clients at risk. Medication doses usually need to be reduced when hypothyroidism presents concurrently with diabetes.

Hyperthyroidism usually causes a worsening of glycemic control and an increased need for insulin. Some of the symptoms of hyperthyroidism, such as rapid or pounding heartbeat, sweating, and tremors, can mimic hypoglycemia.

Clients with diabetes should be screened for thyroid disease soon after diagnosis and on a recurring basis, according to 2026 ADA Standards, and periodically thereafter, even in the absence of symptoms because many cases are subclinical.

Obesity

The majority of obese persons lead sedentary lifestyles. The initial goal is usually to simply increase activity. The 2026 ADA Standards emphasize the importance of utilizing therapeutic language (nonjudgmental, empathetic, and patient-centered) when caring with this population.

The client should be assisted in identifying and overcoming barriers to physical activity. If the client is embarrassed by his or her lack of fitness, solitary exercise or finding a group of people with similar status can be suggested. BMI should be measured annually in patients with obesity in addition to another method for measuring body fat (or more frequently if there is acute weight gain or loss) according to 2026 ADA Standards.

Continuous aerobic activity has the most beneficial effect on weight loss and fat burning. A progressive walking program is suitable for many obese clients. Water exercise is a good option for those with joint or foot pain. However, swimming is less likely to produce aerobic effects and weight loss. Obese clients should avoid high-impact exercises that place too much stress on the joints, such as jogging or high-impact aerobics.

Exercise intensity should start at the lower end of the target heart range. Frequency of exercise should be 3–5 times per week. Goal of weight reduction should be at least 5–7% of initial body weight.

Sleep Apnea

As many as 50% of people with type 2 diabetes also have sleep apnea. Sleep apnea worsens insulin resistance and increases the risk for cardiovascular events, hypertension, and erectile dysfunction.

Symptoms of sleep apnea include:

- Snoring, especially if loudly and frequently
- Breathing cessation or gasping to regain breath while asleep
- Frequent awakening during the night
- Being sleepy during the day
- Having trouble concentrating

Primary prevention of sleep apnea is to achieve and maintain a healthy BMI. Self-treatment options include avoiding alcohol and sleeping on the back. Dental appliances that position the mandible to maintain an open airway are also available. The most effective treatment is the continuous positive air pressure (CPAP) machine.

All patients with diabetes should be routinely screened for sleep apnea. If sleep apnea is suspected, diagnosis can be confirmed with sleep lab studies.

Depression

Depression encompasses several mood disorders characterized by persistent feelings of sadness or lack of interest in usual activities.

- **Major depressive disorder (MDD)** is the most common of these mood disorders. Diagnosis of MDD is based on the presence of 5 out of 9 symptoms that the patient has experienced over a minimum of 2 weeks. These symptoms include sleep disturbance, unintended change in weight, difficulty in making decisions, fatigue, feelings of guilt or worthlessness, and suicidal thoughts or plans.
- **Dysthymic disorder** is a disorder of prolonged depressive symptoms and results in greater impairment of social and vocational functioning.
- **Adjustment disorder with depressed mood** is depression that occurs within 3 months of an identified stressor, such as a death or job loss. This is a shorter-term condition and usually lasts 6 months or less.

Relationship Between Diabetes and Depression

The rate of depression in people with diabetes is approximately three times that of people without diabetes. This condition affects about 15–20% of patients with diabetes. The causal relationship between the two conditions is unclear. It is not fully understood how one condition may cause the other or if there is bidirectional causation.

Depression has a negative impact on diabetes self-management. Studies show that depression is directly related to poor glycemic control and subsequent complications. This may be partly due to the association of depression with obesity, sedentary lifestyle, and poor adherence to treatment recommendations. Diabetes complications shown to have a direct association with depression include retinopathy, neuropathic symptoms, nephropathy, hypertension, and sexual dysfunction.

Depression is also associated with maladaptive coping methods, such as abuse of tobacco and other substances. This further increases the risk for cardiovascular disease, a risk already high in people with diabetes. For these reasons, the ADA recommends screening for depression annually, and should depression be suspected, to make a referral to a mental health provider.

Atypical Symptoms of Depression

Depression is known to have a negative impact on glycemic control and to decrease tolerance to the physical symptoms related to diabetes. It has also been shown that reports of neuropathic pain, gastrointestinal problems and symptoms of hyperglycemia and hypoglycemia are more common among depressed people with diabetes.

Atypical symptoms of depression in the person with diabetes may include:

- Symptoms of hypoglycemia or hyperglycemia despite objective findings of glycemic control
- Physical symptoms that are out of proportion with objective data
- Sexual dysfunction
- Chronic pain
- Worsening of glycemic control
- Decline in self-care behavior
- Poor adaptation to diabetes

If these symptoms are identified, further evaluation for depression by standard means is required for diagnosis of the disorder.

Review Video: Major Depression
Visit mometrix.com/academy and enter code: 632694

Anxiety

It is common for clients to feel anxious about having diabetes. One study demonstrated that anxiety was elevated in 40% of subjects with diabetes. Anxiety is often experienced upon initial diagnosis of diabetes, at the onset of complications and during periods of poor glycemic control. People are often more receptive to outside help and support during these times, so they present an opportunity for providing education. ADA Guidelines recommend screening annually for anxiety in individuals with diabetes.

Diabetes-related anxieties often focus on the fear of hypoglycemia, complications, using insulin, or performing fingersticks. Anxiety can also be manifested by compulsively checking blood glucose.

Depending upon the severity of the anxiety, emotional support, education, and help with problem-solving can often alleviate anxiety related to diabetes. In other cases, referral to a mental health professional is warranted, especially if anxiety interferes with activities of daily living and effective self-care behavior.

Manifestation of Anxiety vs. Hypoglycemia

Anxiety disorders are common in adults in general and even more common in people with diabetes.

Common manifestations of anxiety include:

- Sleep disturbance
- Restlessness
- Muscle tension
- Agitation
- Irritability
- Lack of concentration
- Nervousness
- Poor memory
- Inability to make decisions

Clients with diabetes may exhibit anxiety by demonstrating irrational fears and refusing to perform certain aspects of self-care, such as monitoring blood glucose or injecting insulin.

Some of the symptoms of anxiety are similar to the symptoms of hypoglycemia. Clients who experience any symptoms of hypoglycemia should be instructed to check blood glucose when these symptoms appear. If the symptoms occur in spite of normal blood glucose, anxiety should be suspected as the cause.

Person-Centered Education on Self-Care Behaviors: Problem-Solving

Sick Days

Sick Day Management for the Child with Type 1 Diabetes

Illness in the child with type 1 diabetes presents significant risk for diabetic ketoacidosis (DKA). Colds, flu, and other infections can cause hyperglycemia. In infants, hyperglycemia can also be caused by teething or following routine immunizations.

The primary goal of **sick day management** is to maintain hydration and prevent severe hyperglycemia. Consistent oral hydration with 0.5–1.0 cup of sugar-free fluid every hour is needed.

Urine ketone testing is used to monitor sick day response. Urine ketones should be checked when blood glucose is 300 mg/dL or greater. The presence of moderate to large amounts of ketones requires additional insulin. If the child is not eating, fluids that contain sugar should be given. If hypoglycemia occurs, a glucagon injection may be needed. The FDA recently approved the use of intranasal glucagon and subcutaneously injected glucagon in the treatment of hypoglycemia. This should be on hand for those at risk for hypoglycemia who are unable or unwilling to ingest oral carbohydrates.

Parents and caregivers should know that DKA is a medical emergency and should seek immediate medical care for the following:

- Prolonged vomiting or diarrhea
- Not taking fluids
- Lethargy
- Rapid deep breathing
- Persistent hyperglycemia or ketonuria

Guidelines for Managing Diabetes During Sick Days

The physical stress of illness can trigger a counter-regulatory response resulting in hyperglycemia. This is especially common with colds, flu, and other types of infection. Being ill is a risk factor for the hyperglycemic emergencies of hyperosmolar hyperglycemic state (HHS) and diabetic ketoacidosis (DKA). Both of these conditions can produce profound dehydration and electrolyte imbalance.

Management guidelines for sick days include:

- Continue to take oral diabetes medication and insulin, even if not eating normally.
- Stop taking metformin if dehydrated and contact physician.
- Follow regular meal plan if able. Supplement with a cup of non-caloric fluid every hour.
- If unable to eat, drink 0.5–1.0 cup sugar-containing fluid every hour.
- Check blood glucose every 2–4 hours while awake.
- Notify healthcare provider for:
    - Persistent vomiting or diarrhea
    - Blood glucose consistently over 300 mg/dL
    - Temperature greater than 101°F
    - Small or greater amounts of ketones in the urine

Surgery and Other Procedures

Physiological stressors such as illness, infection, surgery, and trauma can disrupt normal metabolic homeostasis. Counter-regulatory hormone secretion is increased during these times and has the following effects on blood glucose:

- Stimulates the release of glucose from the liver
- Inhibits the action of insulin
- Inhibits the uptake of glucose by the muscle
- Diverts blood from the periphery, possibly affecting the absorption of injected insulin

The subsequent hyperglycemia causes osmotic diuresis and can lead to dehydration and loss of sodium, potassium, phosphorus, and magnesium.

In type 1 diabetes, insufficient insulin and inadequate carbohydrate intake can cause lipolysis and ketogenesis. If ketosis is not treated, diabetic ketoacidosis (DKA) can result. In type 2 diabetes, significant ketosis usually does not develop because endogenous insulin secretion continues. However, severe hyperglycemia, profound dehydration and electrolyte imbalance can result in these clients.

ADA guidelines specify glycemic goals in the context of elective surgery, recommending an A1c goal of <8% within three months of elective procedures and a blood glucose level of 100–180 mg/dL in the perioperative period.

Guidelines for Patients Using an Insulin Pump

For patients using a continuous subcutaneous insulin infusion (CSII) device, also known as an insulin pump, options for surgery and the postoperative period should be discussed with the surgeon and anesthesiologist. If the device is to be used during surgery, the anesthesiologist must demonstrate an acceptable level of comfort with managing it.

When an insulin pump is to be in place during surgery, the catheter should be inserted at a site away from the surgical field and reinforced with extra tape. A new catheter should be inserted 12–24 hours before the surgery to ensure adequate insulin infusion.

If hospital policy allows, patients who are alert and oriented should be allowed to manage their own insulin pump therapy, assuming they have managed well prior to hospitalization.

If the pump is to be discontinued, intravenous or subcutaneous insulin should be given prior to discontinuation.

Preventing Hyperglycemia and Hypoglycemia in Surgical Patients

Because it adversely affects white blood cell function, hyperglycemia is associated with impaired wound healing and increased risk for infection. It also increases platelet aggregation and makes red blood cells more rigid, resulting in decreased circulation through the small vessels. Additionally, high blood glucose interferes with normal protein synthesis, which is essential for healing the surgical wound. For optimal healing, blood glucose should remain at 180 mg/dL or less in the postoperative patient.

Elevated blood glucose increases the risk for ketoacidosis, especially in the patient with type 1 diabetes. Even moderate hyperglycemia can induce ketosis in type 1 patients who are undergoing surgery.

Hyperglycemia significantly increases the risk for electrolyte imbalance and fluid volume depletion in surgical patients with diabetes.

During the operative and the immediate postoperative periods, surgical patients are unable to detect and report symptoms of hypoglycemia, placing them at risk for coma. For this reason, frequent monitoring of blood glucose is required for all anesthetized patients with diabetes.

Implications for Preoperative Patients with Type 1 Diabetes

Preoperative patients with type 1 diabetes should have surgery scheduled for early in the morning to prevent prolonged fasting. If this is not possible, intravenous therapy for those who are not allowed to eat is required to maintain homeostasis. These infusions may include insulin, glucose solution, and electrolytes as needed.

A diabetologist or endocrinologist is usually consulted about intraoperative insulin and fluid management of the surgical patient with type 1 diabetes. Protocols for insulin administration during surgery are used.

People who use an insulin pump may leave the pump attached with a basal rate running during surgery. Supplemental short or rapid-acting insulin is given intravenously as needed.

Frequent blood glucose and ketone monitoring are necessary for these patients. During the operative period, blood glucose is monitored every 30–60 minutes and urine ketones are checked every 4–6 hours.

Subcutaneous insulin must be given 30 minutes prior to discontinuing the intravenous insulin infusion.

Patient Education for Individuals with Type 2 Diabetes Having Surgery

Educating the patient with type 2 diabetes about to undergo surgery includes:

- Follow instructions given by the doctor for taking diabetes medication the day of surgery. Sometimes the oral medications are allowed the morning of surgery and sometimes they are stopped the evening before.
- Chlorpropamide, a longer-acting sulfonylurea, is normally discontinued 48–72 hours before surgery.
- Metformin is usually discontinued the morning of surgery. Instruct the patient not to resume metformin postoperatively until they are eating and drinking normally and urinating sufficiently.
- Many patients with type 2 diabetes who normally use oral diabetes medications need insulin during the perioperative and postoperative periods. Assure patients that this is due to the physiologic stress of illness and surgery and that preventing hyperglycemia promotes healing. Reassure the patient that most people are able to resume their regular medication regimens postoperatively.

Patients should be aware that dextrose is commonly used for people with diabetes having surgery. This can prevent them from thinking there is a mistake in receiving a fluid with sugar.

Changes in Usual Schedule

Management strategies for handling individuals' changes in schedules are most often related to the following influences:

- **Shift work**: For day and evening shifts, individuals should usually maintain the same meal schedules and insulin administration, but switching to night shift can alter circadian rhythms. This can affect blood glucose levels, making individuals more at risk for hyperglycemia or hypoglycemia. Individuals may need more frequent glucose monitoring or continuous glucose monitoring and may need to adjust injection times to correspond with nighttime meal times. Individuals may also need to bring prepared meals rather than relying on snacks if a cafeteria is unavailable.
- **Religious/cultural influences**: Individuals who engage in prolonged fasting, such as that practiced by Muslims during Ramadan, are at risk for blood glucose disruption, such as hyperglycemia after the predawn meal and hypoglycemia during the day. Dehydration can exacerbate hyperglycemia and place the individuals at increased risk of cardiovascular and kidney disease. Early assessment and education are critical. Management includes close monitoring, increased blood glucose testing, and alterations in insulin dosage. Individuals at high risk are advised to avoid fasting.

Travel

People with diabetes should carry medications, insulin, syringes, and testing supplies in their carry-on luggage when traveling by air. Medications and supplies should be protected from temperature extremes.

People at risk need to carry fast-acting carbohydrate to treat hypoglycemia. To prepare for long flights, delays, and cancelled flights, they should also carry a meal. A travel companion should know the signs, symptoms, and treatment of hypoglycemia. Clients should wear medical identification stating that they have diabetes.

The following guidelines are used for making insulin adjustments when traveling across time zones:

- If the time change is 3 or fewer hours, adjust timing of insulin injections by one-half hour ahead or back, depending upon the direction of travel, until resumption of normal schedule.
- If traveling eastbound overseas, reduce basal insulin on the day of travel since it will be a shorter day. Maintain the same bolus regimen.
- If traveling westbound overseas, add injections of short-acting insulin every 4–6 hours, before meals, to compensate for the longer day.

Emergency Preparedness

According to the American College of Endocrinology's emergency preparedness plan for diabetes, an emergency kit is necessary for individuals with diabetes in the event of a natural disaster, such as a hurricane; a pandemic; or a national security risk, such as a bombing. The kit should always be kept up-to-date. The emergency kit should include:

- Information about medical history, a current medication list and regimen (including previous diabetes medications and reasons for discontinuation), names of healthcare professionals and contact information, health insurance cards, living will, power of attorney, and recent laboratory testing results (HbA1c, kidney function tests, and liver function tests)
- If possible, a 30-day supply of oral medications, insulin, and hypoglycemia emergency medications/supplements (glucagon, hard candy, sugar/juice) should be kept on hand and stored appropriately. The ADA recommends at least a week of diabetes supplies rather than 30 days.
- Blood glucose testing supplies with extra batteries and adequate supply of syringes and lancets
- An empty sharps container
- A cooler with 4 re-freezable gel packs to keep insulin cold but not frozen
- A 2-day supply of non-perishable food
- A 3-day supply of bottled water

Assistive and Adaptive Devices for Visual Impairment

Adaptive devices for individuals with diabetes and visual impairment include the following:

- **Audio glucometers** are glucometers that are audio-enabled with voice features that read values out loud. Most also have large buttons for tactile ease of use. Many include alarms that ring at preset times to remind the user to test.
- Some **insulin pens** have audible sounds to help individuals to set the pen for insulin delivery.
- **Continuous glucose monitoring systems** typically include audio alerts for hyperglycemia and hypoglycemia and may have voice features.
- **Handheld and mounted magnifiers** allow individuals with low vision to better see medication bottles, insulin syringes, and insulin vials to ensure proper type of insulin and dosage.

- **Large print diabetes log** facilitates recording of information for individuals with low vision.
- **Disposable lancets (such as twist-top)** allow skin puncture without the need to handle or change lancet blades.

SUBSTANCE USE

Substance use directly impacts diabetes. Education around the use of specific substances should be provided:

- **Alcohol**: Alcohol may result in hypoglycemia because the liver does not release glucose while metabolizing alcohol. Drinks high in carbohydrate may result in hyperglycemia. Individuals must understand risks and be taught to monitor blood glucose frequently and test for ketones. Insulin dosages may need to be adjusted.
- **Marijuana**: Because marijuana increases appetite, individuals may be at risk for hyperglycemia or, if they miss meals, hypoglycemia. Individuals should monitor glucose levels frequently and understand the medical and legal implications of use. Marijuana may increase heartrate and blood pressure.
- **Caffeine**: Caffeine may increase heart rate and blood pressure and have a mild diuretic effect, so individuals need to drink adequate water. Caffeine may cause a short-term increase in blood glucose, especially with type 2 diabetes, and may reduce insulin sensitivity. Intake should be limited to 200–300 mg (2–3 cups of coffee) daily.
- **Opioids**: Some opioids can lead to hyperglycemia, while those that suppress appetite can lead to hypoglycemia. Individuals using opioids need to monitor glucose levels frequently or use continuous glucose monitoring and must be educated about signs of overdose and risk involved in use.

Person-Centered Education on Self-Care Behaviors: Living with Diabetes and Prediabetes

LIFE CHANGES AND TRANSITIONS OF CARE

Life changes associated with living with diabetes and prediabetes include:

- **Diet modifications**: Healthy diet choices should include vegetables, fruits, whole grains, nonfat dairy, lean meats, and limited refined carbohydrates. Meals and snacks should be on a regular schedule, especially if taking diabetic medications.
- **Physical activity**: Individuals should engage in regular exercises for at least 30 minutes a day.
- **Semiannual physical examinations and yearly eye exam**: Regular monitoring of health is essential to prevent progression of disease.
- **Stress management**: Increased stress can lead to hyperglycemia, so stress reduction strategies should be utilized.
- **Smoking cessation**: Because smoking increases risk of cardiovascular and kidney disease, individuals should be referred to smoking cessation programs.
- **Cannabis cessation**: Due to the risk of cannabis hyperemesis syndrome, cannabis cessation should be encouraged.
- **Alcohol limitation**: Women should have no more than one drink per day and men no more than two.

Individuals are particularly vulnerable during transitions of care, especially if they are not adequately educated about self-management or a receiving facility is not provided adequate information about the individuals' plan of care and medication management. Transition planning must include adequate follow-up and consideration of individuals' needs after discharge.

SPECIAL POPULATIONS

OLDER ADULTS WITH DIABETES

Elderly clients with diabetes have a higher risk for failure to thrive and malnutrition than younger adult clients. Glycemic goals should take into account risk factors that can have a negative impact on nutritional status in this age group. These include:

- Decreased energy needs
- Decreased physical function that impairs ability to shop and cook
- Depression
- Cognitive impairment
- Financial constraints
- Poor dentition or tooth loss
- Altered nutrient absorption
- Decreased thirst sensation
- Social isolation

For frail elderly residents with diabetes in nursing facilities, providing adequate nutrition is the primary concern. Glycemic control is best addressed by implementing a meal plan that provides a consistent amount of carbohydrate from day to day. Specific calorie goals, special "diabetic diets" or "no concentrated sweets" diets are no longer considered appropriate for this population.

MEDICATION CONSIDERATIONS

Elderly patients with diabetes are sometimes treated with sulfonylureas. Glipizide is often preferred over glyburide because it is shorter acting and has fewer hepatic metabolites. First-generation sulfonylureas, such as tolazamide, are rarely used in this population because of their long half-life. The risk for hypoglycemia should always be considered in the elderly because they are more likely to have hypoglycemic unawareness.

Metformin use is restricted in many geriatric patients due to renal or hepatic insufficiency but is still the first line treatment for type 2 diabetes.

Use of thiazolidinediones in the elderly has not been widely studied.

Medication regimens should be simplified as much as possible since polypharmacy is a common problem in the older adult population.

Cost of medication may be an issue for seniors with limited income.

The need for insulin to control blood glucose increases with age due to the progressive nature of diabetes. Teaching should be adapted for alterations in function, such as vision loss and arthritis, as well as the slower mental processing that is a normal change with aging.

IMPLICATIONS OF HYPOGLYCEMIA

Elderly people with diabetes have a higher risk for hypoglycemia, are more at risk for hypoglycemic unawareness, and are more likely to confuse hypoglycemia with other disease symptoms.

There are numerous reasons why this population has a higher risk for hypoglycemia. Decreased renal function can alter the clearance of medications that lower blood glucose while the counter-regulatory response to hypoglycemia is blunted. Polypharmacy, inadequate or erratic food intake, and slowed intestinal absorption are additional risk factors.

The elderly and their significant others should learn about the signs and symptoms of hypoglycemia and be cautioned to not confuse these with other disease symptoms, the side effects of medications or normal aging. The 2026 ADA Standards recommend the use of continuous glucose monitoring in older adults with type 1 and type 2 diabetes on any type of insulin as a means to reduce hypoglycemic events. They also encourage the use of automated insulin delivery systems for this population.

Glycemic goals for the elderly are sometimes liberalized to avoid hypoglycemic episodes. Oral agents that do not produce hypoglycemic effects may be preferred for these patients. Older adults at risk for hypoglycemia may need emergency systems in place, such as an emergency pager. They should wear medical identification stating that they have diabetes.

Adolescents

Adherence to diabetes therapy is a challenge for any group, but probably more so for the adolescent. Some of the developmental issues of adolescence that impact treatment adherence include increased awareness of body image and differentiation from adult authority figures.

Strategies to help improve treatment adherence in the adolescent with type 1 diabetes include:

- Focus on what is relevant to the individual. For adolescents, this includes body image and peer relationships.
- Work with the client in establishing his or her own goals and be willing to compromise.
- Establish the primary relationship with the teen, but keep parents involved. Parental involvement is essential in prevention of ketoacidosis.
- Enhance feelings of normalcy.
- Involve the teen in peer support groups and diabetes camp.
- Maintain open lines of communication and explore perceived barriers.
- Provide positive reinforcement.

Social Support

Diabetes educators should be familiar with services tailored to teens that are offered by the American Diabetes Association (ADA), the Juvenile Diabetes Research Foundation (JDRF) and diabetes camps throughout the United States.

Content of diabetes self-management education for the teenager should be relevant to the developmental issues of this stage in life. These issues include peer allegiance, sexuality and contraception, substance abuse, driving issues, and social situations. Because peer influences are important, classes and support groups exclusively for teens are appropriate. These groups are most effective when the learning is centered on an activity that is fun.

Diabetes camps facilitate formal and informal learning among the peer group. Learning and sharing with other teens having the same problems and challenges helps develop feelings of normalcy and facilitates problem-solving.

Peer-centered weight loss groups and camps can also benefit the overweight teen with type 2 diabetes.

Pre-Conception Planning for Women with Diabetes

All women of childbearing age should be tested for diabetes prior to conception if they have risk factors for diabetes.

Starting at puberty, all women of childbearing age with diabetes should be counseled about the potential risks of unplanned pregnancy. Family planning resources should be offered. The importance of preconception care should be incorporated into all routine medical visits for appropriate patients.

For women with pre-existing diabetes, HbA1c levels should be 6.5% or less before conception is attempted. Glycemic control prior to conception and in early pregnancy reduces the risk of birth defects to a level similar to that of the general population.

A preconception workup includes evaluation and treatment, if indicated, for diabetic retinopathy, nephropathy, neuropathy, and cardiovascular disease.

Medication assessment is also important for such patients since many drugs used for the treatment of diabetes are contraindicated or not advised in pregnancy. These include statins, ACE inhibitors, most oral antidiabetic agents, and GLP-1 medications. Women with diabetes who are on GLP-1 therapy and are considering pregnancy should be advised to stop GLP-1 therapy and then meet preconception glycemic goals before conception.

Perinatal Complications Associated with Maternal Hyperglycemia

Perinatal complications can be correlated with the level of maternal glycemic control during pregnancy.

Planned pregnancy is of critical importance in women with diabetes because fetal organ formation takes place in the first 8 weeks of gestation, at which time many women are unaware that they are pregnant. Uncontrolled blood glucose in the first trimester of pregnancy is associated with spontaneous abortion and congenital malformations, such as neural tube defects, heart anomalies, and renal anomalies.

The placenta becomes fully grown and functioning by about 18 weeks gestation, at which time the fetus can develop metabolic complications secondary to maternal hyperglycemia. These complications include macrosomia (abnormally high birth weight), increased risk for childhood obesity and glucose intolerance, stillbirth, respiratory distress syndrome, and hyperbilirubinemia.

Hypoglycemia in the neonate is the most common complication of second and third trimester hyperglycemia in the mother. Neonatal hypoglycemia is defined as:

- 35 mg/dL or less in full-term infants
- 25 mg/dL or less in preterm infants

Maternal Complications Related to Diabetes During Pregnancy

Maternal complications of uncontrolled blood glucose during pregnancy include hypertension, preterm labor and delivery, cesarean section, and pyelonephritis.

Hypertension in such women may include pregnancy-induced hypertension (preeclampsia) and chronic hypertension. For chronic hypertension, the usual antihypertensive medications, such as ACE inhibitors and ARBs, are contraindicated during pregnancy. Calcium channel blockers and labetalol are often substituted. Target blood pressure during pregnancy is <135/85 mmHg.

Hypertension, whether pregnancy-induced or preexisting, is the most significant risk factor for progression of retinopathy in pregnancy.

Women with preexisting early renal disease should be encouraged to attempt pregnancy as early as feasible because pregnancy presents a risk for worsening renal impairment in these patients.

While diabetes is not an absolute indication for cesarean section, the risk is increased in this population. Women with proliferative retinopathy often require cesarean delivery to avoid the Valsalva maneuver, which could cause retinal hemorrhage. High birth weight neonates are at increased risk of shoulder dystocia from vaginal delivery, necessitating cesarean delivery in some cases.

Considerations When Educating Clients About Diabetes and Pregnancy

The 2026 ADA Standards place emphasis on preconception education and care for women with diabetes.

Having diabetes does not appear to affect fertility. The chance of having a child with type 1 diabetes when the mother has type 1 diabetes is 2%. For the child of a father with type 1 diabetes, the risk is 6%.

Glycemic control during pregnancy is correlated with the risk for spontaneous abortion (SA). When the patient has good blood glucose control during pregnancy, the risk for SA is about the same as for the general population.

The risk for congenital birth defects is greatly increased when the mother has markedly elevated HbA1c levels during pregnancy. Maternal serum alpha-fetoprotein screening can detect neural tube defects. Ultrasonography can detect anomalies of the central nervous system, heart, and kidneys. Patients should be made aware that these tests are not 100% sensitive for detecting these problems.

Those planning a pregnancy should consider the possible financial challenges associated with a complicated pregnancy. This may include increased surveillance requiring more medical tests and appointments. The potential need for more missed work days should be taken into consideration.

Risks for Diabetic Retinopathy During Pregnancy

Certain placental hormones cause vascular changes that can accelerate **retinopathy**. Women of childbearing age with retinopathy should be educated about the effect that pregnancy can have on their eyes.

Preconception planning for women with diabetes should include a thorough ophthalmologic exam.

Nonproliferative retinopathy is not a contraindication for pregnancy. While there is significant risk that nonproliferative retinopathy will progress during pregnancy, this is expected to reverse after delivery.

Results of studies are mixed concerning the risk for the progression of **proliferative retinopathy** in pregnant women whose eyes have been stabilized with photocoagulation prior to pregnancy. Those with untreated proliferative retinopathy have the highest risk for progression during pregnancy. Pregnancy in these women is contraindicated until their eyes can be stabilized with photocoagulation. Many women with proliferative retinopathy deliver their babies by cesarean section or vacuum extracted vaginal delivery to avoid pushing during childbirth.

Impact of Pregnancy on Normal Metabolism

Normal pregnancy is a diabetogenic state. Hormones produced during pregnancy, such as progesterone, human placental hormone, and prolactin, lead to an insulin-resistant state. Normally, blood insulin levels double or triple during the third trimester due to increased needs of the placenta. For women with pre-existing insulin resistance or gestational diabetes, the relative amount of available insulin remains insufficient.

In pregnancy, the glycemic response to food consumption results in greater and more prolonged elevation in blood glucose.

During the second and third trimesters of pregnancy, the risk for maternal ketosis increases. This should be avoided since ketones have an adverse effect on the fetus. Education includes advising the client to refrain from fasting and unsupervised weight loss and to check for urine ketones in the later stages of pregnancy.

In the immediate postpartum period, insulin sensitivity increases due to the sudden drop in placental hormones and most women promptly return to their pre-pregnancy insulin requirements.

Gestational Diabetes

Gestational diabetes mellitus (GDM) is broadly defined as a condition of carbohydrate intolerance at the onset or first recognition of pregnancy. This definition includes women with existing but undiagnosed diabetes prior to pregnancy. In the United States, it is estimated that about 2% of women of childbearing age have undiagnosed diabetes. In 2009, new criteria for the diagnosis of GDM were established. The current method for screening and diagnosis of GDM is:

- Screen all women for diabetes risk at first prenatal visit (before 15 weeks gestation).
- Test at 24–28 weeks gestation in all pregnant women of average risk.*
- One step strategy: Use 75-gram oral glucose tolerance test (OGTT) OR
  Two step strategy: 50-gram test followed by a 100-gram test if positive
- Diagnose GDM when:
  - Fasting blood glucose is ≥92 mg/dL (one step) or ≥95 mg/dL (two step)
  - 1-hour post-OGTT result is ≥180 mg/dL (one step and two step)
  - 2-hour post-OGTT result is ≥153 mg/dL (one step) or ≥155 mg/dL (two step)
  - 3-hour post OGTT result (for two step only) is ≥140 mg/dL
- Only 1 of the abnormal values listed above is required for diagnosis for the one step strategy and 2 are required for diagnosis for the two step strategy.

*Women with high risk for diabetes should be tested for GDM as soon as possible. If first test is negative, retest again at 24–28 weeks gestation. Risk factors include:

- History of GDM
- Family history of diabetes
- Obesity
- Glycosuria

Treatment Goals

Regular self-monitoring of blood glucose is highly recommended for all women with GDM. Plasma glucose targets are as follows.

- Fasting: <95 mg/dL
- 1-hour postprandial: <140 mg/dL
- 2-hour postprandial: <120 mg/dL

Medical nutrition therapy (MNT), following a carbohydrate-controlled meal plan, is the initial focus of treatment. Because early glycemic control is important, prompt intervention by a registered dietitian is recommended. The goals of MNT are normoglycemia, adequate nutrition, appropriate weight gain, and absence of ketosis. For obese women with GDM, weight loss is controversial. If attempted, it must be medically supervised and caution must be taken to prevent ketosis.

Unless contraindicated, exercise is recommended to improve glucose tolerance and potentially prevent the need for insulin injections.

When diet and exercise do not produce desired results, insulin is the most commonly used medication to treat GDM. Glyburide and metformin have also been studied and may be used in some cases of GDM.

Postpartum Considerations for Women with Gestational Diabetes

Most women with GDM return to normal blood glucose levels shortly after delivery, although 40–60% will develop type 2 diabetes within 10 years. Client education and medical surveillance are indicated for the prevention and early detection of subsequent type 2 diabetes in women with GDM.

Following childbirth, the patient should continue self-monitoring of blood glucose until normoglycemia is reached. A 75-gram oral glucose tolerance test is indicated at approximately 6 weeks postpartum.

Women with a history of GDM should have a fasting plasma glucose test every year and a 75-gram oral glucose tolerance test every 3 years to screen for type 2 diabetes. They should be educated to request these screening tests if they change healthcare providers.

Education includes the importance of a healthy diet and BMI, using the USDA dietary guidelines, and regular exercise (after medical clearance has been obtained). Since many clients with GDM are overweight or obese, initial weight loss to 5–7% below preconception weight is indicated for the prevention of type 2 diabetes.

Implications of Breastfeeding for the Woman with Diabetes

Many women mistakenly believe that they cannot breastfeed if they have diabetes, whether chronic or gestational. Education includes informing these clients that breastfeeding is not contraindicated but is, in fact, highly recommended. Perceived barriers to breastfeeding should be explored.

Breastfeeding has many advantages for women with previous gestational diabetes (GDM) and should be strongly encouraged in this group. Breastfeeding lowers glucose levels postpartum and reduces the risk for future development of type 2 diabetes. It also mobilizes fat stores and promotes weight loss, which is important for the 50% of GDM patients who are obese.

For women with pre-existing diabetes who use insulin, breastfeeding may enable the insulin dosage to be reduced. These women should self-monitor blood glucose frequently and be aware of the increased risk for hypoglycemia. Sometimes, taking a snack before breastfeeding and an overall increase in daily calorie consumption are recommended.

Implications for Ketone Monitoring During Pregnancy

During pregnancy, the blood glucose value at which women can spill **ketones** is lower, placing them at greater risk for diabetic ketoacidosis (DKA). In rare cases, ketoacidosis occurs in pregnant women with normal blood glucose levels.

The elevated risk for ketosis is caused by increased fat catabolism during pregnancy. Ketones cross the placenta and can pose a risk to the fetus. Fetal exposure to ketones is associated with fetal demise and lower IQ scores.

Routine monitoring of urine and blood ketones is necessary during pregnancy; urine ketones are monitored with the first morning specimen. Indications for additional ketone testing are blood glucose ≥200 mg/dL or significant vomiting with morning sickness or other illness. The most common cause of ketosis is infection.

When ketones are present with normal or low blood glucose, inadequate food intake is suspected. When ketones are concurrent with elevated glucose, ketosis is imminent.

Nutritional Considerations for Pregnant Women with Diabetes

The general goals of nutrition therapy during pregnancy are to provide sufficient nutrition for mother and fetus, to promote appropriate fetal growth and maternal weight gain and to maintain glycemic control.

Nutrients of particular concern during pregnancy include protein, calcium, iron, and folate. Folic acid supplementation of 400-800 μg per day is recommended.

Recommendations for weight gain depend on the preconception weight status of the mother. Obese women are generally recommended to gain only as much as the products of conception, approximately 15 pounds. Weight loss for these women is occasionally recommended but is controversial.

Women of healthy weight are recommended to gain 1 pound per week during the 2nd and 3rd trimesters. Overweight women should gain only 1/2 pound per week during the last 2 trimesters.

Consistency of the timing and amount of food intake is especially important for pregnant women using insulin. Bedtime snacks are often needed to prevent ketosis related to overnight starvation.

Non-nutritive sweeteners, such as aspartame and acesulfame K, are considered safe for use during pregnancy.

Morning Sickness for the Pregnant Woman with Diabetes

Any time a pregnant woman with diabetes is unable to eat or keep food down, there is a risk for the development of ketosis. Careful monitoring of urine and/or blood ketones is recommended when a client has significant morning sickness.

Hypoglycemia can produce morning sickness. Women at risk should be instructed to check blood glucose when nausea appears and to treat low blood glucose promptly and appropriately.

Vomiting presents a challenge for clients who use insulin. If vomiting occurs after taking the short-acting pre-meal insulin, the client should take enough glucagon to raise the blood glucose 30–40 mg/dL to prevent hypoglycemia. The glucagon is effective for 1–2 hours, during which time morning sickness may subside and food can be taken. If the client remains unable to eat and blood glucose declines, additional glucagon is needed until the peak action of the insulin has abated. Clients should contact their healthcare provider if they develop persistent nausea and vomiting.

Psychosocial Wellbeing

Diabetes Burnout

Diabetes burnout results from the frustration of dealing with diabetes on a daily basis and leads to feelings of inadequacy and emotional depletion. Poor self-care practice is a symptom of diabetes burnout.

Ways the diabetes educator can help a client deal with diabetes burnout include:

- Acknowledging that living with diabetes is challenging and that many people with the disease have feelings of burnout
- Developing a supportive and collaborative relationship with the client
- Helping the client identify areas where he or she has been successful, as opposed to only pointing out shortcomings
- Helping the client set reasonable, attainable goals
- Encouraging the client to seek help and support from others and to optimize available resources
- Helping the client develop effective problem-solving skills

Overcoming the Adverse Impact of Diabetes on Social Relationships

Sometimes a support person becomes overly involved in a client's diabetes self-management. The support person might try to dictate and monitor what the person with diabetes should be doing without regard for the rights of the individual. This can be disempowering for the person with diabetes and can lead to power struggles in the relationship.

It is important to remember that the person with diabetes is the one with the rights and responsibilities related to his or her own diabetes care. The empowerment approach to self-care should be supported at every opportunity.

It is also important to recognize that a certain degree of dependency can be beneficial in a relationship. Therefore, the person with diabetes and the support person should openly discuss mutual expectations with regard to the management of diabetes. The feelings of the support person should be acknowledged, as they may include feelings of fear, grief, and resentment. Referral to a mental health specialist is recommended when unhealthy behaviors are noted in a relationship.

Coping Skills

Examples of coping skills include the following:

Assertiveness

- Being able to express feelings, wants, and needs in a direct way
- Being able to say "no"
- Asking for help and clarification when needed

Positive self-talk

- Using positive language and speaking in terms that indicate optimism and hope
- Using language to support self-confidence, such as "I can do it"

Problem-solving

- Able to identify a problem
- Able to brainstorm possible solutions
- Able to select one or more realistic options for solving the problem

Priority setting and time management

- Able to differentiate between higher and lower priorities
- Able to organize and manage multiple priorities

Use of support system

- Can identify sources of help and support
- Able to specify how others can provide support
- **Reframing** is a cognitive technique that can be an appropriate coping skill for people with diabetes. Using this technique, clients learn to identify thoughts and attitudes that trigger maladaptive behavior in challenging situations. Once the self-sabotaging thoughts are identified, the person can learn to restructure thoughts, feelings, and attitudes in a more positive and productive way.
- **Relaxation** techniques can also be effective in coping with the demands of diabetes. These may include progressive muscle relaxation, deep breathing, and guided imagery.
- **Problem-solving skills** are essential in coping with diabetes. Studies indicate that training in problem-solving improves glycemic control.
- The effective use of a **support system** is another appropriate coping skill. Educators can help clients identify sources of support and guide them in specifying what they need from those around them.
- **Relapse prevention**, another coping skill, may include maintaining an environment that supports a healthy lifestyle and having a system of rewards for staying on track.

Motivational Interviewing

Motivational interviewing is a validated behavioral intervention technique that helps clients to explore ambivalence about change and to engage them in talking about change. It is usually most appropriate in one-to-one sessions.

Motivational interviewing elicits "change talk" from the client. The interviewer mirrors ambivalent statements made by the client and asks the client to reinforce the perceived benefits. Thus, by vocalizing one's own reasons for considering change, the client motivates him- or herself to move toward change.

Another premise of motivational interviewing is to "roll with resistance." When a client is reluctant to engage in the recommended behavior, the interviewer explores the reasons for this rather than directly confronting the client.

Example of motivational interviewing: "It sounds like you have some reasons why you don't want to check your blood sugar regularly, yet you've indicated that you should be doing it more. What benefits do you think you would have by checking more often?"

Managing Disordered Eating

Disordered eating is more common in those with diabetes, especially type 1, than in the general population, averaging about 20% overall but with higher percentages among young adult females. Of note, anorexia is less common than binge-eating in this population. Patterns of disordered eating include:

- Restricting dietary intake and calories, leading to malnutrition
- Binge eating
  - Objective binge eating describes when the person eats large amounts and feels eating is out of control.
  - Subjective binge eating describes when the person feels eating is out of control but is not necessarily eating excessively. Subjective binge eating can lead to insulin restriction.
- Night eating syndrome: Binging during the night
- Insulin restriction: Prevention of the metabolism of carbohydrates as a means to increase weight loss

Indications of eating disorders include elevated HbA1c (although it can be normal), fluctuations in fasting blood glucose levels, repeated episodes of ketoacidosis, preoccupation with weight, electrolyte imbalance, anemia, and significant weight changes. Screening questions include asking clients if they feel their eating is out of control, if they alter insulin dosage to lose weight, and if they feel overwhelmed or distressed by their condition. Management includes referral to a specialist in eating disorders and diabetes, referral to diabetes support groups, consultation with an endocrinologist, emotional support, and less-frequent weighing.

Empowerment Approach to Self-Management

Role of the Client

The empowerment approach to diabetes management upholds that the person with diabetes has the rights and responsibilities for his or her care and management. This includes making the decision about when and how the individual will initiate and maintain self-care behaviors.

In adherence with this philosophy, the **client's role** includes:

- Identifying goals and setting an agenda for education
- Utilizing knowledge gained from education to make informed healthcare decisions
- Taking an active role in identifying problems and learning to problem-solve
- Participating in contracts with educators and other healthcare providers
- Identifying a support system and specifying the help needed

It is important to realize that clients have differing levels of comfort with self-care and some may prefer a more passive role. In these cases, it is best to support an incremental approach to developing self-management skills.

Role of the Educator

In adherence with the empowerment approach, the **role of the educator** includes:

- Assisting clients to make informed decisions about their care and self-management
- Approaching education from the client's perspective and offering information relevant to the individual
- Identifying clients' readiness to change and providing stage-appropriate interventions
- Assisting clients to identify problems and helping them develop problem-solving skills
- Helping clients identify thoughts, feelings, and attitudes that have an effect on diabetes self-management
- Assist with goal setting

Collaboration Between the Educator and Client

The empowerment approach to diabetes self-management education and support is built upon a foundation of collaboration between educator and client. In a collaborative relationship, the educator provides expertise and relevant information for safe decision-making on the part of the client. The client chooses how to use the information.

An important aspect of a collaborative client-educator relationship includes jointly setting and agreeing on an agenda. The agenda should start with things that are important to the client but should also include items that the educator feels are important.

Working together to identify and solve problems is an important part of the collaborative relationship. The educator should resist the temptation to solve problems for the client, and instead help him or her identify possible solutions from which to choose.

A collaborative relationship relies on active listening from the educator. This includes asking open-ended questions so that the client can verbalize thoughts, feelings, and attitudes. Reflection and summarizing are also active listening techniques.

Role of the Family

Family support is an important component of successful diabetes self-management. Two important things to consider when involving the family in education are the cultural context of the family and the functional health and stability of family dynamics.

One role of the family is to learn about diabetes self-management along with the client. Ideally, this should begin at diagnosis and be maintained throughout the continuum of care. The educator can facilitate this by inviting family members to attend educational sessions with the client.

Family members' feelings about diabetes should be explored. These may include negative feelings based on erroneous information. The educator should help the family understand what is expected with regard to the client's blood glucose and behavior, so that their expectations will be realistic.

The family's role is to support the client. This may include supporting healthy eating as a family, engaging in physical activity together, and working mutually to solve problems as they arise.

Safety Issues

Driver Safety

Patients who use sulfonylurea medications and insulin are at risk for hypoglycemia and should receive driver safety information. Non-sulfonylurea secretagogues, such as repaglinide, have a lower potential for causing hypoglycemia. Insulin poses the greatest risk.

Hypoglycemia can interfere with vision and mental processing, placing the person at high risk for accidents and injury. People at risk should wear medical identification to avoid being mistaken as driving while intoxicated.

Clients at risk should keep a fast-acting carbohydrate within arm's reach while driving. Good choices for the car include glucose tablets or a disposable juice box or bag.

Studies have indicated that many people underestimate the danger of driving with low blood glucose. Therefore, the educator should ask the client what he or she feels is a safe cutoff point.

The client should be instructed to test blood glucose prior to driving and to not drive if it is below 70 mg/dL.

Sharps Disposal and Medical Identification

Individuals should be taught about the FDA guidelines for disposal of sharps, particularly as it relates to insulin needles and lancets:

- Immediately dispose of needles and sharps (lancets) in an FDA-approved sharps container or heavy-duty plastic container and carry a small portable sharps container when traveling. Do not dispose of sharps in the toilet, sink, or usual trash containers.
- Do not bend, break, or recap needles before placing them in the sharps container.
- Contact local trash disposal company or public health department for guidelines regarding discarding the container in the trash. Seal the container and label according to community guidelines before disposal.
- Keep sharps disposal containers out of reach of children and pets.

After diagnosis, individuals should be fitted with a **medical ID bracelet** and the importance of wearing it at all times, so that first responders will know the individual is diabetic in case of emergency, should be stressed. Medical alert bracelets come in various forms, some that look like jewelry and may be more acceptable to adolescents. Most medical alert bracelets are inexpensive, but the cost is not usually covered by insurance.

Social/Financial Considerations

Economic Burden of Diabetes

Diabetes exacts a heavy economic burden upon the individual and society, with healthcare expenditures for people with the disease averaging 2–3 times that of the general population. In addition, many of those with diabetes have decreased earning potential due to disability imposed by the disease.

The Social Security Disability Insurance (SSDI) program provides assistance to disabled workers and their families. The government reported that there were 122,000 cases in which diabetes was the primary basis for disability in 2002. The economic burden of diabetes has since increased drastically, by 35% between the years of 2012 and 2022 (by 7% between 2017 and 2022).

Costs to the individual are high and include insurance premiums, co-pays, multiple prescription medications, testing supplies, and durable medical equipment. Studies show that many people do not take all of their prescribed medication due to the cost.

Disability, Discrimination, and School Issues

While schools should have trained staff available at school and during field trips, some schools are without school nurses. School staff should be made aware of signs of hyperglycemia and hypoglycemia so they can manage emergencies. The use of CGM and various insulin infusion devices should be supported in the school environment, and students should have appropriate accommodations to allow for these devices. Students may need to carry medication, but this is restricted in most schools. Students may need time to test and inject insulin. Students may be eligible for an IEP if diabetes affects education and a 504 plan to allow for accommodations such as testing time and excuses for doctors' appointments.

Financial considerations associated with diabetes are also prevalent. Those with diabetes have medical expenses, on average, double that of those without diabetes, and the cost of medical care, medications, and supplies can be difficult for those without adequate insurance. Additionally, individuals may lose income because of absenteeism from work. Some people may be eligible for medical and financial assistance.

INSURANCE OPTIONS

FEE-FOR-SERVICE AND MANAGED CARE HEALTH INSURANCE PLANS

Fee-for-service plans, also known as indemnity plans, reimburse the beneficiary after medical expenses have been incurred. Claim forms are typically utilized. The insured usually pays an annual deductible amount for the first expenses incurred during the calendar year. Once the deductible is satisfied, the insurer pays a percentage, often 80%, of the incurred expenses. Indemnity plans offer the consumer free choice of healthcare provider.

Managed care plans are administered by health maintenance organizations (HMOs). They generally require lower premiums because they have greater cost control. Members pay a nominal copayment for services rendered and there are no claim forms or annual deductibles. Managed care plans are more restrictive in choice of provider and some HMOs are provider-owned. This type of plan places more emphasis on preventive services.

Fee-for-service and managed care plans represent two extremes in health insurance coverage. In between, there are other types of plans such as preferred provider organizations (PPOs) and managed fee-for-service plans.

FEDERAL INSURANCE PROGRAMS

Medicare: Provides full medical services to people age 65 and older, people permanently disabled of any age, and all people with end-stage renal disease.

Veterans Administration (VA): Care is provided free of charge to veterans who have service-related medical conditions, served in specific wars, or meet low-income criteria. Veterans not meeting these criteria can also receive medical care with copayments.

Indian Health Services (IHS): Medical services are provided free of charge to Native Americans and Alaska Natives who are members of federally recognized tribes.

TRICARE: Offers healthcare services to active duty and retired military, their families, and their survivors.

Bureau of Primary Health Care: Provides medical services to vulnerable, underserved people who have geographic, financial, or cultural barriers to healthcare. Eligible beneficiaries pay on a sliding scale basis at federally qualified centers, many of which are in rural areas.

MEDICARE

Medicare is the largest federally funded payer of health insurance coverage.

Eligibility criteria include:

- Age over 65
- Disabled, any age
- End-stage renal disease, any age

Parts to Medicare include:

- Medicare Part A covers hospital, skilled nursing, home health, or hospice. Beneficiary pays deductible.
- Medicare Part B covers physician office visits, outpatient services, laboratory costs, equipment, and supplies. Part B is elective and the beneficiary pays the premiums.
- Medicare Part C, also known as Medicare Advantage, covers things not covered by Parts A and B, such as extra days in the hospital. Although not available in all areas, Part C provides an option for some to avoid purchasing "MediGap" insurance to fill gaps in Medicare coverage. Beneficiary pays a monthly premium.
- Medicare Part D is prescription drug insurance that lowers the cost of medications. Beneficiaries pay a monthly premium and choose a drug plan from a participating private company.

Eligibility for Healthcare Services and Supplies

Eligibility: Includes membership criteria, such as age in the case of Medicare, or being a policyholder under private insurance plans. Other eligibility criteria may include being classified in a diagnostic group or requiring a specific type of medical treatment.

Covered benefits: These are the types of services and supplies that the insurance plan covers. Examples of covered benefits may include laboratory services, specific procedures, equipment such as glucose monitors, and medical supplies. The insurers normally have specific criteria under which payment for covered services will be rendered. For example, a carrier may only pay for a specific brand of glucose meter and may stipulate the quantity of testing strips that can be distributed over a specified period of time.

Exclusions: These are items not covered by the insurance plan. Common exclusions are eyeglasses, dentistry, and cosmetic surgery.

Medical necessity: Certain criteria must be met and documentation provided to justify that the services or supplies are necessary.

Legal Rights of the Individual with Diabetes in the Workplace

Diabetes educators must be knowledgeable about clients' legal rights in the workplace and be prepared to advocate for them. The law protects people with diabetes from job discrimination based solely upon having diabetes and includes being allowed reasonable accommodations to enable diabetes management.

The Americans with Disabilities Act Amendments Act (ADAAA) of 2008 protects people with diabetes from discrimination in the workplace. The law requires that people with diabetes be afforded reasonable accommodations to follow a doctor's orders and protects them from being fired as long as they can perform the essential functions of the job. For example, a person on insulin may require a break at a particular time to be able to eat and avoid hypoglycemia.

A letter from a healthcare provide to the employer can explain the client's need for reasonable workplace accommodations and fulfill the requirements of the ADAAA to protect the client's job security. The letter should document how diabetes affects major life activities and describe the reasonable accommodations needed for the client's self-management.

Evaluation, Documentation, and Follow-Up

Evaluating Educational Objectives

Surveys are easy to design and use. Questions can be given in written or oral form. A disadvantage of surveys is that respondents can interpret questions differently, affecting the reliability of data. Telephone and face-to-face surveys often yield a high response rate.

Chart audits can produce objective data such as laboratory results and adherence to recommendations for preventive services. Chart audits involve reviewing records to capture associations between education and outcomes. Disadvantages of this method are the time required to go through records and the variability of different reviewers' skill in collecting data.

Checklists gather concurrent information and can reveal behavior change and implementation of tasks. Reliability of collected data depends upon the consistency and skill of those collecting the data.

Other methods of evaluation include asking participants to take pre- and post-tests or perform return demonstration of skills taught.

Evaluating the Effectiveness of Teaching Self-Management Skills

Behavior modification helps the client learn and practice new skills, such as eating a healthy diet, exercising, and maintaining a healthy weight. Prevention of relapse and providing intervention are important components of a behavior modification program.

It is usually most effective to target a single behavior change at one time and to encourage progress in small steps toward the goal.

Behavioral contracts with clients help establish goals and provide a basis for evaluation. Clients should be assisted in developing goals that they feel are realistic, manageable, and measurable. Examples of measurable goals are:

- I will eat 5 servings of vegetables every day.
- I will walk for 20 minutes 5 days per week.

Clients should set a date for achieving stepwise progress toward a goal. While this should be evaluated at every diabetes visit, intermittent contact can take place over the phone or by email to evaluate clients' self-management skills.

Evaluating the Client's Progress Toward Behavioral Goals

Evaluation of client progress toward behavioral goals should be done in a nonjudgmental manner. Intensive diabetes management is rigorous and even those who are adherent may occasionally relax their standards, such as during times of stress or on holidays and vacations. These relapses are expected and do not signify a failure on the part of the client.

The educator can support the client through a relapse by helping identify the cause of the relapse and exploring optimal ways of dealing with it. The client should be supported and encouraged to resume working toward his or her behavioral goals as soon as feasible.

Lifestyle behaviors, such as diet and exercise, can be difficult to maintain for long periods. Therefore, ongoing monitoring and evaluation of these behaviors is indicated. When needed, adjustment of behavioral goals should be negotiated with clients to fit their preferences and lifestyle needs. Positive reinforcement for making small steps toward behavior change is recommended.

Evaluating the Effectiveness of Education

Educational sessions should be planned to allow adequate time to evaluate client learning. Evaluation of teaching includes asking clients if they have understood the information given and how they could put it into practice. Evaluation can include asking clients if they have further questions or if they found something difficult to understand. Clients can also be asked to summarize the teaching sessions by stating 2 or 3 points that they feel are the most important.

Although tests or quizzes are not inappropriate, they are not always necessary for effective evaluation. Adult learners tend to remember information that is practical and can be readily put to use. Simply asking questions oriented to everyday problem-solving can provide adequate evaluation of learning. An example of a question to evaluate the ability to apply learning could start with "What would you do if..."

Evaluating a Client's Psychosocial Adaptation to Diabetes

Healthy coping is identified by the Association of Diabetes Care and Education Specialists as an outcome of successful diabetes education. Behavioral goals related to this outcome include adaptation to the lifestyle changes required by diabetes and mobilization of an appropriate support system.

Psychosocial adaptation to diabetes involves mastering such behavioral skills as setting realistic goals, solving problems effectively, and attaining self-efficacy.

Methods for measuring healthy coping consist of:

- Depression scores, such as the Zung/Beck Depression Scale
- Quality of life measures, such as the Diabetes Quality of Life Measure
- Self-efficacy scales, such as the Diabetes Empowerment Scale
- Self-report of constructs such as self-efficacy, feeling of empowerment, and stress management

An informal or less-structured way to assess psychosocial adaptation to diabetes is to ask clients how they feel they are coping. Additionally, clients can be given various scenarios and asked how they would handle them.

Documenting the Educational Process

Documentation is a legal requirement of healthcare intervention. It also provides communication between team members and is critical for evaluating outcomes of the diabetes self-management education and support program.

Documentation is ongoing and must occur at every step of the educational process, which includes assessment, planning, implementation, and evaluation of outcomes. Effective documentation is relevant to the individual and his or her goals. Accuracy in documentation ensures legal compliance and effective communication. Documentation should be timely so that results of intervention can be appropriately utilized by other members of the diabetes care team.

Standardized checklists are often used for documenting many of the steps of the educational process. Documentation of each step includes:

- Assessment: identifying the individual's specific learning needs
- Planning: identifying desired outcomes and goals and developing a collaborative plan with the client
- Implementation: describing the educational and behavioral interventions that are designed to help the client achieve the stated goals
- Evaluation: reporting the outcomes of the interventions in relation to the goals

HEALTHCARE PROVIDERS THAT CAN HELP ADDRESS DIABETES-RELATED PROBLEMS

Endocrinologist or diabetologist:

- Education for preoperative patients with type 1 diabetes about fluid and insulin management during surgery

Gastroenterologist:

- Diabetes-related gastroparesis

Gynecologist:

- Diabetes-related female sexual dysfunction

Nephrologist:

- A glomerular filtration rate (GFR) of 30 mL/min or less

Orthopedist:

- Charcot foot, a unilaterally warm and misshapen "rocker bottom" foot

Podiatrist:

- Foot problems or ulcers in conjunction with peripheral neuropathy and/or peripheral vascular disease

Primary Healthcare Provider:

- Exercise prescription (if client is planning more than brisk walking or has complications that may be exacerbated by exercise)
- Preconception counseling

Registered dietitian:

- Medical nutrition therapy (MNT); all clients with diabetes should be referred for MNT
- Celiac disease (intolerance to gluten)

Urologist:

- Male sexual dysfunction

Multidisciplinary Diabetes Team

The person with diabetes is central to the multidisciplinary diabetes team. In addition to the client and healthcare professionals, the team also includes the client's family, spouse, and other significant people. Good communication among team members enhances team cohesion and consensus.

An understanding of the roles of each team member is important. However, role definitions that are rigid and territorial are counterproductive. Members of an interdisciplinary team should allow for shared responsibility and flexibility within a framework of shared expectations. Clients must receive consistent messages and treatment approaches across multidisciplinary lines, requiring team members to share a common philosophy.

Encounters with clients should be carefully documented and otherwise communicated to appropriate team members. Behavioral goals, developed with the client, must be included in communication. Client records often include behavioral contracts that facilitate communication of goals.

Team meetings are an effective method of communication and provide a multidisciplinary approach to problem-solving. If team meetings are not feasible, other methods of communication, such as phone calls and emails, are necessary.

Team Communication

Diabetes education crosses numerous healthcare disciplines. Team members include nurses, physicians, dietitians, mental health professionals, social workers, and psychologists, among others.

The team approach implies that education does not stand alone and that everyone teaches across the continuum. Roles should be defined collaboratively and communicated openly because there is considerable overlap of responsibility. Team members' roles may be defined by credentials, areas of expertise, or job descriptions.

Examples of role responsibility include:

- Client: always the center of the team
- Physician: establishes diagnosis and guides implementation of medical treatment plan
- Nurse educator: coordinates team effort; also provides self-management education and acute problem management
- Dietitian: provides nutrition assessment and MNT
- Mental health and social services professionals: identify psychosocial barriers and sources of support within the community and family

Information from the various team members must be consistent, requiring them to communicate what they have told clients. This is true for both oral and written information. When team members provide consistent messages, the client is able to develop trust.

Standards and Practice

Standards

National Standards for Diabetes Self-Management Education and Support

The National Standards for Diabetes Self-Management Education and Support (NSDMES) (2022) include the following:

- **Support for DSMES services**: Support from sponsor organizations, internal leadership, healthcare teams, individuals, physicians, and diabetes care and education specialist are essential for success of DSMES services.
- **Population and service assessment**: The target population's demographics and perception of risk is key to designing and delivery quality services, which must address population barriers and health inequities.
- **DSMES team**: Teams should be multidisciplinary with diabetes knowledge and documented continuing education, and service should be based on evidence-based knowledge. Teams should be led by a quality coordinator.
- **Delivery and design of DSMES services**: Services will depend on evidence-based content and delivery that utilizes current technology and culturally appropriate curriculum. Both initial DSMES and ongoing follow-up and support are required.
- **Person-centered DSMES**: Each person's education plan should be tailored to individual needs, based on health status, health literacy, lifestyle practices, and psychosocial adjustment.
- **Measuring and demonstrating outcomes of DSMES services**: Ongoing continuous quality improvement efforts should be in place to assess process outcomes, clinical outcomes, psychosocial and behavioral outcomes, individual-centered outcomes, and individual-generated health data.

National Diabetes Prevention Program Standards

As part of the National Diabetes Prevention Program, the CDC established the Diabetic Prevention Recognition Program (DPRP) and standards, which include the following guidelines and recommendations:

- Participant eligibility: ≥18 years, high risk of developing type 2 diabetes, BMI ≥25 kg/m^2 (or ≥23 kg/m^2 if Asian).
- Safety of participants and data privacy: A liability waiver must be signed for required physical activity and HIPAA compliance ensured.
- Location: A suitable venue with privacy for weighing and individual meetings should be selected.
- Delivery mode: Various options should be considered, including in-person, online, distance learning, or a combination.
- Staffing: Organizations are responsible for vetting, hiring, training, and supporting lifestyle coaches and program coordinator.
- Training: Minimum training for lifestyle coach is 12 hours/2 days with additional on-the-job training by program coordinator. Lifestyle coaches must receive 2 hours of advanced coach training annually.
- Change of ownership: Recognition status can transfer to a new organization if requirements are met.

- Required curriculum content: Weeks 1–26 (core phase) involves all curriculum topics being covered in at least 16 weekly sessions, and from weeks 27–52 (core maintenance phase) at least 6 sessions (one each month) are held to review and cover additional curriculum.
- Makeup sessions: These are encouraged but not required.
- Umbrella arrangements: These arrangements occur when an organization with CDC recognition sponsors other organizations.
- Requirement for pending, preliminary, and full recognition: Organizations submit data every 6 months to gain and maintain recognition.

AACE Practice Guidelines and Algorithms

The American Association of Clinical Endocrinologists (AACE) provides a number of clinical practice guidelines and algorithms to guide the care and education of individuals with diabetes. These guidelines are evidence-based and were developed following National Academy of Medicine standards. Guidelines are updated when needed in order to remain current with clinical practice. Guidelines include:

- Comprehensive Type 2 Diabetes Management Algorithm
- Clinical Practice Guideline for Development of a Diabetes Mellitus Comprehensive Care Plan
- Clinical Practice Guideline for the Use of Advanced Technology in the Management of Persons with Diabetes Mellitus
- Position Statement on Transcultural Diabetes Care in the United States

For example, the algorithm for diabetes mellitus type 2 emphasizes individualized care, monitoring, and lifestyle modification, and covers assessment and initial management (diagnosis confirmation, individual history, and lifestyle modifications), glycemic targets (individualized, <7% HbA1c for adults, and <8% for older adults or those with significant comorbidities), pharmacologic therapy (metformin initially, dual therapy for ≥9% HbA1c, add-on, and intensification), comprehensive care (blood pressure and lipid management, cardiovascular risk reduction, monitoring, and screening), individual education and support, and follow-up and adjustment.

Endocrine Society's Clinical Practice Guidelines

The Endocrine Society provides a number of evidence-based practice guidelines for the field of endocrinology, including diabetes mellitus and glucose metabolism. Guidelines are routinely updated and new ones developed. The Endocrine Society collaborates with and endorses clinical guidelines produced by other organizations as well. Guidelines for diabetes mellitus and glucose metabolism include the following:

- **High Risk for Hypoglycemia**: Contains a full guideline with a list of resources, including continuing education courses, summary of essential points, and recommendations.
- **Individual Hyperglycemia Guideline**: Contains a full guideline, brief summary, and list of resources.
- **Treatment of Diabetes in Older Adults**: Contains a full guideline, brief summary, list of resources, essential points, and a list of recommendations:
    - 1.0 Role of the Endocrinologist and Diabetes Care Specialist
    - 2.0 Screening for Diabetes and Prediabetes, and Diabetes Prevention
    - 3.0 Assessment of Older Individual with Diabetes
    - 4.0 Treatment of Hyperglycemia
    - 5.0 Treating Complications of Diabetes
    - 6.0 Special Settings and Populations

Additional guidelines that may be of use for the management of diabetes mellitus include those for obesity management:

- Pediatric Obesity Guideline
- Pharmacological Management of Obesity Guideline

ADCES and ADA Recommendations for Diabetes Education Programs

Goals and Content of Diabetes Self-Management Education (DSMES)

The American Diabetes Association and the Association of Diabetes Care and Education Specialists have set evidence-based standards for the content and outcome of diabetes self-management education and support (DSMES). The goals and objectives of DSMES include enabling people with diabetes to make informed decisions and actively participate as much as possible in their own care. These objectives are met by programs that provide training in self-care behavior, problem-solving, and collaboration with healthcare providers. According to 2026 American Diabetes Association Standards, critical points for DSMES include at the time of diagnosis, annually, when treatment goals are not being met, when new/complicating factors arise, and when there is a transition of care or transition in life. The 2026 ADA Standards also acknowledge that barriers to DSMES exist across all levels, from patient and provider to healthcare systems and healthcare payors. These barriers must be identified early and mitigated/lifted when possible. One newly recommended avenue to help bridge DSMES barriers involving access to education is the use of digital means (smartphones, web-based programs, and telehealth) to provide education, coaching, and self-management interventions to support individuals that have obstacles such as transportation, isolated location, or the dangers of exposure to infectious diseases.

Basic Content Areas

An approved diabetes education program includes **basic content areas** that have been jointly identified by the ADA and ADCES. Content areas were selected based on evidence that knowledge of these topics has helped people with diabetes achieve favorable outcomes.

Educators should select educational content that matches the needs of the individual or group receiving the education. A learning needs assessment determines how a program should be tailored to such characteristics as age, culture, educational level, type of diabetes, and identified learning needs.

Identified content areas for diabetes education include:

- Diabetes disease process and treatment
- Nutritional management
- Physical activity and exercise
- Benefit and use of medication
- Monitoring blood sugar
- Prevention and treatment of acute complications
- Prevention and treatment of chronic complications
- Management of psychosocial issues
- Promotion of health behavior change

Client-Centered Areas of Self-Care Behavior

The Association of Diabetes Care and Education Specialists (ADCES) has identified 7 client-centered areas of self-care behavior needed for successful management of diabetes. This framework for diabetes self-management education is called the **ADCES7**. The self-care behaviors identified by the ADCES7 are:

- Healthy eating
- Healthy coping
- Being physically active
- Monitoring blood glucose and other clinical markers of health
- Taking medication
- Problem-solving
- Reducing risk

The impetus for developing the ADCES7 was to provide an evidence-based structure for facilitating behavior change and measuring the clinical and health-related outcomes of education. Adopting the ADCES7 makes educators accountable for providing interventions that result in measurable improvements in health status, quality of life, and healthcare costs. The ADCES recommends that educators measure the ADCES7 self-care behaviors at both pre-intervention and post-intervention.

Adopting the ADCES7 provides grounds for better communication among members of the diabetes education team, allows for comparative research between different self-management education programs and clarifies the processes and outcomes of diabetes self-management education.

Summary of ADA Standards for Adults with Diabetes

Self-monitoring of blood glucose: Valuable for virtually all clients with diabetes. Those requiring intensive insulin therapy should monitor at least 3 times per day.

HbA1c test: Should be performed at least 2 times per year in clients with glycemic control. It should be performed quarterly in those not meeting glycemic goals and as needed for making decisions about changes in treatment.

Glycemic goal: An HbA1c <7% is the goal for most adults.

Medical nutrition therapy (MNT): Clients with prediabetes and diabetes should receive comprehensive MNT provided by a registered dietitian. Diet should meet recommended dietary allowances for all micronutrients. Diet recommendations must be individualized to the client.

Weight loss for overweight and obese people: Modest weight loss (loss of 5–7% of initial body weight) by following a low-carbohydrate or low-fat, calorie-restricted diet, along with exercise and behavior modification, is recommended. Pharmacotherapy may be indicated for some individuals.

Primary prevention of diabetes: For the prevention of diabetes in those with high risk, modest weight loss, increased physical activity, and a diet with plenty of fiber and whole grain foods is recommended.

Saturated fat intake: Should be controlled and minimized.

Carbohydrate intake: Should be monitored by carbohydrate counting, exchanges, or experience-based estimation.

Non-nutritive sweeteners and sugar alcohols: Are safe when consumed within limitations set by the Food and Drug Administration.

Routine supplementation with antioxidants and chromium: There is insufficient evidence to recommend routine supplementation with vitamin A, vitamin C, carotene, or chromium. The USPSTF has found evidence of harm related to carotene supplementation, so it is not recommended.

Metabolic surgery: Should be considered for individuals with type 2 diabetes who have a BMI ≥30 kg/m^2 (or BMI ≥27.5 kg/m^2 for Asian American individuals), along with lifestyle support and medical monitoring.

Diabetes self-management education and support: A program meeting national standards should be available to all people with diabetes upon diagnosis and as needed thereafter. Education should address psychosocial and emotional needs.

Physical activity: At least 150 minutes per week of moderate intensity aerobic exercise, resistance training, and flexibility/balance training, in 2–3 sessions per week.

Psychosocial assessment and care: This assessment should include a screening of sleep health.

Hypoglycemia: Treatment with 15–20 grams of glucose is preferred, although other forms of glucose-containing carbohydrate may be used. Glucagon should be prescribed for those at risk for severe hypoglycemia. Intranasal and subcutaneous solution forms have recently been FDA approved and are available alternatives. Those with hypoglycemic unawareness should modify glycemic targets to avoid hypoglycemia.

Hypertension: Measure blood pressure (BP) at every routine visit. Goal is less than 130/80 mmHg unless the client has high cardiovascular or kidney risk factors, in which case the systolic goal is less than 120 mmHg, or older adults with specific risk factors who may have a more relaxed goal of less than 140/90 mmHg. Generally, clients with BP greater than 130/80 mmHg should receive pharmacologic therapy, usually beginning with an ACE inhibitor or angiotensin receptor blocker (ARB), and adding a calcium channel blocker or diuretic if blood pressure exceeds 160/100 mmHg.

Dyslipidemia: Measure fasting lipid profile at least annually. Goals are:

- LDL less than 100 mg/dL
- HDL greater than 50 mg/dL
- Triglycerides less than 150 mg/dL

Antiplatelet agents: For primary prevention of cardiovascular disease (CVD), daily combination therapy of aspirin (75–162 mg) and low-dose rivaroxaban should be considered for most men over 50 years of age and most women over 60 who have at least one additional risk factor. Aspirin is used as secondary prevention in people with a history of CVD. Clopidogrel may be substituted in the case of an aspirin allergy.

Smoking/e-cigarette/vaping cessation: Advise clients not to smoke, use e-cigarettes, or vape and provide cessation counseling as part of routine care.

Cannabis use cessation: Cannabis use puts the individual at risk for cannabis hyperemesis syndrome, which can lead to dangerous complications in the individual with diabetes.

Coronary heart disease: Evaluate risk in asymptomatic clients by 10-year risk and treat accordingly. In clients with known CVD, therapy with ACE inhibitor, aspirin, and statin is indicated. Beta blockers should be used for at least 2 years following a cardiovascular event.

Nephropathy: Optimize blood glucose and blood pressure control to reduce the risk or slow the progression of nephropathy. Screen urine albumin and serum creatinine at least annually. Treatment with ACE inhibitors or ARBs is recommended for non-pregnant clients with albuminuria.

Retinopathy: Optimize blood glucose and blood pressure control to reduce the risk or slow the progression of retinopathy. Perform initial dilated eye exam soon after diagnosis of type 2 diabetes and 5 years after onset of type 1. Repeat annually or more often if retinopathy is progressing. Those with glycemic control may repeat dilated eye exam every 2–3 years following 1 or more normal exams.

Neuropathy: Screen for distal symmetrical neuropathy upon diagnosis of diabetes and at least annually thereafter. Screen for cardiovascular autonomic neuropathy upon diagnosis of type 2 diabetes and 5 years after onset of type 1. Treat neuropathic pain with combination therapy (including gabapentinoids, SSRIs, tricyclic antidepressants and/or sodium channel blockers).

Foot care: Annual comprehensive foot exam should include inspection, palpation of pulses, and testing for loss of protective sensation. Sensory testing should include a monofilament test along with vibratory sense, pinprick sensation, and ankle reflexes. Provide foot care education to all clients with diabetes.

ADA Guidelines for Immunizations

Recommended immunizations:

- Annual trivalent influenza vaccine is recommended for all people with diabetes who are over the age of 6 months.
- Pneumococcal vaccination (with Pneumovax) is recommended for all people with diabetes who are age 19–64. Revaccination is recommended for those over age 64 if the initial vaccine was administered over 5 years ago.
- Hepatitis B vaccination is recommended for those under the age of 60 (for those older, discuss this vaccination with a provider).
- Tetanus, diphtheria, pertussis (Tdap) vaccination is recommended for all adults including pregnant individuals, who should receive an additional dose.
- Herpes zoster vaccination (Shingrix) should be administered to all adults greater than or equal to 50 years of age.
- COVID vaccination and booster is recommended for all qualified adults and children as indicated in the guidance for the general population.
- RSV vaccination is encouraged for adults ages 60 and older if they are at high risk, or ages 75 and older if they are at low risk.

ADA Guidelines for Children Regarding Hypertension and Dyslipidemia

Hypertension:

- Blood pressure (BP) consistently above the 90th percentile for age, sex, and height should first be treated with lifestyle modification.
- Pharmacological intervention is indicated if goals are not achieved in 3–6 months. ACE inhibitors or angiotensin receptor blockers (ARBs) are considered first-line therapy.
- BP goal is less than 130/80 mmHg or below the 90th percentile, whichever is lower, for individuals without additional risk factors (such as cardiovascular disease, pregnancy, old age with comorbidities).

Dyslipidemia:

- Fasting lipid profile is indicated for any child greater than 2 years of age with family history of hypercholesterolemia or early cardiovascular event. In the absence of risk factors, screening for dyslipidemia should be performed on any child with diabetes who is 10 years or older.
- Target is LDL less than 100 mg/dL.
- Initial treatment is with lifestyle modification emphasizing the reduction of saturated fat in the diet.
- Treatment with a statin medication is indicated in children greater than 10 years old with LDL greater than 160 mg/dL. In the presence of cardiovascular risk factors, statins are recommended when the LDL is greater than 130 mg/dL.

Measurable Outcomes

Types

Health outcomes are measurable changes in a person's condition resulting from healthcare intervention over time. The Centers for Medicare and Medicaid Services, policymakers, and professional accrediting bodies all rely on outcomes data to assess the quality of interventions and the delivery of healthcare.

Baseline data must be available for interventions in order for them to be evaluated. Without a baseline, change cannot be demonstrated.

There are different types of **measurable outcomes**. These include:

- Clinical outcomes: changes in biological measures such as HbA1c, blood pressure, and lipids
- Education outcomes: changes in knowledge or skills
- Quality of life (QOL) outcomes: changes in measures of QOL, such as the SF-36 and PAID questionnaire
- Behavioral outcomes: changes in such behaviors as physical activity or food choices
- Cost-effectiveness: the cost of the program versus its cost savings from improved health

Program Outcomes

Outcomes demonstrate changes in health status as a result of an intervention. There are different **kinds of outcomes**, such as clinical, educational, and psychosocial. The Association of Diabetes Care and Education Specialists (ADCES) Outcomes Task Force has concluded that health-related behaviors are the unique and measurable outcomes for diabetes education. The ADCES7 identifies the diabetes self-care behaviors as:

- Being physically active
- Healthy eating
- Taking medication
- Self-monitoring
- Problem-solving
- Reducing risk for complications
- Healthy coping

Measurable changes in these behaviors from the baseline demonstrate the effectiveness of a diabetes education program. Recognition of these behavioral outcomes has changed the focus of the diabetes education curriculum from being content-driven to outcomes-driven.

Valid outcomes require a baseline, or pre-program, measurement. This is followed by measurement at regular intervals and post-program. Aggregate population outcomes are pooled outcomes from many different individuals. Aggregate outcomes guide the program and are used in the continuous quality-improvement process.

Continuous Quality Improvement

Continuous quality improvement (CQI) is one of the most widely used methodologies for supporting service excellence and customer satisfaction. It has been adopted by the American Diabetes Association (ADA) Recognition Program as a requirement for accreditation of diabetes self-management education and support programs.

CQI is an overriding business philosophy that applies to daily operations. Successful CQI programs have the buy-in of all staff, not just the managers. CQI is a proactive process that employs systems for preventive management on a daily basis as opposed to relying on crisis management when things are not done right the first time.

Problem identification is an important part of the CQI process. Problems are often considered opportunities for improvement. Data about the problem is systematically collected and analyzed to generate possible solutions. After implementation of a recommended solution, quality outcomes are evaluated and improvement is measured.

HIPAA and Client Confidentiality

HIPAA is a federal law that protects the privacy of consumers' health information. It applies to oral, written, and electronic information and must be followed by health plans and healthcare providers. In the healthcare setting, health information can only be used to the extent that it is needed to provide and coordinate care.

HIPAA requires that healthcare providers have safeguards in place to maintain the security and confidentiality of health information. Employers must provide training programs for employees to demonstrate how information is to be protected.

Insurance companies may legally receive health information in order to settle claims. Public health departments and law enforcement agencies are also allowed access to medical records when appropriate to their duties in protecting and serving society.

Family members and other significant people who are involved in a client's care are allowed access to information only when the client has given permission.

Review Video: What is HIPAA?
Visit mometrix.com/academy and enter code: 412009

Diabetes Education Programs

Gathering Assessment Data on Target Populations

In order for a diabetes education program to be relevant, it is important to assess the specific needs of the target population. An effective assessment identifies the high priority problems pertinent to the population and addresses their unique characteristics, lifestyle issues, and challenges. Thorough assessment reveals the group's barriers to education and self-care, allowing for appropriate program modifications.

Assessment information can be gathered from clients, medical records, focus groups, community forums, or the referring healthcare providers.

Examples of items to include in a **target-population assessment** include:

- Psychosocial attributes
- Cultural characteristics and primary language
- Age and developmental stage
- Physical limitations (e.g., older age or immobility)
- The practice setting (e.g., inpatient, community clinic, HMO)
- Functional limitations
- Educational level
- Economic characteristics
- Barriers to access (e.g., working hours, transportation issues)

Components of Curriculum Development

Curriculum development begins with assessing the needs of the target population. The information gained can be synthesized to create a program relevant to the needs of the participants.

Curriculum development involves prioritizing those needs to fit the timeframe allowed. Safety and survival skills should always be taught first when time is limited.

Curriculum development includes attention to the cultural characteristics of the learners. Language needs should be addressed. Written materials should not only be translated, but also modified to be culturally appropriate.

Principles of adult learning should be incorporated into programs for this population. Adults prefer information that is practical and immediately useful. Therefore, the curriculum should emphasize application of knowledge over theoretical information.

Targeting outcomes is an essential element of program development. According the Association of Diabetes Care and Education Specialists (ADCES), behavior change is the focused outcome measurement of diabetes self-management education. Therefore, learning objectives should be stated in measurable behavioral terms.

Considerations of the Practice Setting as It Relates to Goals of the Program

The goals of a diabetes self-management education program must be individualized to the client and relevant to the practice setting where education will take place.

For a patient who is hospitalized with a new diagnosis of diabetes, the goals of education will concentrate on immediate "survival skills" and discharge planning. These skills include:

- Self-monitoring of blood glucose
- Using insulin, as appropriate, and knowing about insulin actions
- Preventing, detecting, and treating hypoglycemia
- Meal planning

For a patient who has had repeated hospitalizations for diabetic ketoacidosis (DKA) or a history of poor glycemic control, the goals of education are based on the results of a targeted assessment that identifies the areas of need for the individual.

Appropriate program goals for clients who are stable and seen on a continuing outpatient basis are comprehensive. In addition to mastery of survival skills, comprehensive program goals are related to physical activity, weight management, prevention of complications, problem-solving, coping skills, cardiovascular health, and other topics for long-term management.

Required Resources and Materials for a Diabetes Education Program

Most diabetes education programs take place in group settings, requiring accessible and adequate classroom space. At least one family member or significant other should be allowed to attend classes with the client, so space is needed to accommodate guests. Rooms can be set up in classroom, horseshoe arrangement, or another style according to the space available and the needs of the class.

Financial resources will dictate the choices available for audiovisual teaching aids. Slide show presentations using a computer and LCD projector can be effective audiovisual tools. Other options include overhead projectors, videotapes, flipcharts, and whiteboards with markers.

Other teaching supplies may include participant books, supplemental handouts, pens, notepaper, food models, posters, and other teaching models.

A diabetes education program also requires office resources for program planning, storage, communications, and documentation. Some programs require an area for seeing clients individually.

Marketing a Diabetes Education Program

The first step in marketing a program is to identify the primary customers. Although there may be several types of customers, the marketing plan should focus on the customer who has the greatest potential to provide referrals. Key customers may include healthcare providers, insurers, private-paying clients, organizations, and others.

The needs of the primary customer must be identified and marketing messages should match those needs.

Many vehicles for promoting programs are available. Newsletters for physicians, hospitals and communities may be in print form or online. General mailings can be sent to physicians and other key customers. Brochures can be placed in physicians' offices, hospital staff lounges, waiting rooms and local markets and pharmacies. Permission should be obtained prior to leaving brochures in these settings. Personal presentations at hospital staff meetings, physician meetings, and professional meetings can be used to promote a program. A website is valuable for marketing and has become increasingly important for business marketing.

Adapting to Clients with Physical Disabilities

The educator should not assume that clients with physical disabilities are less capable of diabetes self-management or that they are learning disabled. Many people with disabilities are able to effectively manage their diabetes when given the appropriate adaptations in education and equipment. Community and professional organizations can help with planning educational programs adapted to specific disabilities. Examples include the Amputation Coalition of America, the National Association for the Deaf, and the American Council for the Blind.

The Americans with Disabilities Act was established to ensure that people with disabilities have the same opportunities and access to services as those without disabilities. For an educator, this means that diabetes self-management education must be accessible to people with disabilities. This may include wheelchair access to classrooms or providing American Sign Language interpreters for educational sessions. Provisions for including those who assist the disabled person should also be incorporated into the teaching plan.

Maintaining Accreditation for Diabetes Self-Management Education Programs

The American Diabetes Association's Education Recognition Program (ERP) and the Association of Diabetes Care and Education Specialists' Diabetes Education Accreditation Program (DEAP) are the two accrediting bodies approved by the Centers for Medicare and Medicaid Services (CMS) for the accreditation of diabetes self-management education and support programs. Both programs are based on principles of the National Standards for Diabetes Self-Management Education and Support. The accreditation process is similar for both organizations, but each organization has slightly different requirements.

Among other criteria, both the ADA and ADCES's programs require tracking and documentation of program and site demographics. The total number of clients who receive education during the data period must be documented, along with the average number of hours of instruction received per client. Follow-up and limited consultation hours must also be documented. Accredited programs must track and document population statistics such as age, types of diabetes, race, and special needs. Program setting and service area characteristics are also included in demographic data. This includes documenting the type of service provided and information about the academic instructors' experience, academic credentials, and education.

Population Health, Advocacy, and Prevention

Population Health Strategies

Population health strategies associated with diabetes mellitus include the following:

- **Public health campaigns**: These campaigns combat common contributors to diabetes and advocate for diabetes awareness. Common topics include obesity, smoking, lack of exercise, and general information about diabetes.
- **Community screening**: Community-based diabetes screening should be conducted regularly, especially in areas with high-risk populations.
- **Healthcare provider training**: Distribute information to healthcare providers that includes the tools they need in diabetes prevention and management. Increase information about diabetes in medical and nursing school curricula.
- **Wearable devices**: Encourage self-monitoring through electronic devices that help track dietary habits, exercise, and blood sugar.
- **Data collection**: Conduct epidemiological studies regarding prevalence and risk factors, and use data to identify trends and guide policies.
- **School interventions**: Encourage healthy eating through food offerings and engage in physical exercise campaigns to prevent obesity.
- **Workplace interventions**: Offer wellness programs and health screenings.
- **Healthcare system**: Implement integrated care models and team-based care.
- **Self-management**: Educate individuals and families about diabetic management.
- **Social determinants**: Increase government food programs, such as SNAP, to ensure access to nutritious food and house the homeless.

Public Screening for Diabetes

The appropriateness of performing random fingerstick blood glucose testing to screen for diabetes at community health fairs, shopping malls, and other public places is questionable. Blood glucose results collected in this way are difficult to evaluate and may not be accurate or reliable. Further, this practice has not been demonstrated to be cost-effective. For these reasons, the American Diabetes Association (ADA) does not recommend community blood glucose testing to screen for diabetes.

However, public screening for diabetes risk by other means is advocated. This involves risk-factor assessment by a health professional to identify those at high risk for type 2 diabetes and cardiovascular disease. High-risk people can be made aware of their risk and referred to a healthcare provider for blood glucose testing. As a public health benefit, this may result in early detection and treatment and promotes preventive strategies.

Advocacy Efforts for Individuals with Diabetes

Advocacy for people with diabetes includes raising awareness of critical needs to manage the disease and providing the support needed through research, programs, and policy. Advocacy efforts should include:

- **Access to treatment, medications, and supplies**: Provide information on support programs that provide financial assistance for low-income individuals and encourage expansion of telehealth services to increase access to care. These programs provide individuals with information about pharmacy assistance programs, non-profit organizations (e.g., Diabetes Foundation Diabetes assistance program, RxAssist, Insulin for Life USA), Medicaid, community health programs, and discount pharmacies (e.g., GoodRx, Walmart's ReliOn brand, and Costco member prescription plan), as well as state-specific and hospital or clinic-based programs.
- **Institutional care**: Provide staff with education on diabetes management, advocate for standardized diabetes care plans, provide comprehensive individual/family education, utilize multidisciplinary teams, educate individuals about their rights, and provide healthy dietary options.
- **Policies**: Conduct public awareness programs; lobby policymakers; support organizations, such as the American Diabetes Association and World Diabetes Foundation, that help formulate public policies; advocate for programs to ensure affordable care for all individuals with diabetes; and support funding for diabetic research.

PRIMARY AND SECONDARY DIABETES PREVENTION STRATEGIES

Diabetes prevention strategies include both primary (prevention of the disease) and secondary (prevention of the progression of the disease with screening measures):

Primary (to prevent prediabetes)	Secondary (to prevent progression)
• Engage in an exercise regimen. • Maintain a healthy diet low in refined carbohydrates. • Replace saturated fats with unsaturated fats. • Avoid sedentary activities, such as video games. • Limit alcohol intake. • Encourage smoking cessation. • Carry out public health campaigns. • Ensure access to healthy foods.	• Monitor fasting blood sugar regularly. • Assess risk factors and symptoms. • Use medications, such as metformin, at first indication of symptoms. • Continue to maintain a healthy diet. • Provide diabetes education. • Encourage participation in support groups. • Examine feet, eyes, and kidney function regularly.

Evidence-Based Practice

SCIENTIFIC METHOD OF RESEARCH

Research is a systematic process that utilizes the scientific method to answer questions. Research findings generate new knowledge and guide clinical practice.

Rigor in research refers to a method that moves in an orderly fashion, applies scrupulous attention to detail, and imposes control on the research situation to maximize validity. Research evidence is collected in such a way that it can be reviewed and replicated by others.

The first step of the scientific method is to devise research objectives, questions, and hypotheses. The subsequent tasks of the scientific method are to collect and analyze data and report results.

Although rigorous, the process of scientific research is considered flexible and circular. As the study progresses, researchers often have to rework a problem several times. This may be due to new findings from other research or identifying a problem with the initial research design.

QUANTITATIVE VS. QUALITATIVE RESEARCH

Quantitative research translates data into numbers for statistical analysis. It seeks to explain cause-and-effect relationships. Quantitative studies are classified according to the level of control applied and the likelihood that the findings occurred by chance. For example, level 1 research evidence means that the study used a highly controlled and randomized design, while level 5 means that the evidence is based on a descriptive study or expert opinion.

Qualitative research uses the subject's own words or the researcher's narrative summary of an observed phenomenon. An example of a qualitative study would be to investigate the concept of "becoming diabetic" by analyzing interviews and journals on the subject and extracting common themes.

Both types of research should be conducted with rigorous methods such as attention to detail and strict accuracy. When both types of research are blended to collect data, it is referred to as **multi-method research**.

Studies on Diabetes Glycemic Control

The Diabetes Control and Complications Trial (DCCT) demonstrated a 60% reduction in the development of microvascular complications in intensely-treated people with type 1 diabetes. Over 6.5 years, the mean HbA1c of the intensive treatment group was 7%, compared to about 9% in the standard treatment group.

The United Kingdom Prospective Diabetes Study (UKPDS) followed newly diagnosed people with type 2 diabetes for 10 years. With intensive glycemic control, yielding a median HbA1c of 7%, the risk for microvascular complications was significantly reduced. UKDPS also suggested that intensive control can reduce the incidence of heart attack and stroke in people with type 2 diabetes.

The Action to Control Cardiovascular Risk in Diabetes (ACCORD) study compared the effects of intensive glycemic control on cardiovascular outcomes in people with type 2 diabetes. One arm of this study terminated early due to findings that intensive glycemic control (HbA1c goal <6%) was associated with increased mortality of participants. The potential explanations for this are still being studied. Other arms of ACCORD, studying lipid and blood pressure control, continue.

Infection Control Practices

Handwashing facilities should be available in areas where insulin injection or fingerstick techniques are being practiced. Occupational Safety and Health Administration (OSHA) and Joint Commission requirements should be consulted for procedures to appropriately clean areas where blood products are used.

Clients do not usually need to use alcohol swabs to disinfect the skin prior to pricking the finger or injecting insulin. Handwashing and good personal hygiene are normally adequate. Alcohol may be used to cleanse the skin when handwashing facilities are not available or when the insulin injection site is unclean.

Educators should be knowledgeable about local requirements for syringe and lancet disposal. Many areas have regulations requiring that medical sharps be disposed of as hazardous waste. Disposing of containers with used sharps in bins designated for recycling is prohibited.

While manufactures do not recommend the reuse of needles and lancets, the American Diabetes Association (ADA) does not forbid it. Clients with acute concurrent illness, compromised immunity, or poor personal hygiene should not reuse needles.

Addressing Disparities and Diversity

Impact of Disparities on Diabetes

Disparities in diabetes care can significantly impact individuals affected. Disparities include:

- **Economics**: According to the CDC, individuals with income less than 100% of the federal poverty level have the highest prevalence of diabetes. Individuals may lack insurance and are often unable to afford routine medical care or medications. Additionally, with poorly managed disease, individuals may have difficulty maintaining employment.
- **Access**: Individuals may lack transportation to healthcare facilities or be unable to access care that is only available during working hours. Access to advanced treatments and monitoring, such as insulin pumps and continuous glucose monitors, may not be available to all individuals, and the quality of care may vary widely.
- **Gender**: Internationally, diabetes affects over 17 million more males than females, and males are often diagnosed at a younger age; however, at the time of diagnosis of type 2 diabetes mellitus, females tend to have more risk factors (such as obesity).
- **Ethnicity**: Some ethnic groups, such as African Americans, Hispanics, Native Americans, and Alaskan Natives, have higher rates of diabetes than others, putting them at greater risk.
- **Geography**: Rural and underserved communities may lack easy access to medical care and specialists and may have to travel long distances for care.

Principles of Diversity, Equity, and Inclusion in Diabetic Care

Incorporating principles of diversity, equity, and inclusion (DEI) is an important step in ensuring that all individuals receive culturally competent and equitable diabetic care:

- **Diversity**: Carry out assessments to understand the cultural, ethnic, gender, age, linguistic, religious/spiritual, disability, and socioeconomic needs of individuals. Train staff members in cultural competence and addressing the needs of the community and target populations. Develop community outreach programs to reach underrepresented populations.
- **Equity**: Develop educational materials that reflect the language, cultural practices, and dietary preferences of the community members. Provide access to screening and individual care in easily accessed local community areas, such as religious centers, community centers, and schools. Provide telehealth services and sliding scale fees to increase access.
- **Inclusion**: Maintain a culturally diverse individual care team that reflects the community and target populations when possible. Include community members in planning and primary prevention strategies and encourage collaboration. Offer translation services and individual feedback mechanisms. Develop policies that promote inclusion.

CDCES Practice Test #1

Want to take this practice test in an online interactive format?
Check out the online resources page, which includes interactive practice questions and much more: **mometrix.com/resources719/certdiabedu**

Refer to the following for questions 1 - 6:

B. Jones, a 78-year-old African American male newly diagnosed with type 2 diabetes, is accompanied by his daughter for his initial DSMES assessment visit. He admits that he has poor eyesight (at least close-up) and sometimes forgets things. He states that he is willing to learn about his diabetes and is willing to make some minor changes in his lifestyle if it will help him have more energy to play golf and play with his grandchildren. He does not do much cooking (he leaves that to his daughter or eats out); presently he walks for 15 minutes each weekday and plays 9 holes of golf every weekend. His BMI is 25 kg/m^2, BP is within normal limits, and HbA1c at this time is 8.2%. He states that has no known diabetes-related complications; his daughter confirms this and his patient medical record lists none either.

1. Based on his statements, Mr. Jones most fits which transtheoretical model stage of change?

a. Precontemplation
b. Contemplation
c. Action
d. Maintenance

2. Which of the following would be an appropriate behavioral objective (both in terms of the goal itself and how it is stated) for Mr. Jones?

a. "I will choose items from the restaurant menu that fit with my healthy eating plan, including vegetables, low-fat meat, and 3 servings of carbohydrates."
b. "I will understand the reasons that I need to monitor my blood sugar."
c. "I will know the difference between my diabetes medications."
d. "By modifying eating patterns, taking medication, and increasing frequency of self-monitoring, my HbA1c will be within less than 8% within six months."

3. Which question below is the best example of an appropriate patient empowerment question the diabetes educator might ask Mr. Jones?

a. "You do not want to end up on dialysis, do you?"
b. "What do you think your HbA1c should be?"
c. "What effect do you think changes such as taking your medication and eating better might have on your daily life?"
d. "I think that we need to set a goal for you to lose some weight. Ten pounds would put you closer to a normal BMI. How does that sound to you?"

4. Which of the following is an example of an instructional method that would be LEAST appropriate for Mr. Jones?

a. Group discussion on choosing healthy food options at a restaurant
b. One-on-one, hands-on BG meter training
c. Role-playing on how Mr. Jones would react if he accidentally took a double dose of his diabetes medication
d. Printed material (e.g., the package insert) from the manufacturer regarding the side effects of the medications

5. Which of the following options below is the BEST example of an appropriate SMART (specific, measurable, attainable, relevant, time-bound) behavioral goal for Mr. Jones?

a. Lose ten pounds by October 31 (3 months) by increasing walking to 25 minutes per day and limiting second helpings to just vegetables.
b. Reduce HbA1c to 6% by October 31 (3 months) by checking blood glucose twice daily and starting insulin.
c. Improve diabetes and overall health by doing the things he learned in the diabetes class.
d. Take good care of himself for the rest of his life by eating better, taking medicine consistently, checking blood sugar, getting good rest, checking feet daily, and keeping all medical appointments.

6. Mr. Jones's provider has prescribed him Januvia (sitagliptin) QD and a sulfonylurea BID, with a note in the chart to possibly initiate insulin if the patient's HbA1c is not less than 8% in six months. Which of the following items is LEAST important in the initial education plan for this patient?

a. How to use an insulin pen
b. Preventing, recognizing, and treating hypoglycemia
c. Making appropriate food choices
d. Preventing diabetes-related complications

7. A client is advised to eat fruits with a low glycemic index. Which of the following fruits would be the best choice?

a. Pineapple
b. Banana
c. Strawberry
d. Watermelon

8. What is the distinction between *assessment* and *evaluation*?

a. Assessment is clinical in nature, whereas evaluation is typically administrative.
b. Assessment is always done at the beginning of a process or procedure, whereas evaluation is performed at the end.
c. Assessment implies gathering and interpreting data for the purpose of directing action, whereas evaluation is to determine the extent to which an action or process was successful.
d. In relation to diabetes program management, there is no significant difference between assessment and evaluation; the two are used interchangeably.

9. If a person is diagnosed with latent autoimmune diabetes in adults (LADA), a typical characteristic is:

a. Central obesity
b. Metabolic syndrome
c. Family history of type 2 diabetes
d. No or mild insulin resistance

10. Which one of the following organizations is the most comprehensive resource for education for persons with diabetes?

a. International Diabetes Federation (IDF)
b. Centers for Disease Control and Prevention (CDC)
c. American Diabetes Association (ADA)
d. Diabetes Research Institute Foundation (DRIF)

11. A 72-year-old client with type 2 diabetes has had stable blood glucose levels with daily glipizide and metformin. She has just started taking trimethoprim/sulfamethoxazole (Bactrim) for a mild urinary tract infection. She complains of a dry mouth, thirst, and cold hands and feet. Her blood pressure is 90/58 mmHg, and her heart rate is 106. These are indications of:

a. An adverse response to the antibiotic
b. Diabetic ketoacidosis
c. Hyperosmolar hyperglycemic state
d. Hypoglycemia

12. In which of the following situations would the procedure most likely be canceled or rescheduled?

a. Glucose >550 mg/dL; appendectomy
b. DKA; knee replacement
c. HHS; tibia compound fracture repair
d. Type 2 diabetes on insulin; elective gastric bypass surgery

13. In speaking with a group of new inpatient nurses, the diabetes educator discusses the American Association of Clinical Endocrinologist (AACE) and American Diabetes Association (ADA) consensus statement recommendations of inpatient blood glucose targets for critically ill individuals who do not have diabetes. Which of the following statements accurately reflects those recommendations?

a. Pre-meal BG target for non-critically ill patients: <100 mg/dL
b. Random BG target for non-critically ill patients: <140 mg/dL
c. Target (all times) BG for critically ill patients: 100–130 mg/dL
d. Target (all times) BG for critically ill patients: 140–180 mg/dL

14. The CDCES has been working with a Chinese client with type 1 diabetes. She speaks English as a second language. The CDCES has explained blood glucose monitoring and the importance of collecting a fasting sample, and the client has practiced. The client repeatedly indicated that she understood the directions and had no questions. However, when the CDCES returns a few days later, the client has carried out only haphazard testing, mostly postprandial. What is the most likely reason for this?

a. The client forgets to perform her fasting blood glucose tests.
b. The CDCES was unclear in the instructions.
c. The client chooses to ignore the CDCES's instructions.
d. The CDCES's education was not tailored to the client's needs.

15. A diabetes educator is assessing a patient's blood glucose monitoring technique by having her demonstrate a blood glucose test. Which of the following actions is indicative of IMPROPER technique?

a. Cleaning her hands with warm water and soap instead of alcohol
b. Setting the lancet device to her preference
c. Milking the lanced finger at the tip to acquire a sufficient blood sample
d. Recording the reading in her notebook rather than on the clinic-provided sheet

16. A patient comes in for a return visit one month after starting basal bolus insulin therapy. She tells her educator that she will have to stop taking half of her insulin because her insurance does not pay for Apidra insulin, only Lantus, and she cannot afford to pay out of pocket for it. Assuming that there may be other insulin brands in this class that her insurance does cover, which of the following insulins below would be the most appropriate replacement for Apidra that the educator might suggest to this patient's provider?

a. NPH/regular (Novolin 70/30)
b. Insulin detemir (Levemir)
c. NPH insulin (Humulin-N)
d. Insulin lispro (Humalog)

Refer to the following for questions 17 - 20:

Mrs. M, a 52-year-old Hispanic woman, was diagnosed with type 2 diabetes three weeks ago while hospitalized for dehydration and a bladder infection. She presents for her initial visit with the diabetes educator. Her lab data sent from her PCP show an HbA1c of 8.9%, BMI of 29 kg/m^2, and blood pressure controlled with medication. Her PCP has instructed her to take 500 mg metformin twice a day. She states that she has been good about taking her morning dose but forgets about half the time to take her evening dose.

She was given a blood glucose meter in the hospital but is not sure that she is using it correctly. She is not sure when she is supposed to check her blood sugar, so she has been doing it every morning, just before breakfast, when she takes her morning metformin.

Mrs. M seems very sociable and open minded, but admits that she is concerned about this new diagnosis. Her main concern is that she does not want to give up everything she loves to eat, nor have to stop cooking foods her family enjoys. At the advice of her PCP, she is scheduled for a retinal exam next week, but is not sure why because she sees very well, and only needs glasses to see small print.

17. Which of the following DSMES topics should be discussed at this visit with Mrs. M?

a. Diabetes-related complications and how to prevent them
b. The meaning of the HbA1c results
c. How to safely administer insulin
d. Proper use of an individualized schedule for blood glucose monitoring

18. Based on the information provided so far, which education plan makes the most sense for Mrs. M?

a. Group classes to include comprehensive diabetes self-management education and support
b. One-on-one education sessions, at least until all of her personal concerns are resolved
c. Printed information on diabetes, including a list of reputable diabetes websites
d. All of the above are equally appropriate for this patient, provided she has no scheduling conflicts.

19. Keeping in mind that Mrs. M has not yet had any diabetes education beyond survival skills, the diabetes educator suggests that she set a preliminary behavioral goal, which is discussed. Based on Mrs. M's current situation, which of the following self-care behavior goals would be appropriate?

a. Lose 10 pounds by the next visit (3 months from now).
b. Take metformin as directed, with fewer missed doses, over the next three months.
c. Reduce HbA1c to less than 8% by the next three-month visit.
d. Significantly reduce the risk of diabetes-related complications.

20. What referrals, if any, should be made at this time for Mrs. M?

a. Mental health (to address her anxieties)
b. Ophthalmology (since she has just been diagnosed with type 2 diabetes)
c. Registered dietitian to address her meal concerns and weight management
d. No referrals are warranted until she has at least completed initial DSMES.

21. When assessing for risk of hypoglycemia in relation to exercise, which element of the patient record is most important to consider?

a. The patient's typical signs and symptoms with hypoglycemia
b. Current patient physical/glycemic status (weight, BMI, HbA1c)
c. Timing and content (i.e., carb content) of meals in relation to the activity
d. Medication regimen: types, dose, and timing

22. What fasting plasma glucose (FPG) and oral glucose tolerance test (OGTT) results are diagnostic of diabetes?

a. FPG ≥156 mg/dL, OGTT ≥220 mg/dL
b. FPG ≥126 mg/dL, OGTT ≥200 mg/dL
c. FPG ≥120 mg/dL, OGTT ≥180 mg/dL
d. FPG ≥110 mg/dL, OGTT ≥170 mg/dL

23. A diabetes educator is instructing insulin-requiring patients on how to treat hypoglycemia. To treat hypoglycemia that occurs immediately before a meal, which of the following is the best course of action?

a. Skip insulin because blood sugar is already too low. If the glucose is normal or high before the next meal, then take the recommended dose at that time.
b. Eat a meal now but take the dose of mealtime insulin about an hour after the meal.
c. Treat the blood sugar as one would any low blood sugar, and then once it is in the normal range, take the regular dose of insulin and eat the regular meal.
d. Take the insulin right away, then prepare the meal and eat as one normally would.

24. Which of the following elements is NOT part of the standard exercise prescription?

a. Commencement (when the patient will begin the activity program)
b. Intensity (how difficult and challenging the activity will be)
c. Frequency (how often the activity will be performed)
d. Duration (how long the activity will last for each session)

25. In response to low patient satisfaction scores for a class on medications, the diabetes educator redesigns the class content outline to contain more information on the mechanism of action of each class of oral medication. After receiving approval from the continuous quality improvement (CQI) team, the educator implements the new content. She is surprised when the patient satisfaction scores for the class are even lower the next month. What is the most likely explanation for the failure of this change to better satisfy participants?

a. The educator most likely failed to thoroughly explain her idea to the CQI team.
b. The educator did not collect and analyze information on why the patients did not like the class before deciding on the change.
c. The evaluation method used to gauge patient satisfaction is most likely not a valid or reliable tool.
d. The educator was not creative in her solution to the problem.

26. A client with type 1 diabetes has had repeated episodes of dangerous hypoglycemia because of hypoglycemia unawareness. Many episodes of hypoglycemia have occurred during the night. He takes a long-acting basal insulin (glargine) and mealtime boluses of rapid-acting insulin (aspart) depending on his blood glucose levels. His premeal fasting blood glucose target is 80–130 mg/dL (4.44–7.22 mmol/L). What intervention is most indicated?

a. Add a bedtime snack.
b. Decrease the dosage of the boluses.
c. Change to a different type of insulin.
d. Increase the fasting blood glucose target.

27. A client with type 2 diabetes takes metformin and glipizide. She reports switching from three meals and a bedtime snack to the same diet but with 16-hour fasting, restricting food intake to the hours between 8 a.m. and 4 p.m. The CDCES should stress that this may result in:

a. Fluctuating blood glucose levels
b. Better glycemic control
c. Increased insulin resistance
d. A need for decreased medication dosage

28. A 59-year-old single female patient with type 2 diabetes admits that she only takes half of her recommended Januvia (sitagliptin) tablet, but does take her full metformin tablet. She later tells the educator that she has added more vegetables to her meals, but only canned vegetables. Based on these brief statements, what barrier does the diabetes educator believe is MOST likely a concern for this patient?

a. Transportation barrier
b. Cultural barrier
c. Cognitive ability barrier
d. Financial barrier

29. Some dietary supplements are packaged in containers with a "USP-verified mark." What is the role of the US Pharmacopoeia (USP) and thus indicated by this label?

a. To verify that the products listed on the label are accurate and pure
b. To market herbal products that have been FDA approved
c. To verify that the clinical claims made by the products are accurate
d. To ensure that herbal supplements will not interact with other medications

30. A client with type 1 diabetes is instructed to check his blood glucose levels before meals and at bedtime. His recordkeeping appears meticulous; the blood glucose levels recorded are all within his target range; and he takes the lowest dosages of insulin or no insulin, based on the recorded blood glucose levels. However, when his fasting blood glucose is checked by the laboratory, it is 240 mg/dL (13.3 mmol/L), and his HbA1c is 9.5%. What should the CDCES suspect?

a. The person's glucose monitor is defective.
b. The person is falsifying recordkeeping.
c. The person is experiencing the Somogyi effect.
d. The person has undetected postprandial hyperglycemia.

31. For persons with type 2 diabetes, there is some evidence that caffeine may:

a. Have little or no effect
b. Help stabilize glucose levels
c. Decrease insulin resistance
d. Increase insulin resistance

32. The Association of Diabetes Care and Education Specialists' Policy and Advocacy group has identified six goals. Which of the following choices is NOT one of the identified goals?

a. Influencing the future of diabetes education and the role of the diabetes educator in healthcare
b. Limiting the specialized skill of providing evidence-based diabetes education to healthcare professionals who are certified as diabetes educators
c. Advocating for policies that improve access to diabetes self-management training
d. Attaining and maintaining reasonable reimbursement for diabetes educators

33. The FDA has approved six nonnutritive sweeteners for use in moderation: acesulfame-K, aspartame, neotame, saccharin, sucralose, and stevia. Which of these should be AVOIDED by women who are pregnant or breastfeeding?

a. Aspartame
b. Stevia
c. Neotame
d. All have been shown to be safe, even for pregnant or breastfeeding women.

34. With type 1 diabetes, hyperglycemia occurs when what percentage of beta islet cells are destroyed?

a. 60–70%
b. 70–80%
c. 80–90%
d. 90–100%

35. What blood glucose range is classified as mild hypoglycemia?

a. 90–100 mg/dL
b. 70–90 mg/dL
c. 54–70 mg/dL
d. 48–54 mg/dL

36. A client is taking insulin to control his diabetes and monitors his glucose prior to exercising. If his blood glucose is 98 mg/dL (5.4 mmol/L), he should:

a. Proceed with moderate exercise
b. Skip exercising until his blood glucose level is higher
c. Ingest 15–30 mg of carbohydrate
d. Ingest 30–60 mg of carbohydrate

37. A patient has had type 2 diabetes for the past twelve years. He controls his diabetes with diet, exercise, and oral medication. Similarly, he watches his fat intake because of occasional borderline LDL (currently WNL). His last three HbA1c labs were all less than 7%. He has no apparent co-morbidities. According to the American Diabetes Association Standards of Practice, which of the following screenings is NOT indicated to be performed annually for this patient?

a. HbA1c
b. Comprehensive foot exam
c. Dilated eye exam
d. Fasting lipid profile

38. A continuous glucose monitor (CGM) shows that a client's glucose level is 92 mg/dL and falling. The correct response is to:

a. Ingest rapid-acting carbohydrates.
b. Monitor again in 30 minutes.
c. Take no further action.
d. Eat a high-protein snack.

39. For a patient with type 2 diabetes, who is mostly sedentary and who has a BMI of 26 and no contraindicative comorbidities, which option below is the BEST example of a goal that is relevant and attainable?

a. Purchase a pair of walking shoes and walk to and from the mailbox every day.
b. Participate in the half marathon at the end of the month.
c. Enroll and attend all the daily spin classes at my local health club.
d. Walk briskly for 25 minutes every day following dinner.

40. Which of the choices below is the BEST example of a behavioral goal/objective that is specific?

a. Decrease intake of regular soda from three cans to one can per day by December 1.
b. Decrease the risk for diabetes-related cardiovascular complications by 25%.
c. Improve glycemic control by the next diabetes care visit.
d. Improve overall health by eating better, moving more, and getting better rest.

41. A patient is beginning a physical activity regimen to include moderate intensity exercise 5 days a week for 30 minutes each day. He wants to know how to tell if he is exercising at the right intensity. From previous encounters with the patient, the diabetes educator is aware that he has some literacy/numeracy challenges, and decides to suggest the original rating of perceived exertion (RPE). How would the educator explain this intensity guide to the patient?

a. The RPE lets you estimate how intense your physical activity is by counting the number of breaths per minute and comparing it to the number at rest. Moderate/vigorous intensity is equal to an increase of 2–4 breaths per minute.
b. The RPE estimates intensity by how easy it is to have a conversation during the activity. For moderate/vigorous intensity, you should be breathing harder but still be able to talk while performing the activity. If you are breathing too heavily to talk, then the activity is too intense.
c. The RPE has you estimate the intensity of your activity based on how much your heart rate has increased (from resting). For every 10 beats per minute, you go up one number in the scale. You should be between a "5" and an "8" (or 50–80 bpm increase) for moderate/vigorous-intensity activity.
d. The RPE helps you estimate the intensity of your activity by focusing on how tired you feel and how difficult the activity seems. It uses a scale of 6 ("extremely light") to 20 ("beyond extremely hard" or "maximal exertion"). Moderate/vigorous-intensity activity is about 12–16 ("somewhat hard" to "hard") on the scale.

42. If a patient with type 1 diabetes usually takes a long-acting and a short-acting insulin in the morning, what does the CDCES expect the patient will be advised to take the morning of a surgery?

a. Only the long-acting drug
b. Only the short-acting drug
c. Neither drug
d. Both drugs

43. As part of the initial comprehensive DSMES assessment, the educators ask their patient to describe his meals and snacks from the past 24 hours. He states that he cannot recall what he ate yesterday. What action or response would be MOST appropriate?

a. Note "patient does not recall" in the documentation and move on to the next question.
b. Invite his wife, who has accompanied him, to help recall what he ate yesterday.
c. Give the participant a 24-hour dietary log sheet and ask him to return it completed by next week.
d. Encourage him by prompting, "Now, honey, I can't believe that a man as smart as you can't come up with anything."

44. According to the Academy of Nutrition and Dietetics, what percentage of the caloric intake for a person with diabetes should be protein?

a. 45–60%
b. 30–45%
c. 20–35%
d. 15–20%

45. Which of the following options is an outcome of personal recordkeeping in relation to physical activity, according to recent studies?

a. Those who keep logs of physical activity are more adherent to other elements of therapy (e.g., diet, medication).
b. Those who keep exercise logs are more likely to enroll in organized exercise programs (e.g., gym memberships, classes).
c. Keeping a physical activity log is associated with a higher level of self-efficacy.
d. The obligation of recordkeeping has been identified as a barrier to exercise by study participants.

46. The primary factor in the development of diabetic foot ulcers is:

a. Treatment noncompliance
b. Anatomic abnormalities
c. Obesity
d. Peripheral neuropathy

47. The Somogyi effect is believed to result from:

a. Prolonged fasting
b. An excessive basal dose of insulin
c. Natural surge of hormones
d. Rebound reaction to hypoglycemia

48. In relation to safe driving, which of the following advice would the clinician LEAST likely recommend?

a. Always wear medical identification when driving.
b. When driving long distances, stop every one to two hours to check blood glucose.
c. Always eat something with carbohydrates within the hour before you drive.
d. Keep some form of glucose or quick carb handy in the vehicle at all times.

49. A person has been diagnosed with prediabetes because of signs and symptoms of metabolic syndrome, which is characterized by:

a. Fasting blood glucose ≥100 mg/dL
b. Blood pressure ≥145/90 mmHg
c. Male waist circumference >35 inches
d. Triglyceride level >120 mg/dL

50. A patient who is reluctant to attend DSMES class states the reason as, "I already know all this stuff." In light of his learning readiness, what would be the MOST appropriate action?

a. Tell him that if he changes his mind, he may call at any time. Document his refusal to participate.
b. Give him a pop quiz with challenging diabetes knowledge questions to help him see that he does not know everything.
c. Acknowledge his reluctance and ask if he might be willing to share some of his knowledge and experiences with the other class members.
d. Change the subject to minimize conflict and then speak with his wife to see if she might have better luck convincing him.

51. Which of the following statements regarding preconception care and diabetes is true?

a. Only about half of all female patients of childbearing age with diabetes receive preconception counseling.
b. Preconception care should include weight management as the first priority so that those women who become pregnant are as close to ideal body weight as possible.
c. The rate of congenital malformations for diabetic women whose HbA1c is less than 7% prior to and at conception is similar to rates for women without diabetes.
d. An important part of preconception counseling may be to initiate lipid management medication (such as a statin), since lipid levels tend to increase during the first part of pregnancy.

52. Which of the following statements below is a recent evidence-based practice recommendation and an example of translating research into practice?

a. Low-carbohydrate diets are recommended for persons with type 2 diabetes because of studies showing greater weight loss and improvements in lipid levels compared to other diets.
b. Unvaccinated adults with diabetes who are aged 19 through 59 years should receive hepatitis B vaccination.
c. Routine antioxidant supplementation, including vitamins A and C and carotene, is recommended for adults with type 2 diabetes.
d. Glycemic goals for critical-care hospitalized patients with diabetes should not exceed 120 mg/dL and should not be less than 80 mg/dL.

53. According to the recently published ADA Nutrition Therapy Recommendations, which of the following statements regarding outcomes of low-carbohydrate diets is true?

a. The glycemic effects of low-carb diets are mixed; therefore, no definite conclusions can be drawn regarding the effects of low-carb diets on HbA1c.
b. Low-carb diets were found to raise LDL and triglyceride levels in most studies.
c. Studies suggest that low-carb diets are effective because compliance with these diets is high.
d. Low-carb diets are the safest option for a patient with renal disease.

54. A 23-year-old client presents with moderate hyperglycemia but is of normal weight and shows no evidence of metabolic syndrome or ketoacidosis. She complains of increased thirst and urination and reports that multiple generations of her family had been diagnosed with diabetes prior to age 25. What type of diabetes should be suspected?

a. Type 1
b. Type 2
c. Maturity onset diabetes of the young (MOBY)
d. Latent autoimmune diabetes in adults (LADA)

55. A client is taking a sulfonylurea for control of her type 2 diabetes and wants to engage in running for exercise. If she takes the medication at 8 a.m., when should she begin exercising?

a. Immediately after taking the medication
b. At least 2 hours after taking the medication (after 10 a.m.)
c. At least 4 hours after taking the medication (after noon)
d. At least 6 hours after taking the medication (after 2 p.m.)

56. A person with type 2 diabetes complains that she often feels stressed and worries obsessively about how she will manage her disease and what complications may occur, and this sometimes keeps her awake at night. What stress reduction technique may be the most helpful?

a. Mindfulness-based meditation
b. Physical activity and exercise
c. Self-help books and videos
d. Hobbies or other creative outlets

57. Which dietary strategy is the primary recommendation for those with prediabetes?

a. A meal plan that focuses on moderate carbs, including carb monitoring/counting
b. A low-carbohydrate diet (i.e., Atkins diet or similar)
c. A calorie-reduced diet with reduced intake of dietary fat
d. A low glycemic-index/glycemic-load diet

58. Which of the following is NOT considered a social determinant of health that places individuals at greater risk for diabetes, according to 2026 ADA Standards?

a. Low level of health literacy
b. Food insecurity
c. Limited time to see the provider
d. Homelessness

59. A patient who has just been prescribed two oral medications for type 2 diabetes also takes many other medications for chronic conditions, including Crohn's disease, COPD, hypertension, anemia, and vitamin deficiencies. She is very concerned about medication dose timing, contraindications, and side effects and requests an educational appointment to address her concerns. Which team member would be the best professional to meet with this patient?

a. The doctor(s) who originally prescribed each medication
b. A mental health professional to help her with anxiety
c. The pharmacist assigned to the patient's healthcare team
d. The registered dietitian, who is also a certified diabetes educator

60. For persons with diabetes, their low-density lipoprotein (LDL) level should ideally be kept at less than:

a. 120 mg/dL
b. 100 mg/dL
c. 90 mg/dL
d. 70 mg/dL

61. A patient suffers from obesity, type 2 diabetes, hypertension, and hyperlipidemia. He recalls his dinner from last night: a low-fat turkey and cheese sandwich with mustard, a side salad with low-fat Italian dressing, pickles, a small serving of baked chips, and one can of club soda. Based on assessment, which of the patient's conditions is at GREATEST risk due to his food choices?

a. Hyperlipidemia
b. Type 2 diabetes
c. Obesity
d. Hypertension

62. The diabetes educator is teaching a group class on diabetes and healthy meal planning. All four participants have provided an example of what they consider to be a healthy, well-balanced meal for someone who has diabetes. Which example would be cited as the BEST example of an appropriate meal choice?

a. A turkey and cheese, lettuce, and tomato sandwich with an apple, a small serving of baked chips, and a diet soda.
b. A bowl of chicken broth, pickle, sugar-free Jell-O, 2 celery sticks, water, and a multi-vitamin.
c. A medium chef salad with lettuce, eggs, cheese, chicken, celery, and Italian dressing, and a glass of water.
d. Whole-grain pasta (about 2 cups) with low-fat cream sauce, 1 slice of garlic bread, 1 cup of cooked green peas, and skim milk.

63. In the last few years, professional diabetes organizations including the ADA have adopted the HbA1c test as a diagnostic tool. In order for a valid diagnosis to be made using an HbA1c of 6.5% or greater, which of the following stipulations or qualifiers must also be present?

a. HbA1c must be accompanied by a fasting glucose test of over 126 mg/dL.
b. The patient must also have symptoms of hyperglycemia.
c. The patient must also have at least one episode of random plasma glucose over 180 mg/dL.
d. The HbA1c test must be NGSP-certified and standardized to the Diabetes Complications and Control Trial (DCCT); a repeat test is recommended.

64. According to the ADA, which diet is recommended if the goal is to reduce HbA1c, lower blood pressure, lose weight, lower triglycerides, and increase HDL?

a. Low carbohydrate
b. Low fat
c. Mediterranean
d. Vegetarian

65. With a continuous glucose monitor (CGM), the target time in range is usually:

a. 50%
b. 60%
c. 70%
d. 80%

66. For a person with diabetes and predialysis chronic kidney disease (stages 1–4), what is the recommended daily intake of protein?

a. 0.8 g/kg per day
b. 1 g/kg per day
c. 0.5 g/kg per day
d. 1.4 g/kg per day

67. Using the ADCES7 Self-Care Behaviors Goal Sheet, a diabetes educator and a patient are working on individualizing self-care behavior goals. The educator documents that the patient has checked the box labeled "make better food choices" under the "Healthy Eating" category. Which of the following statements is the best example of individualization of this goal?

a. Make better food choices to reduce HbA1c to less than 7.5%.
b. Make better food choices over the next 6 months (by October 31).
c. Switch to diet soda and sugar-free ice cream.
d. Report to educator each Monday on the previous week's food choices.

68. A client has glycemic variability that is not evident in her HbA1c and is not always captured with blood glucose monitoring. Therefore, she is to temporarily use a CGM system. To monitor a person with glycemic variability, CGM use is recommended for at least:

a. 48 hours
b. 5 days
c. 7 days
d. 14 days

69. A person with diabetes has been home sick with the flu. His condition has worsened, and he has been unable to keep down fluid and foods. He should go the emergency department if he is unable to keep fluids down for more than:

a. 2 hours
b. 4 hours
c. 8 hours
d. 12 hours

70. The dietary requirement of protein to promote wound healing is:

a. 0.25–0.4 g/kg/day
b. 0.5–0.75 g/kg/day
c. 0.76–1.24 g/kg/day
d. 1.25–1.5 g/kg/day

71. A client with type 2 diabetes has good fasting glucose numbers in the morning (100–115 mg/dL) but has much higher postprandial numbers after dinner (250–320 mg/dL). She likely needs to:

a. Increase the dosage of the oral medications.
b. Switch from oral medications to insulin.
c. Decrease her carbohydrate intake at dinner.
d. Eat the large meal earlier in the day.

72. A person with type 2 diabetes has diabetic neuropathy affecting the feet. What type of exercises should he engage in to help slow its progression?

a. Low-impact
b. Plyometrics
c. High-intensity interval training
d. Moderate-intensity aerobics

73. When reading the Nutritional Facts food label to assess the sodium content of a food item, what percentage of the daily value (DV) is considered high?

a. 15% or more
b. 20% or more
c. 25% or more
d. 30% or more

74. A person with type 2 diabetes controlled with metformin has been monitoring their blood pressure with a new wrist monitor, and readings have been very inconsistent—high at times and low at others—even though the person has a long history of stable blood pressure readings. The CDCES should suspect:

a. Unstable cardiovascular condition
b. Improper use of the monitor
c. Defective monitor
d. Adverse response to medications

75. The most common sexual dysfunction associated with diabetes in males is:

a. Decreased libido
b. Erectile dysfunction
c. Premature ejaculation
d. Anorgasmia

76. Jeff is a 26-year-old with type 1 diabetes; he wears an insulin pump. He reports that he has noticed a pattern of hypoglycemia two to three hours after lunch and dinner. When asked, he states that before meals, and even after breakfast, he seems to have no problem. Which of the following pump setting changes would be recommended?

a. Reducing his basal rate by 10% between lunch and bedtime
b. Changing his insulin-to-carb ratio from 10 to 12 for lunch and dinner only
c. Modifying his correction/sensitivity factor to give less insulin
d. Changing his insulin-to-carb ratio from 10 to 8 for lunch and dinner only

77. A diabetes educator has been asked to provide a 90-minute diabetes education activity at a senior center for 6–12 residents, all of whom have diabetes. Group members will have different levels of pre-existing diabetes knowledge. Which instructional strategy below would be MOST appropriate? Assume that the educator has access to or will be provided with any equipment and furniture that may be needed.

a. Conversation maps
b. Computer/web-based DSMES (with access to six laptops)
c. Printed diabetes materials to address a variety of topics; use activity time to go over what each publication addresses
d. Slide show lecture addressing basic diabetes principles

78. Which of the following behavioral goals is measurable?

a. "Improve diabetes control by managing my portion size."
b. "Increase cardiovascular endurance by January 1."
c. "Run 20 minutes at least three times per week."
d. "Minimize the risk of diabetic eye disease by keeping my ophthalmology appointments."

79. For an insulin pump, which type or types of insulin are typically used?

a. Rapid-acting
b. Rapid-acting and long-acting
c. Intermediate-acting
d. Long-acting

80. What is the blood pressure threshold at which patients with diabetes should be advised on lifestyle changes to reduce blood pressure?

a. ≥150/90 mmHg
b. ≥140/80 mmHg
c. ≥130/80 mmHg
d. >120/80 mmHg

81. An older patient is not completing her assessment paperwork along with other group members. She moves slowly and squints at the signs on the door. Her hands shake as she retrieves an item from her handbag. Based on what has been briefly observed, which of the following learning barriers does the diabetes educator MOST likely suspect may be present?

a. Visual and tactile/dexterity
b. Hearing and literacy
c. Financial and visual
d. Mobility and cultural

82. Which of the following reflects 2026 ADA Standards related to blood pressure measurements at a single healthcare visit for hypertension diagnosis?

a. A blood pressure reading of ≥180/110 mmHg at a single healthcare visit is sufficient for hypertension diagnosis.
b. A blood pressure reading of ≥170/100 mmHg at a single healthcare visit is sufficient for hypertension diagnosis.
c. Blood pressure measurement from a single healthcare visit is not sufficient for hypertension diagnosis and should be confirmed with a second blood pressure measurement one week after the first.
d. A blood pressure reading of ≥140/90 mmHg on both arms at a single healthcare visit is sufficient for hypertension diagnosis.

83. The primary focus in coaching should be on:

a. Pointing out the learner's areas of weakness or errors
b. Watching the learner carry out return demonstrations
c. Developing goals for the learner
d. Using questioning to help the learner recognize their problem areas

84. According to the National Standards for Diabetes Self-Management Education and Support, what is the most important action on the part of the person with diabetes?

a. Adherence to a diet plan
b. Outcome tracking
c. Behavioral change
d. Knowledge acquisition

85. Assuming each of the patients below are currently consuming an average amount of protein daily (about 0.8–1.0 g per kg body weight per day), which of the patients may need to REDUCE his or her daily protein intake?

a. A pregnant woman, normal weight, in second trimester
b. A 60-year-old male with diabetes and stage 4 kidney disease, normal BMI
c. A female with type 2 diabetes and a slow-healing lower-extremity wound
d. None of the above should be switched to a low-protein diet

86. Every teaching strategy has both advantages and limitations that impact the setting in which it can be most effectively used. Group size is one of the most significant factors to consider when deciding whether to use a given strategy. Select the series of teaching strategies that is placed in order by the group size for which it is ideally suited (from individual to large group).

a. Games, printed materials, demonstration, case studies
b. Web-based activities, role-playing, group discussion, lecture
c. Printed materials, lecture, demonstration, Web-based activities
d. Games, lecture, printed material, group discussion

87. A 53-year-old male with type 2 diabetes has a stocky build and is overweight, with a BMI of 32 kg/m². His fasting blood glucose levels are in the 128–134 mg/dL range. He works as a travel agent 40 hours a week and assists in managing his household. The client states that he sleeps 8 hours during the night but often feels sleepy during the day and tends to fall asleep during the evening when he sits down to watch television. He has frequent morning headaches. His spouse reports that he snores loudly. The most likely cause for his sleepiness is:

a. Hyperglycemia
b. Obstructive sleep apnea
c. Hypertension
d. Stress/overwork

88. A client with long-term type 2 diabetes has good blood flow to his feet but markedly reduced sensation. He twisted his ankle, and 3 days later developed sudden swelling and redness of his entire foot but has continued to walk without difficulty or pain. These may be indications that he is at risk for:

a. Charcot arthropathy
b. Amputation
c. Gout
d. Deep vein thrombosis

89. For most females with type 2 diabetes, the LDL and HDL targets are:

a. LDL <100 mg/dL (2.6 mmol/L) and HDL >50 mg/dL (1.3 mmol/L)
b. LDL <100 mg/dL (2.6 mmol/L) and HDL >40 mg/dL (1.0 mmol/L)
c. LDL <70 mg/dL (1.8 mmol/L) and HDL >50 mg/dL (1.3 mmol/L)
d. LDL <70 mg/dL (1.8 mmol/L) and HDL >40 mg/dL (1.0 mmol/L)

90. If a person with diabetes tests positive for urine ketones, this generally means that the blood glucose level is greater than:

a. 200 mg/dL (11.1 mmol/L)
b. 240 mg/dL (13.3 mmol/L)
c. 280 mg/dL (15.6 mmol/L)
d. 300 mg/dL (16.7 mmol/L)

91. A client with diabetes complains that her legs and feet feel cold and that the skin on her lower legs appears shiny and smooth. This is an indication of:

a. Chronic venous insufficiency
b. Deep vein thrombosis
c. Raynaud's phenomenon
d. Peripheral arterial disease

92. Eating disorders are more common in those with diabetes than in the general population, and are more prevalent in women than in men. Recent studies have been focused on women with type 1 diabetes who restrict insulin in order to avoid weight gain. Which of the following statements is NOT a finding of these studies?

a. Withholding insulin to prevent weight gain is associated with problems in other diabetes self-care areas.
b. Withholding insulin to prevent weight gain is associated with higher levels of diabetes-specific stress.
c. Women who withheld insulin to prevent weight gain have higher mortality risk, which correlates with the frequency of withholding the insulin.
d. Women who have had diabetes for shorter duration are more likely to restrict insulin than those who have had diabetes for longer duration.

93. Which of the following is a secondary diabetes prevention strategy?

a. Closely monitoring blood glucose values
b. Adopting a healthy diet and losing weight
c. Exercising routinely
d. Stopping smoking

94. Which of the following goals set by a client fits the SMART format?

a. "I will improve my blood sugar levels over the next 3 months."
b. "I will limit my carbs to 50 g daily for the next 6 weeks in order to control my glucose levels."
c. "I will never eat any sugar or processed foods from now on."
d. "I will walk 30 minutes a day 5 or 6 days a week for the next 90 days to improve my glucose control."

95. Which class of oral medications for type 2 diabetes has a mechanism of action that relies on the kidneys to excrete glucose through the urine, and should therefore not be used in those with eGFR of less than 20 mL/min or by those on dialysis?

a. Sulfonylureas (i.e., glyburide)
b. Biguanides (i.e., metformin)
c. SGLT2 inhibitors (i.e., canagliflozin)
d. DPP-4 inhibitors (i.e., sitagliptin)

96. What is *acanthosis nigricans* and what does it suggest?

a. Darkening and thickening of the skin, typically on the back/sides of the neck or the axillae; indicative of insulin resistance
b. A pattern of deep, labored breathing; indicative of acidosis, common in advanced DKA
c. Darkening of the toe nails; indicative of poor pedal circulation
d. Blackening around the edges of an ulcer; indicative of tissue ischemia due to poor circulation and oxygenation

97. Blood pressure readings for a pregnant patient (26 weeks gestation), who has gestational diabetes, at her last three visits were as follows: 134/92 mmHg, 144/90 mmHg, and 142/96 mmHg. She is already on a low-sodium diet and says she follows it consistently. Which of the treatment options below would be appropriate for this patient?

a. Methyldopa
b. A low-dose of an ACE inhibitor (i.e., lisinopril)
c. A low-to-moderate dose of a diuretic (i.e., furosemide)
d. No medical treatment is necessary, as these levels are mostly within target for pregnancy. Reinforce lifestyle modification, including a low-sodium diet and regular walking.

98. Which of the following is NOT among the top treatment fears for patients who are being prescribed insulin?

a. Nausea and subsequent weight loss
b. Worsening of their diabetes
c. Needles
d. Hypoglycemia

99. When teaching a person with diabetes about reading and interpreting food labels, it is especially important for the person to focus on:

a. Percentage of vitamins
b. Total carbohydrates
c. Serving size
d. Total calories

100. The CDCES is planning classes for six clients with diabetes to teach them about monitoring their glucose levels. Which educational approach is most indicated?

a. One-on-one instruction
b. Educational workshop
c. Lecture
d. Discussion

101. A diabetes educator is reading the patient chart of a 30-year-old African American female newly diagnosed with diabetes (type is unspecified). Her BMI is recorded as 17.5 kg/m^2. Her BMI falls into which category?

a. Underweight
b. Normal weight
c. Overweight
d. Obese

102. The CDCES has been working with an older adult who was treated with oral medications for many years but now needs to take insulin. The client is able to give herself injections without difficulty and is mentally alert, but she is very inconsistent in filling insulin syringes with the correct dosage. Her family lives within 5 miles of her home. The best solution is to arrange for:

a. Daily home health agency visits
b. Further instruction
c. Prefilled insulin syringes
d. A family member to fill the syringes

103. A 50-year-old client is diagnosed with prediabetes because her blood glucose levels are in the 110–115 mg/dL (6.1–6.38 mmol/L) range, although her HbA1c is 5.6%. Her BMI is 30. The woman works as a computer programmer and engages in little physical activity. She routinely skips lunch and snacks late into the evening. She states that she feels stressed about her workload and often sleeps poorly. Although the woman is worried about developing diabetes, she is unsure where to start improving her health. Which initial changes in lifestyle should the CDCES recommend?

a. Intensive exercise program and strict adherence to a healthy diet
b. Participation in a prediabetes support group
c. Change of employment or decreased workload
d. Moderate exercise and improved nutrition

104. A housebound client is very distressed about her diagnosis of diabetes, has little in the way of social support, and calls the clinic every day asking simple questions. What may be the best solution to help her become less dependent on the clinic staff?

a. Schedule routine calls three times weekly.
b. Tell her to avoid calling unless it is an emergency.
c. Provide resources for education about diabetes.
d. Provide information about message boards, such as the Diabetes Daily forums.

105. Which of the following lab findings is MOST closely associated with hypertriglyceridemia?

a. High HDL
b. Elevated fasting plasma glucose
c. Low HDL
d. Small-sized LDL-C particles

106. Which of the following is the LEAST likely to result in low blood glucose?

a. Decreased food intake
b. Increased insulin
c. Increased level of stress
d. Increased intake of alcohol without carbohydrates

107. Which theoretical approach to learning and health behavior change maintains that individuals learn from their personal experiences as well as from observing the actions and experiences of others?

a. Social cognitive theory (SCT)
b. Health belief model (HBM)
c. Theory of planned behavior (TPB)
d. Transtheoretical model (TTM)

108. Which of the following personal characteristics has proven to positively affect behavioral outcomes through healthy coping with one's diabetes?

a. Stubbornness
b. Affluence
c. Optimism
d. Consistency

109. Which of the following is NOT a standard recommendation for those with mild-to-moderate chronic kidney disease (stages 1 through 4)?

a. Restricting foods high in vitamin K (e.g., some leafy green vegetables)
b. Good glycemic control (as tight as can be achieved without hypoglycemia)
c. Blood pressure management using an ACE inhibitor or ARB medication
d. Abstaining from use of nonsteroidal anti-inflammatory drugs (NSAIDs)

110. A diabetes educator has been asked to teach a diabetes class to a small group of patients, all of whom are hearing impaired. The educator has secured an American Sign Language (ASL) interpreter to interpret for the class members. What other modification should be made to meet the needs of this particular audience?

a. Write medication names and other "proper" nouns on the white board.
b. Modify some of the handouts to include more pictures and less text.
c. Arrange the chairs in a circle so class members can clearly see each other.
d. Provide each class member with a pad of paper and pen to facilitate written communication.

111. When calculating the impact that sugar alcohols, such as mannitol and xylitol, have on blood glucose levels, what percentage of grams of sugar alcohols should be subtracted from the total carbohydrate count?

a. 25%
b. 50%
c. 75%
d. 100%

112. Which of the following options below is the MOST appropriate example of a learning objective for a diabetes education class?

a. Learner will select an appropriate, balanced meal choice from a restaurant menu.
b. Learner will know what it means to eat healthily.
c. Learner will improve HbA1c through better food choices.
d. Learner will understand the difference between glycemic index and glycemic load.

113. Which of the following is a difference between medication administration using a disposable insulin pen device to inject insulin and medication administration using a pen device to inject a GLP-1 analog medication such as exenatide (Byetta)?

a. Insulin pen devices require a new pen needle each time, but with GLP-1 receptor agonist pen devices, the same needle can be used repeatedly.
b. Insulin injections require site rotation, but GLP-1 receptor agonist injections can be given in the same spot since they are typically given less frequently.
c. When using an insulin pen device, the patient should prime the pen (perform an "air shot") before each use, whereas with a GLP-1 agonist medication, the priming is only done as part of new pen setup (before first use of each pen).
d. GLP-1 agonist medication must be kept refrigerated until immediately before use, whereas an in-use insulin pen may be kept at room temperature until the use limit (i.e., 28 days for insulin aspart or insulin glargine).

114. Which of the following patient statements should alert the diabetes educator to a LACK of understanding about the purpose of self-monitoring of blood glucose?

a. "I test my blood sugar whenever I feel bad, even if it is not my regularly scheduled time to test."
b. "I test two to three times per day and schedule my testing times for when I think my numbers will be the best."
c. "I wake up at 3:00 in the morning and test for a couple of days whenever my doctor changes my dose of basal insulin."
d. "I try to test a couple of hours after a meal to see if my mealtime insulin dose was too little or too much."

115. According to the ADA, people who are prediabetic or at risk for diabetes can lower their risk of developing diabetes by 58% by exercising and losing:

a. 7% of body weight
b. 10% of body weight
c. 15% of body weight
d. 18% of body weight

116. A 58-year-old male client has a history of type 2 diabetes and alcoholism. Which of the following laboratory findings may be indicative of hepatic damage?

a. ALT 400 U/L
b. GTT 32 U/L
c. Prothrombin time 12 seconds
d. Ammonia 30 μg/dL

117. What is the MAIN purpose of personal recordkeeping with regard to dietary habits?

a. The patient is able to look back and feel proud of the positive changes that have been made, thus promoting patient empowerment.
b. A food record allows the patient and educator to review, evaluate, and reassess choices, which can be used to set or modify nutritional goals.
c. Insurance providers need to see evidence of the impact of medical nutrition therapy (MNT) and the food record can be admitted as part of the official patient record.
d. Keeping a food record forces the patient to pay more attention to what he or she is eating, and promotes the important diabetes life skill of recording daily activities.

118. The CDCES has been working with a client with type 1 diabetes on self-management tasks, such as glucose monitoring and insulin injections. The best method to determine if he has developed adequate skills is to:

a. Ask him to talk through and demonstrate tasks.
b. Ask him theoretical questions about management.
c. Give him a self-evaluation survey to complete.
d. Review his glucose monitoring and insulin records.

119. Which of the following patients would be classified as "morbidly obese"?

a. A 50-year-old white male who is 49 lb (22 kg) overweight and has already suffered one heart attack
b. A 26-year-old Hispanic female with a BMI of 41 kg/m^2
c. A 48-year-old African-American male who is consulting a specialist for possible bariatric surgery
d. A 60-year-old white male who weighs 225 lb (102 kg)

120. A middle-aged client with type 2 diabetes is also struggling with depression and anxiety, impacting his ability to manage diabetes. His education plan should emphasize emotional support and:

a. Small, achievable goals
b. A physical exercise program
c. Adherence to glucose monitoring and a healthy diet
d. Prevention of complications

121. A person with type 2 diabetes living in a rural area has little access to transportation and has chosen to participate in remote learning. The biggest challenge of remote learning is typically:

a. Maintaining the motivation to learn
b. Using technology correctly
c. Having an unreliable internet connection
d. Dealing with distracting environments

122. During the honeymoon period of type 1 diabetes, persons may:

a. Show no symptoms
b. Experience sudden changes in their condition
c. Develop a false sense of security
d. Require no insulin

123. Which of the following marketing strategies has been found to be the most reliable and cost-effective method of bringing new patients into a diabetes education program?

a. Radio ads
b. Personal outreach to referring providers
c. Word of mouth (current participants, employees, etc.)
d. Finding and contacting patients who were previously hospitalized and experienced hyperglycemia

124. An elderly man with type 2 diabetes reports the following exercise plan for six days per week: 40 minutes of jogging on M/W/F and 40 minutes of strength training on T/Th/Sa. As part of the assessment, the CDCES should consider whether which type of physical activity recommendation is being addressed?

a. Aerobic exercise
b. Toning exercise
c. Flexibility exercise
d. Resistance exercise

125. A diabetes educator assesses a patient's self-administration of insulin with a non-refillable insulin pen device and a 5-mm pen needle. The patient performs the following actions: cleans the end of the pen with alcohol, attaches the pen needle, dials the dose, inserts the needle into the skin and fully presses the button, withdraws after 10 seconds, detaches and disposes of the needle, and replaces the pen cap. What is incorrect about the way the patient performs this skill?

a. He needed to clean the skin with alcohol.
b. He needed to pinch the skin before injecting.
c. He needed to withdraw the needle after 5 seconds.
d. He needed to prime the needle before dialing the dose.

126. A 48-year-old client with diabetes is eligible for Social Security disability benefits if diabetes complications:

a. Include DKA
b. Include HbA1c averages >9%
c. Require frequent blood glucose monitoring
d. Prevent the person from working

127. In a group class on nutrition, a diabetes educator shows a sample breakfast menu and asks participants to modify the meals to include about 60 grams of carbohydrate. One patient shares her modified menu: 1 scrambled egg, 2 oz ham, 2 pieces of wheat toast, half of a large grapefruit, 1 cup skim milk. Which evaluation below best describes this meal?

a. The meal has significantly too few grams of carbohydrates.
b. The meal has approximately 60 grams of carbohydrate.
c. The meal has significantly too many grams of carbohydrates.
d. It is impossible to estimate the number of grams of carbohydrates without seeing the grapefruit and the type of bread.

128. A patient with long-term type 2 diabetes has developed chronic abdominal distension and a feeling of fullness long after meals. The person has lost weight and has episodes of nausea and vomiting. These are likely indications of:

a. Gall bladder disease
b. Gastroesophageal reflux disease
c. Gastroparesis
d. Peptic ulcer disease

129. Which hypothetical situation would a diabetes educator pose if they wanted to assess a patient's ability to deal with a glucose emergency?

a. "You are shopping for items for a special birthday meal that will also fit into your diabetes meal plan. What would you choose?"
b. "What actions would you take if you were traveling out of state and realized on your trip that you were almost out of insulin?"
c. "Say you are driving your car and you begin to feel shaky, sweaty, and confused. What would you do?"
d. "How would you deal with a colleague who found out you have diabetes and proceeded to give you advice you knew to be incorrect?"

130. It is important to assess potential barriers to self-monitoring of blood glucose, especially for patients who are not adhering to their plan of care recommendations. Which of the following barriers was NOT cited by patients in recent studies?

a. Cost of testing supplies
b. Discomfort of finger sticks
c. Lack of instruction and support
d. Misplacement of small items

131. If a client with type 1 diabetes admits to being a regular marijuana user, she should be aware that marijuana:

a. May increase her risk of diabetic ketoacidosis
b. May increase her risk of hypertension
c. May reduce her need for insulin
d. Likely has no effect on her diabetes

132. Which active-learning instructional strategy listed below does the educator have the MOST control over content?

a. Group discussion
b. Conversation maps
c. Lecture with visual aids (i.e., slides)
d. Demonstration

133. A 20-year-old female with type 1 diabetes has had repeated bouts of hyperglycemia and diabetic ketoacidosis (DKA) and is losing weight despite insisting that she is staying on her recommended diet and taking her insulin as prescribed. Her HbA1c is 9.2%. What type of disordered eating does this suggest?

a. Diabulimia
b. Restrictive eating
c. Binge eating disorder
d. Bulimia nervosa

134. Which diabetes medication class is generally contraindicated for patients with congestive heart failure (CHF)?

a. DPP-4 inhibitors (i.e., sitagliptin)
b. TZDs (i.e., pioglitazone)
c. Sulfonylureas (i.e., glipizide)
d. GLP-1 receptor agonists (i.e., exenatide)

135. The prescribed meal plan for a patient is based on a 2000-calorie requirement. The patient's total fat intake should not exceed what threshold?

a. Calories from fat for this patient should not exceed 30% of the diet.
b. Fat intake for this patient should not exceed 500 calories per day.
c. Fat intake, for all persons with diabetes, should not exceed 60 g per day, regardless of total calorie need.
d. There is no recommendation for an ideal percentage (or number) of calories from fat for all people with diabetes.

136. After exhausting other medical options, a patient's physician prescribes insulin for his hospitalized patient, and recommends that the regimen be continued at home after discharge. The patient has a very limited income as well as very poor eyesight; the patient is unable to drive to follow-up visits or to pick up prescriptions at the pharmacy. Which healthcare (hospital staff) team member should the diabetes educator most likely consult to assist the patient?

a. Pharmacist
b. Registered dietitian
c. Inpatient social worker
d. Ordering physician

137. The nurse notes that clients in a rural area who fail to return to the clinic to have laboratory tests or other follow-ups for diabetes are most often those who lack insurance. This is likely related to the issue of:

a. Population health
b. Geographic health
c. Social determinants of health
d. Health literacy

138. A client with type 2 diabetes had to get reading glasses and is terrified that this means he will go blind. To reassure him, the best information to share is that:

a. Only 5–10% of people with diabetes lose their vision.
b. Good diabetic management and preventive eye care reduces the risk of blindness by 95%.
c. Blindness is related to diabetic retinopathy, which affects one in three people with diabetes.
d. After 20 years, 60–80% of those with type 2 diabetes have retinopathy.

139. Which of the following items are considered Standards of Care for adults with type 1 or type 2 diabetes?

a. Annual eye exam and annual echocardiogram
b. Annual influenza vaccination and dilated eye exam every six months (more often if needed)
c. Hepatitis B vaccination for adults less than 60 years and annual influenza vaccination for all patients
d. Annual C-peptide lab test and HbA1c lab test every six months (more often if not to goal)

140. A female patient with type 2 diabetes has a body mass index (BMI) of 31 kg/m^2. She drinks one glass of wine daily, takes cannabidiol to help control her arthritic pain, and complains of stress related to her recent retirement. Her lipid panel is as follows:

Cholesterol	234 mg/dL
HDL	50 mg/dL
LDL	156 mg/dL
Cholesterol:HDL ratio	4.7
Non-HDL cholesterol	184 mg/dL
Very low-density lipoproteins (calculated)	30 mg/dL
Triglycerides	155 mg/dL

What lifestyle change or changes are most indicated for this patient?

a. Lower saturated and trans fats, eat a high-fiber diet, and exercise.
b. Eliminate alcohol and cannabidiol.
c. Eat a low-calorie vegetarian diet.
d. Perform stress management techniques, such as yoga and meditation.

141. Which of the following patient attributes (skills/experiences) is NOT considered a prerequisite for continuous subcutaneous insulin infusion (i.e., insulin pump) therapy?

a. Patient must have a diagnosis of type 1 diabetes
b. Patient must be proficient at counting carbohydrates
c. Patient should have previous experience with multiple daily injection (MDI) therapy
d. Patient exhibits a pattern of consistent, frequent blood glucose monitoring

142. A diabetes educator calls to follow up with a patient who was diagnosed with diabetes six weeks ago. The patient admits that after she used all her blood glucose test strips, she quit checking her blood sugar because she has no insurance and they are too expensive for her very limited income. Which of the following resources would be LEAST helpful to this patient?

a. Partnership for Prescription Assistance (a national program sponsored by pharmaceutical research companies)
b. A low-interest medical loan from her local bank
c. The local or state health department low-income prescription program
d. Needymeds.com (a non-profit organization that centralizes information and applications for pharmaceutical drug assistance programs)

143. The clinic has invested in an interactive virtual reality game to teach clients about managing diabetes. Clients in which age group are most likely to want to engage in this type of education?

a. Middle childhood (6–11 years old) and adolescence (12–18 years old)
b. Adolescence and young adulthood (19–30 years old)
c. Middle adulthood (31–60 years old)
d. Older adulthood (60+ years old)

144. Which class of diabetic medications for the treatment of type 2 diabetes promotes the greatest loss of weight?

a. Alpha-glucosidase inhibitors
b. GLP-1 agonists
c. SGLT-2 inhibitors
d. DPP-4 inhibitors

145. A patient with uncontrolled type 2 diabetes, a sedentary lifestyle, and multiple co-morbidities tells her diabetes educator that she wishes to begin an exercise program to lose weight and improve her overall health. She states she wants to start slowly (walking and mild weight training), but eventually work up to where she can run a mile with her husband. Her co-morbidities include severe non-proliferative retinopathy (according to ophthalmologist notes from 7 months ago), stage 2 renal disease with microalbuminuria, cardiac autonomic neuropathy, and peripheral neuropathy that is manifested by reduced sensation in her feet. Which of the following statements is most accurate and complete regarding pre-exercise evaluation and referrals for this patient?

a. Because the patient is starting slowly (i.e., walking and mild weight training), no referral or extensive pre-exercise physical evaluation is needed.
b. The patient should receive an electrocardiogram stress test since she is currently sedentary. No other referrals are warranted at this time.
c. This patient should be referred for an ECG stress test and a retinopathy exam. In addition, the provider should perform a thorough physical exam and the patient may need to modify the exercise regimen to prevent exacerbation of her complications.
d. This patient should have referrals to ophthalmology, neurology, cardiology, nephrology, and possibly to an exercise physiologist. All team members will need to confer on this patient to devise the best activity regimen; it is likely that exercise will be contraindicated due to the extensive high-risk co-morbidities.

146. The systematic process by which the worth or value of something, teaching or learning in the case of DSMES, is judged is known as which of the following?

a. Evaluation
b. Documentation
c. Planning
d. Implementation

147. According to the practice guidelines of the Endocrine Society, rapid-acting insulin should be used rather than short-acting insulin for:

a. All persons on basal-bolus therapy
b. Adult persons on basal-bolus therapy with a high risk of hypoglycemia
c. Adult and pediatric persons on basal-bolus therapy with a high risk of hypoglycemia
d. Adult and pediatric persons on basal-bolus therapy with a high risk of hyperglycemia

148. What is the first step in the process of diabetes self-management education?

a. Assessment
b. Goal setting
c. Diagnosis
d. Referral

149. Extended-release metformin should generally be taken once daily at what time?

a. Before breakfast
b. With breakfast
c. With the evening meal
d. Before bedtime

150. If a client with type 1 diabetes drinks excessive amounts of alcoholic beverages, such as vodka and whiskey, and skips meals, this can result in:

a. Hyperglycemia
b. Hypoglycemia
c. Ketoacidosis
d. Hyperinsulinism

151. A person with type 2 diabetes has smoked two packs of cigarettes daily for more than 20 years. She has been advised to stop smoking. What approach to smoking cessation is likely to be the most successful?

a. Immediate cessation (i.e., go "cold turkey") and join a support group
b. Tapered dosages of nicotine-replacement therapies
c. Behavioral therapies, such as cognitive behavioral therapy or support groups
d. Combination therapy

152. A person's hemoglobin A1c (HbA1c) has been staying at approximately 7%, representing an average blood glucose of 154 mg/dL. If the person's HbA1C increases to 8%, this means that the average blood glucose has increased by approximately:

a. 8–10 mg/dL
b. 18–20 mg/dL
c. 28–30 mg/dL
d. 38–40 mg/dL

153. A patient tells the diabetes educator that she is very worried about "dropping too low" at night and therefore eats a bowl of ice cream every night and only takes a half dose of her nighttime basal insulin. Because this results in high fasting morning blood sugars and she is not willing to increase her basal insulin anyway, she has stopped testing in the morning. What mental health issue does this patient exhibit?

a. Depression
b. Eating disorder
c. Denial
d. Anxiety

154. Which of the following aggregate patient outcomes are required to be collected and reported as part of DSMES program recognition and accreditation?

a. Patient attendance rates for educational appointments
b. Overall change in patient HbA1c (pre/post education)
c. Percentage of patients achieving behavioral goals
d. The ADCES and ADA do not specify which outcomes must be tracked.

155. Which of the following accurately describes the best policy for disposing of sharps, such as insulin syringes, lancets, and infusion set needles?

a. Used sharps should only ever be put into official biohazard (sharps) containers, which can be purchased at a pharmacy.
b. It is okay to put sharps in a hard plastic container (such as a laundry detergent bottle) and, when it is full, tape the lid on and throw it away in the regular garbage.
c. Sharps may be put in a hard, non-permeable container, but should be taken to the pharmacy for final disposal, and never put in the regular garbage collection.
d. Since medical waste disposal laws vary from state to state, patients and educators need to determine the specific policies for their areas.

156. A patient underwent a craniotomy for a brain tumor and was placed on high dosages of glucocorticoids because of cerebral edema, resulting in hyperglycemia and insulin-dependent diabetes. What is the most likely outcome when the steroids are reduced and discontinued?

a. Continued treatment for type 1 diabetes with the same insulin requirements
b. Transition to a diagnosis of type 2 diabetes and a need for continued treatment
c. Continued treatment for type 1 diabetes with reduced insulin requirements
d. Resolution of hyperglycemia and no further treatment needed

157. For an Asian American woman to reduce her risk of developing diabetes, she should aim to exercise and lose weight until her waist circumference is no more than:

a. 29 inches
b. 31 inches
c. 35 inches
d. 37 inches

158. If a client with diabetes is a kinesthetic learner and is learning about different delivery systems for insulin, the CDCES should allow the client to:

a. Read the instruction manuals for the recommended devices.
b. Handle and manipulate the recommended devices.
c. Watch a video presentation of the recommended devices.
d. Listen to an audio recording describing the recommended devices.

159. A person with diabetes presents with hyperventilation and complains of nausea, vomiting, weight loss, abdominal pain, lethargy, and excessive thirst, urination, and hunger. The CDCES notes that the patient's breath has a fruity odor. The most likely cause is:

a. Diabetic ketoacidosis
b. Hypoglycemia
c. COVID-19 infection
d. Acute pancreatitis

160. Which of the following HbA1c targets would be MOST appropriate for a 69-year-old woman with long-standing type 1 diabetes who has cardiovascular disease, advanced kidney disease, retinopathy, and autonomic neuropathy?

a. <9.5%
b. <8%
c. <7%
d. <6.5%

161. Which of the following over-the-counter medications may result in an increase in blood glucose levels?

a. A decongestant
b. Diphenhydramine
c. Aspirin
d. A laxative

162. The ADA recommends the following daily limits on alcohol for males and females:

a. Males and females, ≤2 drinks daily
b. Males and females, ≤1 drink daily
c. Males, ≤2 drinks daily; females, ≤1 drink daily
d. Males, ≤3 drinks daily; females, ≤2 drinks daily

163. A patient takes basal insulin with a sulfonylurea. The diabetes educator meets with him to consider adjustment to his current regimen, at the patient's request. His most recent HbA1c was 8.9%. At the appointment, he states that he is not sure where the problem lies, and he expresses frustration that his insurance will only cover 4 bottles of test strips (200 test strips) every two months. Which self-monitoring regimen below would be the MOST appropriate for this patient?

a. Test right before and two hours after a single meal per day, rotating the meal. Do this for two to three weeks and then bring in results.
b. Monitor fasting glucose every morning and then test again just before bed every night for one month, then bring in results.
c. Because this patient takes insulin, he needs to test before each meal, every day, indefinitely.
d. Due to his limitation on test strips, he should save them for when he feels that his blood glucose may be high or low, and rely on other records, such as food and exercise logs, to pinpoint the problem.

164. A patient comes into a clinic to sign up for diabetes education classes. He tells the diabetes educator that he has had diabetes for 12 years but did not want to face his diagnosis. Now, after seeing how he is unable to keep up with his grandchildren, he has realized the need to make some changes and control his blood sugar. What stage of change in the transtheoretical model most accurately describes this patient's state?

a. Precontemplation
b. Contemplation
c. Preparation
d. Action

165. A patient with gestational diabetes (GDM) is convinced she developed GDM from eating too much of her favorite food—popcorn—early in her pregnancy. She insists that if she does not eat any again during her pregnancy, she will not have to start insulin and her blood glucose values will return to normal. What emotional stage associated with chronic disease diagnosis (similar to the Kübler-Ross stages of grief) does the diabetes educator assess in this patient?

a. Denial
b. Anger
c. Bargaining
d. Frustration and depression

166. Which one of the following conditions is associated with insulin resistance?

a. Nonalcoholic fatty liver disease
b. Type 1 diabetes
c. Celiac disease
d. Anorexia nervosa

167. In a discussion on meal planning, a patient states, "My whole family is from Mexico, and they get offended when I don't want to eat our traditional foods." What type of barrier is this patient is facing?

a. Physical barrier related to problem solving
b. Interpersonal barrier related to healthy eating
c. Personal independence barrier related to healthy coping
d. Financial barrier related to personal independence and family relationships

168. The diabetes educator is reviewing recent lab data for a new patient with diabetes but with no other documented co-morbidities. Which lab value is of the greatest concern?

a. Hemoglobin HbA1c of 7.8%
b. LDL of 101 mg/dL
c. HDL of 88 mg/dL
d. Serum creatinine of 2.8 mg/dL

169. Mr. D drops by the clinic on his way home from work to obtain a copy of his wife's most recent lab results. Mr. D regularly comes to appointments with his wife and assists in her diabetes self-management. What is the appropriate action for the diabetes educator to take?

a. Politely explain that it is a HIPAA violation to provide any private health information to anyone but the individual or personal representative (someone legally appointed to make healthcare decisions).
b. Provide Mr. D with a blank copy of the Release of Information form and tell him that if his wife will sign it, only then will the diabetes educator be able to comply with his request.
c. Suggest that the lab result is not needed at this time and that it can be discussed with the provider or educator in person at Mrs. D's next appointment.
d. Since Mrs. D has identified her husband as a participant in her care, the diabetes educator may provide Mr. D with a copy of the lab result, provided that it does not violate the policies of the workplace.

170. Which of the following accurately describes an association between celiac disease and diabetes?

a. Celiac disease is associated with insulin resistance, and therefore has a greater prevalence among those with type 2 diabetes compared to the general population.
b. Because celiac disease is an immune-mediated disorder, there is a greater prevalence among those with type 1 diabetes compared to the general population.
c. Because wheat-free diets are naturally lower in carbohydrates, the celiac diet is a recommended meal plan option for those with type 2 diabetes, even without diagnosed celiac disease.
d. Because celiac disease occurs with much greater frequency in the diabetic population (as compared to general population), screening for celiac disease is recommended for all persons with diabetes.

171. When developing an education plan for an individual with diabetes, which of the following is an achievable goal?

a. "I will lose 20 pounds in the next 30 days."
b. "I will decrease my HbA1c by 1% within 6 months."
c. "I will limit my carbohydrates to 50 g a day."
d. "I will lower my blood glucose levels to normal within 7 days."

172. The "talk test" is used to determine if a person:

a. Can describe lifestyle changes needed to control diabetes
b. Is experiencing an episode of hypoglycemia
c. Can tolerate a level of exercise
d. Can describe the steps to glucose monitoring

173. If an adolescent has diabetes, hormonal fluctuations may result in:

a. Rapid changes in medication requirements
b. Increased insulin resistance
c. Increased complications such as hypertension
d. Improved glucose control

174. A person is trying to lose weight and practices the four Ds of dealing with food cravings: (1) delay, (2) distract, (3) deep breathe, and (4):

a. Detox
b. Drink water
c. Deny
d. Define

175. During a visit with a 68-year-old man with type 2 diabetes, he and the diabetes educator discuss a physical activity goal that was set six months ago. His goal was to begin a walking program starting at 10 minutes per day and advance until he is walking 30 minutes per day at the six-month point. He rates his progress towards his goal at a "0" and says that he has not done anything since he set the goal at his visit six months ago. What is BEST next step to take with this patient?

a. Suggest that he not dwell on this failed goal and focus on a different aspect of self-management.
b. Offer the patient more time to work on his goal.
c. Discuss with the patient his motivations and barriers to achieving the goal.
d. Suggest that the goal be revised to begin with less time walking and increase the time at a slower rate.

Answer Key and Explanations for Test #1

1. B: Contemplation, characterized by a person recognizing a problem and potential benefits, yet remaining hesitant due to concerns over what the change will mean, is the stage of change that best describes this patient. He has stated that he is ready to make minor adjustments if it will help him to achieve his goal. He also qualifies that he wants to learn but is hesitant because he does not see or remember well, and he has little perceived control over his food choices. In precontemplation, patients do not yet recognize the problem or the need to make changes. In action, the person is actively engaged in the change process. In maintenance, the person works to sustain the change and help it become habit. None of these last three options apply to Mr. Jones.

2. A: "I will choose items from the restaurant menu that fit with my healthy eating plan, including vegetables, low-fat meat, and 3 servings of carbohydrates" is an appropriate, well-written behavioral objective. Behavioral objectives should begin with an action word: *choose* as opposed to *understand* or *know*. In addition, they should reflect the desired behavior, rather than the clinical outcome (e.g., lab values). Finally, they should be customized and meaningful to the patient.

3. C: Open-ended questions that cause the patient to ponder pros and cons of behavior changes empower the patient to make those changes based on good understanding. Choice A is a redundant and patronizing question. No patient wants to end up on dialysis; therefore, the purpose of this type of question is not to gain actual information from the patient or to empower, but rather to warn or badger. This type of question is likely to make the patient feel childlike and not in control. Furthermore, it is not open-ended; it is inappropriate. Choice B is a probing question that might be helpful in assessing the patient's knowledge but does not empower him to make changes. Choice D is not the best answer because it did not originate from the patient. While the goals may be appropriate, they are the educator's and not the patient's. Collaboration is important, but empowerment comes from self-identification of challenges, emotions, and solutions that lead to change.

4. D: Printed material from the drug manufacturer regarding the side effects of medications is the least likely to be helpful to Mr. Jones. First, he admits that he has poor near-sight vision and so reading may be difficult. In addition, while printed information is valuable to reinforce instruction, it does not yield the retention of more active teaching methods, including group discussion, hands-on demonstration/return demonstration, or role-playing, whether individually or in a group.

5. A: "Lose ten pounds by October 31 (3 months) by increasing walking to 25 minutes per day and limiting second helpings to just vegetables" is the best example of a SMART behavioral goal for this patient. This goal is measurable (in pounds and in minutes walked), it is attainable (not too ambitious at less than 1 pound per week), and has a time limit element (3 months). In addition, it is relevant to the patient. He states that he wants to be able to play more golf and play with his grandchildren. Modest weight loss will have a direct impact on his ability to be able to do the things he wants to do. Choice B does not speak to behavior; it is likely to be a healthcare provider goal and does not extend to what the patient wants out of life. In addition, 6% HbA1c may not be appropriate for a man his age in many cases. Choice C is too vague (improve diabetes and overall health) and too all-encompassing (doing everything learned in diabetes class). The same is true for choice D, which packs too many behaviors into one goal. It would be better to work on just one or two behaviors at a time.

6. A: Use of an insulin pen does not need to be addressed in initial DSMES; DSMES is dynamic and changes as patient needs change. The patient is newly diagnosed and is not starting on insulin. If at six months, he needs insulin, then insulin administration should be discussed at that time. Due to the risk for hypoglycemia with sulfonylureas, a hypoglycemia education should definitely be provided. Likewise, making appropriate food choices applies to anyone with diabetes, even if he claims that he does not have much control over his food since he does not cook. In addition, preventing diabetes-related complications is important information for anyone with diabetes, regardless of age or health status. Prevention topics should include checking feet daily, having regular eye exams and screening labs, monitoring blood glucose, and many others.

7. C: The glycemic index ranks foods that contain carbohydrates according to the effect that they have on blood glucose levels. Low-glycemic-index foods (scores of 55 or less) cause blood glucose levels to increase slowly, while high-glycemic-index foods (scores of 70 or greater) cause a rapid spike in glucose levels. Fruits with a low glycemic index include strawberries and other berries, cherries, grapefruit, apricots, apples, pears, oranges, plums, peaches, and grapes. However, just because a food has a low glycemic index, it does not mean that the food is healthy; for example, foods high in fat have a low glycemic index.

8. C: Assessment implies gathering and interpreting data for the purpose of directing action, whereas evaluation is to determine the extent to which an action or process was successful. Both assessment and evaluation can be clinical or non-clinical in nature. Assessment is done in initial stages of diabetes management, and it is also often performed after interventions, such as to assess a patient's progress towards a goal or assess his or her skill in checking blood glucose. The data gathered will then dictate the next steps the educator might take.

9. D: Latent autoimmune diabetes in adults (LADA, also known as type 1.5 diabetes or slow diabetes) has similarities to types 1 and 2 diabetes. Like type 1, the insulin-producing beta cells are destroyed—but more slowly—so it is usually 2–4 years before insulin is needed. This slower progression and adult onset (ages 30–50) often result in persons with LADA being misdiagnosed as having type 2 diabetes. However, LADA is usually characterized by no or mild insulin resistance, no central obesity, and no metabolic syndrome. Researchers believe that up to 20% of persons diagnosed with type 2 diabetes actually have LADA.

10. C: The American Diabetes Association (ADA) is the most comprehensive resource for education for persons with diabetes because it provides information about type 1, type 2, and gestational diabetes. The ADA provides the Patient Education Library with downloadable (PDF) guides on many topics, with titles such as "Types of Physical Activity" and "Your Mental Health and Diabetes." Information is available about diabetes, living with diabetes, diabetes and heart health, health and wellness, food and nutrition, medication management, and tools and resources.

11. C: Hyperosmolar hyperglycemic state, or very high blood glucose, is a complication of diabetes that is most common with type 2 diabetes. It usually develops over a period of days or weeks and results in intense dehydration because of increased osmolarity, but usually presents without ketoacidosis. It can be triggered by a mild infection, some medications, or more serious disorders such as heart attack. Symptoms include dry mouth, thirst, cold hands and feet, hypotension, tachycardia, nausea and vomiting, leg cramps, and mental changes (e.g., confusion, slurred speech). Management includes IV fluids and insulin and treatment for the trigger as needed.

12. B: Generally, a diabetes diagnosis (when controlled) is not a contraindication for any procedure, but it can increase some risks around surgery (infection, etc.) that must be monitored. However, high glucose readings (>550 mg/dL) such as those that occur in DKA and HHS, are indicators that non-emergency procedures should be delayed in order to first stabilize the patient's glucose and associated complications that arise secondary to the high glucose levels.

13. D: The target for critically ill patients should be between 140 and 180 mg/dL. While lower targets may be appropriate in some cases, targets less than 110 mg/dL are no longer recommended, due to evidence that lower glucose levels resulted in increased mortality among critically ill patients. For non-critically ill patients, the recommended pre-meal target is <140 mg/dL (not <100 mg/dL); targets for random BG (non-critically ill) <180 mg/dL (not <140 mg/dL). Again, lower targets may be advisable for certain patients, but targets less than 100 mg/dL are not recommended.

14. D: It is essential to tailor education to a person's needs, especially if there are cultural differences. Those in many Asian cultures, including Chinese, commonly defer to those in authority, such as healthcare providers, and they may avoid questioning or admitting that they do not understand, as an act of respect. The CDCES should never accept agreement or lack of questioning as understanding, but should instead ask the client to explain and return demonstrate to ensure that she comprehends. Additionally, if there are language barriers, the CDCES should provide a translator.

15. C: Milking the lanced finger at the tip can obstruct blood flow. In addition, it may skew the results by increasing the amount of interstitial fluid in the sample. A patient should milk the finger closer to the base of the finger and move towards the tip, or milk the finger before lancing. All other choices are acceptable actions. Soap and water is preferred over alcohol, as alcohol is unnecessary and may actually skew the sample. Puncture depth may be set to the patient's preference as long as a sufficient drop is produced. The shallower the depth setting, the less pain there will be. Patients should be encouraged to use a system of recording results that fits them best.

16. D: Apidra (insulin glulisine) is classified as rapid-acting insulin. It is designed for mealtime insulin coverage and to correct hyperglycemia. The only other choice that is in this class and designed for these purposes is insulin lispro (Humalog). Novolin 70/30 is a mix of NPH and regular (an intermediate and a short-acting insulin). Levemir (detemir) is a long-acting insulin, which is in the same class as the patient's Lantus (glargine) insulin. Because her insurance will cover Lantus, there is no need to switch her at this point to detemir. Humulin-N (NPH) is an intermediate-acting insulin. It is very different from Apidra and is not typically recommended for mealtime and correction proposes.

17. D: The proper use of the blood glucose meter along with a personalized monitoring schedule would be the priority item to discuss at the visit. Mrs. M has already expressed concern that she is not sure if she is using the meter correctly and that she is not sure when she should test. She has demonstrated by her actions that she is willing to monitor, and is ready for guidance in this area. Discussing diabetes-related complications is too broad and potentially overwhelming for a first discussion. Because the patient has not questioned the meaning of her HbA1c results, it is a topic that could be reserved for comprehensive diabetes education at a later time. Insulin administration does not apply to this patient at this time.

18. A: Based on the given information, group diabetes self-management education makes the most sense. Education plans should be individualized. While any of the first three options are valid ways to provide diabetes education, Mrs. M is a "sociable" person, and does not have any conditions or characteristics that would warrant one-on-one education. Group education is cost-effective, and also allows for interaction with group members as well as the educator, unlike printed information.

In addition, research shows that group education can be just as satisfying and clinically effective as one-on-one education, if not more so.

19. B: The patient has admitted that she misses her evening dose of metformin about half the time. Reducing the number of missed doses is a goal that targets a specific behavior—taking medication. The educator can help her devise ways to remember to take her medication and set up a plan for reporting her progress. In addition, it is a goal that is not overwhelming. Other options, such as losing 10 pounds, reducing HbA1c, and reducing the risk of complications, are outcomes that come from achieving specific behavioral goals, such as reducing portion sizes, taking medication more consistently, scheduling appropriate screening appointments, walking 150 minutes per week, etc.

20. C: A referral to a registered dietitian for medical nutrition therapy is recommended as a standard of care for all persons with diabetes. The American Diabetes Association recommends that individuals who have prediabetes or diabetes should receive individualized medical nutrition therapy (MNT) as needed to achieve treatment goals, preferably provided by a registered dietitian familiar with the components of diabetes MNT. It is recommended that this referral be made as part of the comprehensive diabetes evaluation. In additional to being a recommended standard of care for all, MNT is particularly appropriate for this patient because she is overweight and has expressed concern about changes to her diet. A dilated eye exam with an ophthalmologist is definitely warranted because she has been diagnosed with type 2 diabetes, but the patient has already scheduled a retinal exam. Finally, mental health referral at this point is premature. Mrs. M's reactions and concerns are normal and expected. There is no indication that her psychological state is interfering with her abilities to learn about her diabetes or perform self-care activities. However, it would be wise to conduct a depression screening at this and future visits, especially if she exhibits signs that her mental and psychological health are suffering.

21. D: The medication regimen is the most important factor to consider when assessing risk for hypoglycemia in relation to exercise. Insulin and insulin secretagogues are the greatest risk factor; in the absence any of these medications, risk for hypoglycemia with exercise is low. For patients who use these medications, food intake may be adjusted and careful consideration should be given to preventing, predicting, recognizing, and treating hypoglycemia.

22. B: Tests used to confirm a diagnosis of diabetes include:

Test	Normal	Prediabetes	Diabetes
HbA1c	<5.7%	5.7–6.4%	≥6.5%
FPG	<100 mg/dL	100–125 mg/dl	≥126 mg/dL
OGTT	<140 mg/dL	140–199 mg/dL	≥200 mg/dL
Random plasma glucose	Any time with symptoms		≥200 mg/dL

23. C: "Treat the blood sugar as one would any low blood sugar, and then once it is in the normal range, take the regular dose of insulin and eat the regular meal" is the correct option. Choice A is the course patients often take, but not only does this *not* address the immediate need to treat the hypoglycemia, it leads to hyperglycemia later because the meal consumed still requires insulin. Choice B is incorrect for the same reason. In addition, taking insulin after a meal puts a person at risk for hypoglycemia hours later when the food has metabolized but the insulin is still peaking. Choice D is incorrect because no one should ever take insulin while experiencing a hypoglycemic reaction. The first priority is always to treat the hypoglycemia.

24. A: Commencement, which involves determining when the exercise plan should start, is not part of the standard exercise prescription, although it is important when helping patients set physical activity goals. The five components of an exercise prescription are: mode (what type of activity will be performed), intensity, frequency, duration, and progression. The exercise prescription is a plan the patient follows to improve physical fitness. The challenge for the clinician is to design a plan that meets the patient's desired fitness goals.

25. B: A systematic process is required for effective continuous quality improvement (CQI). Once a problem has been identified, the next step is to analyze the data to determine what the root of the problem may be. In this case, the educator made the assumption that participants wanted more information on the mechanisms of action of oral medications. In fact, it may have been that there was too much information, the information was not applicable, the class was too long, or any other of a large number of reasons. Without further analysis, time, effort, and other resources may be spent in the wrong way. There is no indication that incomplete explanation of the idea to the CQI team resulted in poor satisfaction. Likewise, most patient satisfaction tools that simply ask participants to share in some way how satisfied they were presents an accurate reflection of this metric. Finally, the educator's proposed change may have been the correct solution for dissatisfaction that resulted from not enough information on medication mechanisms of action. While creativity is very valuable in some circumstances, sometimes the solution can be straightforward if the cause of the problem is clearly identified.

26. D: One of the most common reasons for hypoglycemia unawareness is repeated low blood glucose levels. This person is on a strict glucose control regimen, so the most appropriate intervention is to increase the fasting blood glucose target, for example, from a high of 130 mg/dL to 140 mg/dL or more. This may involve a change in the dosage of the long-acting insulin. With fewer episodes of hypoglycemia, people tend to become more aware of acute symptoms when they do occur.

27. A: Persons with diabetes should normally avoid 16-hour fasting because it can result in fluctuating blood glucose levels, hyperglycemia during eating hours (especially if the person overeats carbohydrates), and hypoglycemia during fasting hours. Since the person is taking glipizide, a sulfonylurea, this increases the risk of episodes of hypoglycemia. Studies regarding the benefits of fasting regimens vary, but any person considering fasting should be advised to talk with a physician and dietician before starting. Persons participating in fasting should check their blood glucose levels frequently.

28. D: A financial barrier is the most probable obstacle facing this patient, based on the limited information available. The patient takes her medication consistently, but cuts the expensive name-brand pill in half. She was willing to add more vegetables, but not the pricier fresh vegetables. Of course, the clinician should never assume a barrier without having an honest, frank discussion with the patient first. A transportation barrier might be the case since she only uses canned vegetables (perhaps to not need to travel to the store as often), but this does not explain why she cuts only one of her medicines in half. There is no evidence of a cultural or cognitive barrier in the information provided, although again, these should not be ruled out without talking to the patient first.

29. A: The US Pharmacopoeia, through their Dietary Supplement Verification Program, verifies that the products listed on the label are accurate and pure. The mark does not indicate FDA approval, efficacy, or safety from drug interactions.

30. B: If there is a large discrepancy between a person's recorded blood glucose levels and insulin and the results of laboratory tests, the CDCES should suspect that the person is falsifying recordkeeping by recording a target blood glucose level when, in fact, the real level was higher, or the person is recording blood glucose levels but not actually checking them. The person may be careless, lack a good understanding of the importance of diabetic control, or be avoiding the use of insulin for various reasons, such as to lose weight or to avoid taking injections.

31. D: Some studies have indicated that caffeine increases insulin resistance in persons with type 2 diabetes, leading to an increase in the blood glucose level by as much as 8%. This occurs because caffeine stimulates the release of hormones, such as epinephrine, that inhibit the effects of insulin. Despite this, some studies suggest that people who routinely drink black coffee may have a decreased risk of developing type 2 diabetes. Persons with diabetes should be advised to have a moderate intake of caffeine.

32. B: "Limiting the specialized skill of providing evidence-based diabetes education to healthcare professionals who are certified as diabetes educators" is not an advocacy goal identified by the Association of Diabetes Care and Education Specialists. In fact, the ADCES recognizes five levels of diabetes educators, only the top two of which are certified as professional diabetes educators. Levels 1 through 3 include non-healthcare professionals such as volunteers that may assist with support groups, healthcare professionals not functioning in roles as diabetes educators, and non-credentialed diabetes educators, respectively. Choices A, C, and D are three of the six advocacy goals. The other goals are: providing ADCES members with tools and resources to stay engaged in public policy and be better equipped to advocate on their own behalf, supporting programs and initiatives that detect diabetes or serve to prevent more people from developing the disease, and educating Congress, state legislators, and other professional organizations and stakeholders about ADCES's advocacy priorities.

33. D: Aspartame, neotame, and stevia have all been shown to be safe, and are approved for use even during pregnancy/breastfeeding, according to the FDA. There is no contraindication for pregnant/breastfeeding women for aspartame, saccharin, neotame, or any others of the approved nonnutritive sweeteners.

34. C: With type 1 diabetes, when 80–90% of beta islet cells in the pancreas are destroyed, the person develops hyperglycemia. Without adequate insulin, there is no inhibition of the conversion of glycogen to glucose by the liver or the synthesis of glucose from amino acids and fats, so the blood glucose levels continue to increase. Common symptoms occurring at this point include polydipsia, polyuria, high urinary frequency, and unintentional weight loss. Typically, glucose begins to spill into the urine when the blood glucose level is greater than 200 mg/dL.

35. C: Hypoglycemia is classified as level 1 (mild), level 2 (moderate), or level 3 (severe) according to the following:

Level	Blood Glucose	Symptoms	Treatment
1	54–70 mg/dL (3.0–3.9 mmol/L)	Sweating, shaking, hunger	Rapid-acting carbohydrates
2	<54 mg/dL (3 mmol/L)	Confusion, changes in behavior, difficulty speaking	Rapid-acting carbohydrates, monitor, call for help if needed
3	Characterized by symptoms	Severe cognitive impairment, seizures, loss of consciousness, coma	Call for help immediately, glucagon or IV glucose

36. C: The safe range for exercise is generally a blood glucose level of 100–250 mg/dL (5.6–13.9 mmol/L). If the person's blood glucose is lower than 100 mg/dL, there is a risk of developing hypoglycemia, so 15–30 mg of carbohydrate should be eaten before the beginning of exercise. If the blood glucose level is greater than 250 mg/dL (13.9 mmol/L), then exercising may not be safe, and the urine should be checked for ketones. If ketones are present, then there is insufficient insulin and a risk for ketoacidosis.

37. A: The HbA1c screening is recommended at least twice annually for patients who meet glycemic guidelines, in this case less than 7%. The other screenings listed—a comprehensive foot exam, dilated eye exam, and fasting lipid profile—are indicated once yearly for a patient with these characteristics. A lipid profile may be performed every two years for those with very low risk, but since this patient has had borderline LDL levels, the screening should be done annually.

38. A: A glucose level of 92 mg/dL by itself is not alarming; however, if the continuous glucose monitor (CGM) indicates that the trend is falling, then the person is at risk of developing hypoglycemia and should immediately ingest rapid-acting carbohydrates, such as candy, glucose tablets, or fruit juice. If the device shows that the trend is level or rising, no immediate response is needed. If the person fails to take action, he or she may become confused or dizzy or may even lose consciousness and not be able to respond adequately.

39. D: "Walk briskly for 25 minutes every day following dinner" is a behavioral goal that is relevant and attainable for most patients with the above health history. Position statements and ADA recommendations stipulate that 150 minutes (spread over three days with no more than 2 consecutive days without exercise) of moderate intensity, such as brisk walking, is the minimum goal for patients with type 2 diabetes. Choice A is such a low bar that it fails to be relevant for the patient. Choices B and C are too aggressive and are likely not attainable for a patient with the characteristics of someone who is sedentary and overweight.

40. A: "Decrease intake of regular soda from three cans to one can per day by Dec. 1" is a specific behavioral objective/goal because it stipulates the details of what will be done, including going from what amount to what amount and by what date. Choices B, C, and D all have elements that could be considered ambiguous: what will be done to decrease cardiovascular risk; how glycemic control will be measured; and how overall health, better eating/rest, and movement will be measured, respectively.

41. D: The rating of perceived exertion (RPE) is a subjective rating in which the patient estimates their exertion level based on feelings of effort and fatigue. The original scale rates perceived exertion from 6 to 20, with moderate/vigorous intensity equating to a 12 to 16 on the scale. Choices A and C are not actual intensity estimation tools. If these were tools, they would not be "perceived" since the estimate would be based on actual measurements. An actual method that is similar is the heart rate reserve (HHR), which uses a formula to calculate 55 to 90 percent of the maximum heart rate. This method can be very confusing for those with limited literacy/numeracy abilities. Choice B actually describes the "talk test," which would be another appropriate intensity estimation method to use with this patient.

42. A: Because a patient with type 1 diabetes needs to fast before a surgery, the short-acting insulin is typically omitted or reduced significantly on the morning of a surgery, while the long-acting drug is continued to prevent hyperglycemia from occurring. For patients taking oral diabetic medications, the dose is usually held the morning of surgery. It is especially important to verify with diabetic patients what medications they have taken before being admitted to the presurgical area.

43. B: Inviting the client's wife to help recall what he ate yesterday would be appropriate in this case. Family members can often be helpful when gathering information for the assessment. If the educator was testing his diabetes knowledge and the patient was unable to answer a question, then "patient does not recall" should be noted and choice A would be appropriate, but the educator is seeking to find out what the client actually ate. A 24-hour dietary recall is an appropriate tool in some cases, but the initial assessment is more of an overview, and the information can be provided by means less burdensome to the patient. Finally, choice D would not ever be appropriate because of the use of a patronizing title and question.

44. D: The Academy of Nutrition and Dietetics recommends the following guidelines for macronutrients for diabetic diets:

- Carbohydrates: 45–60% of daily calories, focusing on complex carbohydrates with fiber and carbohydrate counting to manage blood glucose levels. Carbohydrates have the most impact on blood glucose levels.
- Proteins: 15–20% of daily calories with protein at every meal. Protein has minimal effect on blood glucose levels.
- Fats: 20–35% of daily calories, focusing on unsaturated fats and limited saturated fats and trans fats. Fats have no direct effect on blood glucose levels.

45. C: Keeping a physical activity log was associated with a higher level of self-efficacy in a small-scale 2006 study. Those in the recordkeeping group did not have significantly higher levels of physical activity than those who did not keep a record over the six-week intervention period. They did, however, report feeling positive about recordkeeping, stating that it helped them to think more about personal activity and that it was not overly time-consuming. There is no evidence that activity recordkeeping is associated with increased regimen adherence, gym membership or class enrollment, or perceived barriers to physical activity.

46. D: The primary factor in the development of diabetic foot ulcers is peripheral neuropathy. Patients may experience pain in the foot, but they also often have reduced sensation or numbness, which can result in injury that goes undetected, allowing ulceration. Neuropathy can also affect the mechanics of walking so that one's weight is distributed unequally, leading to anatomic changes. Other factors that can lead to diabetic foot ulcers include trauma and anatomic abnormalities.

47. D: The Somogyi effect is believed to occur when an evening dose of insulin is too high, hypoglycemia occurs, and this results in a rebound of hyperglycemia in the morning because the hypoglycemia stimulates the release of hormones (e.g., adrenaline, corticosteroids, growth hormone) as a compensatory mechanism, causing the liver to convert stored glycogen to glucose and to release it into the bloodstream. The Somogyi effect is considered to be just a theory, although there is evidence to support it; it must be differentiated from the dawn phenomenon.

48. C: It is not necessary for a person with diabetes to eat every time he or she drives. However, if the person is at risk for a hypoglycemia reaction, such as by recently exercising or if his or her insulin is scheduled to peak, then this may become an important action. Patients should always check their glucose before operating a vehicle; they should never operate a vehicle if a reading is close to hypoglycemic. Other safety precautions include wearing medical identification, stopping every one to two hours to monitor, and carrying testing supplies and a source of glucose.

49. A: Prediabetes is a condition in which blood glucose levels are higher than they should be but the person lacks symptoms of diabetes. Persons with prediabetes often have signs of metabolic syndrome, which is characterized by:

- Insulin resistance/increased blood glucose: fasting blood glucose ≥100 mg/dL
- Abdominal obesity: waist circumference >40 inches (102 cm) for males and >35 inches (88 cm) for females
- Hypertension: blood pressure >130/85 mmHg (or taking medications to decrease blood pressure)
- Dyslipidemia: triglycerides ≥150 mg/dL (or taking medication to decrease the level) and/or high-density lipoproteins (HDLs) <40 mg/dL for males and <50 mg/dL for females

50. C: Acknowledge his reluctance and ask if he might be willing to share some of his knowledge and experiences with the other class members. By acknowledging his emotional state, the educator validates his feelings, which will help him feel that the educator is not his opponent. By asking him to share his knowledge, the diabetes educator invites him to participate in a way that does not contradict his perception but will still allow him to experience the class. Choice A is sometimes appropriate if the patient insists that he will not attend (if choice C fails), but the patient should not be dismissed so easily. Choice B puts the person on the defensive, and may possibly embarrass him. This will damage rapport between the patient and the clinician and he will be less likely to want to attend. Choice D is avoiding/deflecting the clinician's responsibility and puts the spouse in the middle of the educator patient-relationship.

51. C: It is true that the risk of complications such as congenital abnormalities and spontaneous abortions decreases if the woman with diabetes has optimal glycemic control at the time of conception. If the HbA1c level is less than 7%, the rates are similar to that of the non-diabetic population. All other choices are untrue. Far less than half of all women with diabetes (one study showed 37%) receive preconception counseling. The first priority of preconception counseling for patients wishing to conceive is glucose control, although achieving healthy pre-pregnancy weight may be a goal as well. Some medications, including statins, are contraindicated in pregnancy. Therefore, preconception counseling should include a careful review of medications and discontinuation of any medications that are teratogenic.

52. B: A recent evidence-based practice recommendation and an example of translating research into practice is that unvaccinated adults with diabetes who are aged 19–59 years should receive hepatitis B vaccination. For those aged 60 and over, vaccination may be considered but was not found to be as cost-effective, so it is left to the discretion of the patient's physician. All of the other answer choices are not current recommendations, according to the ADA Standards of Care, due to insufficient evidence.

53. A: Some published studies comparing lower levels of carbohydrate intake (ranging from 21 g daily up to 40% of daily energy intake) to higher carbohydrate intake levels indicated improved markers of glycemic control and insulin sensitivity with lower carbohydrate intakes. However, four randomized, controlled trials found no significant differences in glycemic markers with a lower-carbohydrate diet compared with higher carbohydrate intake levels. In addition, several trials resulted in improvements in lipid levels, but many trials also suffered from low retention. Safety of low-carb, high-protein diets for those with renal dysfunction is not known and should therefore not be recommended.

54. C: Maturity-onset diabetes of the young (MOBY) is a rare hereditary (autosomal dominant) type of diabetes that is often misdiagnosed as type 1diabetes, sometimes resulting in unnecessary insulin administration, or type 2 diabetes, resulting in ineffective treatment with metformin. Onset is at age 25 years or younger. Typical characteristics are mild to moderate hyperglycemia but an absence of obesity, metabolic syndrome, or ketoacidosis. There are six subtypes: MOBY 1 and 3 are sensitive to sulfonylureas, MOBY 2 often requires only lifestyle changes, MOBY 4 and 5 usually require insulin, and MOBY 6 may respond to both insulin and oral hypoglycemic agents depending on its severity.

55. C: Like insulin, a sulfonylurea can cause postexercise hypoglycemia, so persons taking the medication should avoid exercising before or during its peak action, which is 2–4 hours after ingestion. Additionally, a 15–30 g carbohydrate snack should be eaten before exercising—or even more if the exercising session lasts for more than 1 hour. A physician may recommend splitting the sulfonylurea dose into smaller amounts or decreasing the dosage altogether on the day of exercise. If episodes of hypoglycemia persist, then an alternative medication may be considered.

56. A: Because this person's stress reaction is to worry to such an extent that it is interfering with her sleep, the best stress reduction technique is likely mindfulness-based meditation. It may be the most useful technique listed because it helps one focus the mind and become aware of the mind's activity without judgment in order to alleviate obsessive thoughts and worries. Meditation may focus on a single object, all thoughts and feelings, kindness to self, or body awareness. Mindful walking, listening, or breathing may also be practiced.

57. C: A reduced-calorie, reduced-fat diet is the primary recommended dietary strategy for those with prediabetes. Not only has this strategy been shown effective for modest weight loss, but the reduction in fat may also improve insulin sensitivity. Low-carb diets for the primary prevention of diabetes are not recommended at this time. Carbohydrate monitoring is a strategy that is recommended for persons with diabetes but not at this time for those with prediabetes. Glycemic index/glycemic load strategies remain unproven at this time and are not recommended as a diabetes prevention strategy.

58. C: The ADA's 2026 Standards emphasize the consideration of social determinants of health when creating treatment plans for patients with diabetes. Of focus were food insecurity, homelessness/housing insecurity, migrant and seasonal agricultural workers, language barriers, health literacy, and social capital/community support. While limited time to see the provider may be a barrier to care, it is not considered a social determinant of health. As an effort to identify and address these determinants of health, the ADA recommends that the diabetes educator assess for these elements and then apply the findings to the patient's treatment plan.

59. C: Medications are the specialty of pharmacists. They are trained to consider the dose, timing, drug interactions, side effects, and contraindications of all prescription medications, including those for diseases other than diabetes, as well as over-the-counter drugs and supplements such as vitamins. If this patient has a healthcare team with an assigned pharmacist, then the pharmacist would be the best person to address this patient's medication-related concerns. That team member can then communicate any problems with the regimen to the rest of the team. Most likely, many providers have prescribed the medications in this patient's regimen, which would make it difficult to address all of her concerns at once. Without a physical complaint or a follow-up, an "educational" appointment may be difficult to have covered by insurance. A mental health visit is not indicated either, as her concerns are very appropriate under the circumstances and no anxiety treatment is likely necessary. While an RD/CDCES is likely informed about the diabetes regimen medications, he or she may not be able to answer all of the patient's questions about how they interact with the medications for the other conditions. If the concern were primarily dietary, then this may be the best choice. However, other team members should be made aware of the patient's concerns as well as any changes made to the regimen.

60. B: Persons with diabetes should maintain their low-density lipoprotein (LDL) level at less than 100 mg/dL. In some cases, if the person has cardiovascular disease, statins may be prescribed to lower the LDL level to 70 mg/dL or less. A high LDL level contributes to the buildup of plaque in the arteries and to endothelial damage, which furthers inflammation and plaque buildup, resulting in atherosclerosis, which increases the risk of cardiovascular disease, including myocardial infarction, coronary artery disease, and stroke. High-density lipoprotein (HDL) levels should be maintained at or above 40 mg/dL for males and at or above 50 mg/dL for females. Triglyceride levels should be less than 150 mg/dL.

61. D: Hypertension is the condition that will suffer the most from the patient's meal due to the high sodium content. Choice A, hyperlipidemia, is addressed due to the low amount of saturated fat. Choice B, type 2 diabetes, is addressed due to the moderate amount of carbohydrates (about 50 grams). Choice C, obesity, is also addressed by the reasonable number of total calories in the meal.

62. A: A turkey and cheese, lettuce, and tomato sandwich with an apple, a small serving of baked chips, and a diet soda is the best example of a *well-balanced* meal. This choice has an appropriate balance of carbohydrate, fat, and protein; the serving sizes are appropriate and fruits and vegetables are included. The sample meals in choices B and C may be healthy in some ways (low fat, low calorie, etc.), but are not well balanced, as they contain almost no carbohydrate. Conversely, the meal choice in option D is almost entirely carbs (with more than 120 grams of carbohydrate).

63. D: The American Diabetes Association recommends a diagnosis of diabetes be made when a person's HbA1c level is ≥6.5% only when "performed using a method that is certified by the NGSP and standardized or traceable to the Diabetes Control and Complications Trial (DCCT) reference assay." In addition, it is recommended that any lab test used to diagnose be repeated to rule out lab error.

64. A: The ADA stresses that there is not one diet that fits all persons with diabetes; rather, there are seven different approaches, depending on the dietary goal: Mediterranean, vegetarian/vegan, low fat, very low fat, low carbohydrate, very low carbohydrate, and the Dietary Approaches to Stop Hypertension (DASH) diet. The low-carbohydrate diet helps reduce the patient's HbA1c, facilitate weight loss, lower blood pressure, lower triglyceride levels, and increase HDL. This diet encourages the use of healthy fats (such as olive oil), nonstarchy vegetables, protein, and limited quantities of carbohydrates, which are restricted to 26–45% of total calories.

65. C: The target time in range for CGMs is usually 70%, meaning that the glucose readings should stay within the desired range 70% of the time. The target glucose range is typically 70–180 mg/dL (3.9–10.0 mmol/L). Instead of measuring the glucose in the blood, CGMs measure glucose in the interstitial fluid; however, the level of glucose in the blood and in the interstitial fluid is usually very similar. With most CGMs, the sensor, applied to an arm or on the abdomen, contains a tiny filament that is inserted under the skin and transmits data to a smartphone.

66. A: Persons with diabetes and kidney disease should focus on maintaining a low intake of high-quality proteins, such as lean meats, plant-based proteins, fish, and eggs; they should also carefully balance carbohydrate and protein intake to maintain adequate blood glucose levels. Those on hemodialysis and peritoneal dialysis require a higher protein intake.

Diabetes-Related Kidney Disorder	Protein Intake (Grams/Kilogram/Day)
Predialysis CKD (stages 1–4)	0.6–0.8
Hemodialysis	1.0–1.2
Peritoneal dialysis	1.2–1.3
Acute kidney injury	0.8–1.5
Post kidney transplant	1.0–1.2 postoperatively; 0.8–1.0 maintenance

67. C: The best choice of an example of individualization of making better food choices is to switch to diet soda and sugar-free ice cream. Individualizing can be accomplished by asking a patient, "What specifically does this statement mean to you?" Making better choices to reduce HbA1c may describe the ultimate purpose for the behavioral goal, just as "over the next six months" specifies the time-specific aspect, but they do not speak to what "making better food choices" will mean to the patient's current eating routine. Reporting to the educator is a good example of breaking the goal down and helping the patient to be accountable, but again, it does not describe the behavioral goal in personal terms. Goals should be individualized so that the patient knows just what actions to take. Furthermore, individualized goals should be documented in the most patient-specific terms to facilitate adjustment to the education and plan of care, communication between healthcare team members, and to demonstrate adherence to the guidelines.

68. D: CGM is especially important for persons with type 1 diabetes but should also be used by persons with type 2 diabetes on insulin, because of the risk of complications due to glycemic variability. A person may stay within a target HbA1c and still have episodes of hyperglycemia, hypoglycemia, and glycemic variability, and regular blood glucose monitoring may not detect these fluctuations. Therefore, the HbA1c and blood glucose results should be compared to the results of at least 14 days of CGM use with the monitoring occurring at least 70% of the time.

69. B: According to the CDC, persons with diabetes should go to the emergency department if:

- They are unable to keep fluids down for more than 4 hours or unable to keep food down for more than 24 hours.
- They lose 5 or more pounds during the course of the illness.
- They have severe vomiting and diarrhea for more than 6 hours.
- Their blood glucose level is less than 60 mg/dL.
- Their temperature stays higher than 101 °F (38.3 °C) for more than 24 hours.
- Their urine is positive for ketones.
- Their breathing has become difficult.

70. D: Protein is critical for wound healing, and because one's metabolic rate increases in response to a wound, protein needs also increase. Dietary protein requirements for wound healing are higher than normal—in a range of 1.25–1.5 g/kg/day. A patient weighing 150 lb (68 kg) would usually require approximately 60 g of protein daily, but that need increases to 85–102 g daily for wound healing, so the patient would need to markedly increase his or her intake of high-protein foods or take dietary supplements.

71. C: If a person's fasting glucose numbers are good in the morning but spike after dinner, then he or she likely needs to decrease carbohydrate intake at dinner. Glucose levels should be monitored before and after dinner a few times to determine how much of the spike relates to the meal. As an alternative to decreasing carbohydrates at dinner, the person may consider engaging in exercise, such as a brisk walk—for at least 30 minutes—after dinner.

72. A: Low-impact exercises improve circulation and help patients manage their blood glucose levels without placing an excessive strain on their feet and legs or increasing the risk of injury. Low-impact exercises that are appropriate for persons with diabetic neuropathy include:

- Walking: Persons should wear properly fitted shoes and begin with a short distance.
- Swimming/water aerobics: Water provides resistance but reduces pressure on the feet and legs. Water shoes should be worn.
- Cycling: Persons with balance problems should use a stationary bicycle; cycling provides non–weight-bearing movement for the legs and feet to improve circulation.
- Yoga, Tai Chi: These provide low-impact and gentle exercise.

73. B: The daily value (DV) of sodium is based on the maximum allowance of 2,300 mg per day for a healthy adult. When reviewing the food label for a product, those with 5% or less of the DV are considered low in sodium while those with 20% or more of the DV are considered high in sodium. For example, if a product has 25% of the DV for sodium, this translates into 575 mg of sodium for just that one serving, and if the serving size is smaller than the average person eats or drinks, then the actual sodium content may be much higher.

74. B: Wrist blood pressure monitors can be accurate if they are positioned and used correctly; however, they are more difficult to use than upper-arm monitors. If the wrist is below the heart, the blood pressure reading will be too high; and, if the wrist is above the heart, the blood pressure reading will be too low. It can be difficult for some people to keep the wrist at heart level during monitoring. The first thing the CDCES should do is observe the person measuring their blood pressure and ask about the usual positioning. Automated upper-arm monitors are the most accurate and are recommended for persons with diabetes. Finger monitors are the least accurate.

75. B: Erectile dysfunction is the most common sexual dysfunction associated with diabetes in males, occurring in 35–75% of males with diabetes, with risk increasing with age. It occurs up to 15 years earlier in males with diabetes than in males in the general population. Prevention includes good control of blood glucose levels, blood pressure, and cholesterol levels, as well as maintaining a healthy diet and engaging in regular exercise. Males should avoid smoking—which in itself is a significant risk factor for erectile dysfunction—and limit alcohol intake to reduce their risk.

76. B: Changing Jeff's insulin-to-carb ratio from 10 to 12 for lunch and dinner only is the correct option. Because his episodes of low blood glucose do not occur before meals, it is not likely that the basal rate is too high. Likewise, the sensitivity factor would be modified if the patient reported hypoglycemia after correcting for high glucose. Finally, changing the insulin-to-carb ratio from 10 to 8 would actually give the patient more insulin at mealtime, which would likely make the pattern of post-meal hypoglycemia worse.

77. A: Conversation maps would be the best choice for this situation for several reasons. Group interaction activities, such as conversation maps, have proven to facilitate learning to a greater extent than passive-learning strategies. In all likelihood, most of the residents can still participate in a discussion-type activity without too much trouble, even with deficits in sight, mobility, or dexterity. A strategy such as this allows those with varying amounts of knowledge/experience to participate equally. Choice B assumes that all participants will be familiar with how to use laptops. If this proves not to be the case, then the diabetes educator will spend much of their time on computer training. Choice C might be good to leave for follow-up, but will not yield the learning that discussion does, and participants won't have the option of bringing up their individual concerns. Choice D does not engage participants and does not allow for much adaptation to the individual needs within the group.

78. C: "Run 20 minutes at least 3 times per week" can be measured by the patient, both in terms of minutes per run and number of runs per week. To achieve goals, patients need to be able to track progress in a measurable way. Choice B is not stated in a way in which the achievement can be measured. It could be re-written to be measurable, though, by including minutes on a treadmill or number of miles run. Similarly, choice A, "improve diabetes control by managing my portion size," needs to be specified in terms that can be measured (e.g., no more than 60 grams of carbohydrate per meal), as does choice D, "keeping my ophthalmology appointments," which should include information such as how many appointments or how often.

79. A: Insulin pumps typically use only rapid-acting insulin, such as aspart, glulisine, and lispro. Rapid-acting insulin is used to provide basal insulin and boluses because the goal is to mimic the natural release of insulin from the pancreas. Insulin is administered continuously at preset rates. Boluses are administered for meals depending on the patient's insulin-to-carbohydrate ratio and the planned carbohydrate intake. Insulin pumps depend on either frequent glucose monitoring or a CGM system.

80. D: According to American Diabetes Association Standards of Care, patients with blood pressure greater than 120/80 mmHg should be advised on lifestyle changes to reduce blood pressure. Patients with confirmed blood pressure ≥130/80 mmHg should "have prompt initiation and timely subsequent titration of pharmacological therapy to achieve blood pressure goals." People with diabetes should be treated to a blood pressure of <130/80 mmHg, but some persons (such as younger patients) may benefit from lower targets. Choice A, ≥150/90 mmHg, is higher than the indicated threshold for hypertensive pharmacological treatment and much higher than the recommended threshold of 120/80 mmHg for lifestyle change recommendations.

81. A: Visual and tactile/dexterity issues are a possible concern for this patient. She squints and is not attempting to complete the written paperwork, which may indicate that she cannot see well. Her shaking hands indicate that small movements, such as those needed to check blood sugar, administer insulin, or even hold a pen, could be tricky. Choice B is not the best choice because the diabetes educator has no reason to suspect a hearing impairment based on these observations. Likewise, she has not given indications thus far of a financial barrier or a cultural barrier. While the educator should not rule out the possibilities of other learning barriers, choice A is the best choice because the educator has already seen indications that these may be present.

82. A: 2026 ADA standards include the possibility for a diagnosis of hypertension with a reading of ≥180/110 mmHg at a single healthcare visit. Otherwise, an elevated blood pressure of ≥130/80 mmHg requires confirmation with a second visit on a separate day in order to qualify for a diagnosis of hypertension. Guidelines recommend screening blood pressure at every healthcare visit, in addition to advising all patients with hypertension to self-monitor their blood pressure at home.

83. D: The primary focus in coaching should be on using questioning to help learners recognize their problem areas. Coaching can include specific training, providing career information, and confronting issues of concern. Other effective methods of coaching include:

- Giving positive feedback, stressing what the learner is doing right
- Providing demonstrations and opportunities for question/answer periods

- Providing regular progress reports so the learner understands areas of concern
- Assisting the learner to establish personal goals for improvement
- Providing resources to help the learner master the material

84. C: According to the National Standards for Diabetes Self-Management Education and Support, behavioral change is essential for persons with diabetes to manage their disease. One of the primary roles of the CDCES is to facilitate behavior change through education, monitoring, and support. Persons with diabetes need to develop healthy habits in relation to diet, exercise, adherence to the medication regimen, and blood glucose monitoring. The CDCES must recognize the emotional burden of living with diabetes that can make self-management difficult and should provide ongoing support.

85. D: None of the patients described require reduced-protein diets. Protein intake of 0.8–1.0 g/kg/day is in the normal range. Pregnant women are recommended to have a protein intake of 1.1 g/kg/day, so the current intake may actually need to be increased. Similarly, those with serious wounds should have a protein intake of 1.0–1.5 g/kg/day. Finally, according to ADA Nutrition Therapy Recommendations, for people with diabetes and diabetic kidney disease, reducing the amount of dietary protein below the usual intake is not recommended because it does not alter glycemic measures, cardiovascular risk measures, or the course of glomerular filtration rate (GFR) decline.

86. B: Web-based activities, role-playing, group discussion, and lecture is a series of appropriate strategies that are ranked in terms of smallest group (individual) to largest. Choice A is not the best choice because games usually involve more than one person, and demonstration is difficult to do in a large group. Choice C lists lecture before demonstration; lecture is not usually the best choice for a small group, while demonstration is. Choice D also lists lecture before printed material. Again, lecture is best used when the group is too large to provide more interaction, and printed materials are designed for one person (as reinforcement) rather than group instruction.

87. B: This person fits the typical profile of a person with obstructive sleep apnea:

- Middle age (40–70): 53 years old
- Gender: Incidence is two to three times higher in males than in females.
- Overweight (BMI >30 kg/m^2): BMI 32 kg/m^2
- Upper airway anatomy (i.e., having a thick neck): Stocky build
- Snoring: As noted by the spouse
- Daytime sleepiness: During the daytime and when sedentary. Client reports 8 hours of sleep per night, but persons with obstructive sleep apnea are often unaware that they awaken repeatedly during the night.
- Morning headaches: Frequent
- Comorbid condition: Type 2 diabetes

88. A: Charcot arthropathy is a progressive joint disorder of the foot and ankle triggered by neuropathy that reduces sensation to the feet, and is often associated with diabetes. If a minor injury occurs, the person may not be aware or may avoid treatment because of the lack of pain. The initial symptoms are typically edema and erythema, but fractures and dislocations can develop, which can result in severe deformities, including the typical "rocker-bottom" foot. The three stages of Charcot arthropathy are:

- Pain, redness, and swelling, potentially continuing to fracture, dislocation
- Reduced symptoms, early signs of healing
- Residual deformity

89. A: LDL and HDL cholesterol levels are especially important to monitor for diabetics:

- LDL: Should be less than 100 mg/dL (2.6 mmol/L) for most persons with diabetes. However, if persons are at a high risk for cardiovascular disease, such as those with a history of heart disease, hypertension, or smoking, then the LDL should be maintained at less than 70 mg/dL (1.8 mmol/L) to further reduce the risk of plaque buildup.
- HDL: Males should maintain HDL levels at greater than 40 mg/dL (1.0 mmol/L) and females at greater than 50 mg/dL (1.3 mmol/L) to help remove excess cholesterol in the blood.

90. B: Ketones typically appear in the urine if a person's blood glucose level is greater than 240 mg/dL (13.3 mmol/L). At this point, the body begins to break down fat to use for energy in place of carbohydrates because of inadequate insulin, which can lead to ketoacidosis. However, if persons are on a very low carbohydrate diet, they may develop nutritional ketosis because of the diet rather than because of inadequate insulin. In this case, the blood glucose level remains controlled.

91. D: Peripheral arterial disease (PAD) occurs in 20–30% of persons with diabetes, especially those with type 2 diabetes. Diabetes is associated with the buildup of plaque and atherosclerosis, which narrows the arteries in the legs and feet, reducing their blood supply. Indications of PAD include a sensation of cold and shiny, smooth skin on the legs and feet. As PAD advances, it can result in intermittent claudication and the development of ulcers (increasing the risk of amputation) as well as weakness, skin discoloration (i.e., pale, cyanotic), weak or absent peripheral pulses, numbness and tingling, hair loss on the legs and feet, and thickened toenails.

92. D: A 2008 study (with 2011 follow-up) found no connection between duration of diabetes and the likelihood of restricting insulin. Restrictors were more likely to be younger, had higher HbA1c values, and reported lower self-care scores and higher levels of diabetes-specific stress. During the initial 11-year study period, the women who restricted insulin were more than three times more likely to die (age of death 45 vs. 58 years) and had increased rates of DKA and some other diabetes-related complications.

93. A: Primary prevention strategies are those that aim to prevent a disease from occurring. These can include adopting a healthy diet, losing weight, exercising routinely, and stopping smoking. Secondary prevention strategies, on the other hand, are those that are used once disease occurs to prevent progression or complications. Secondary strategies can include screening to identify previously undiagnosed diabetes, adhering to medication regimens, closely monitoring blood glucose levels, close follow-up with healthcare professionals, and routine HbA1c assessment.

94. D: "I will walk 30 minutes a day 5 or 6 days a week for the next 90 days to improve my glucose control" fits the SMART format:

S	Specific	Details specific actions that will be taken
M	Measurable	Includes quantifiable parameters
A	Attainable	Can be accomplished
R	Relevant	Relates to improved health and well-being
T	Time-bound	Includes a clear time frame for completion

95. C: SGLT2 inhibitors, such as canagliflozin, work by preventing the reabsorption of glucose in the kidneys. The result is that more sugar leaves the body through the urine and less stays in the bloodstream. Because the mechanism of action is dependent on normal (or close to normal) renal function, this class of medications is contraindicated for those with severe kidney disease (<20 mL/min or on dialysis). Sulfonylurea medications work on the pancreas to release more insulin into the bloodstream. Because the action of endogenous insulin is prolonged with decreased kidney function, the dose may need to be adjusted or even discontinued for those with renal impairment. Biguanides work primarily by reducing hepatic glucose. Because biguanide medications are broken down by the kidneys, they are contraindicated for those with renal impairment. Use of biguanides with renal impairment may result in excess of the medication in the body, which could result in lactic acidosis. DPP-4 inhibitors may be used with renal impairment, but a reduced dose may be needed, depending on the degree of renal impairment.

96. A: Acanthosis nigricans is a darkening and thickening of the skin, typically on the back/sides of the neck or the axillae; it is indicative of insulin resistance. Choice B describes Kussmaul breathing. Darkening of the toenails is not a recognized condition, except in subungual hematoma (which occurs when a nail is traumatized and blood forms under the nail). Choice D is eschar.

97. A: Methyldopa is one of the recommended mediations for treating a hypertensive disorder during pregnancy. Other suggested medications include: labetalol, diltiazem, clonidine, and prazosin. This patient meets criteria for preeclampsia: systolic blood pressure ≥140 mmHg or diastolic blood pressure ≥90 mmHg, diagnosed after the 20th week of pregnancy. Preeclampsia must be addressed as safely as possible to prevent maternal and fetal injury. ACE inhibitors and angiotensin receptor blockers (ARBs) are contraindicated in pregnancy. Chronic diuretic use is also not recommended in pregnancy, as it has been associated with restricted maternal plasma volume, which could reduce uteroplacental perfusion. Lifestyle modification should be reinforced, but since the patient has had three blood pressure readings above target and states that she is already following lifestyle recommendations, it is time for the next step.

98. A: Nausea and subsequent weight loss are not chief fears of patients who are being prescribed insulin, as they are not common side effects. It is, however, a common side effect for some GLP-1 agonist injectable medications. Other common concerns include the idea that taking insulin will actually make diabetes worse or lead to complications (even though the opposite is true), fear of needles, and fear of hypoglycemia. Other commonly reported concerns include social stigma and possible weight gain.

99. C: Everything on a food label provides good information, but it is especially important to focus on the serving size rather than just the total calories or carbohydrates because the serving size may be far smaller than the average person would eat or drink. For example, a label for a blueberry muffin may say that there are 90 total calories, but if the serving size is one-quarter of the muffin, the entire muffin is 360 calories. Listing small serving sizes is especially common on snack foods, processed foods, and candies.

100. B: Educational workshops are usually conducted with small groups, allowing for maximal participation; they are especially good for demonstrations and practice sessions, such as for patients learning to monitor their blood glucose levels. One-on-one instruction is especially helpful for targeted instruction in procedures for individuals but is time-intensive and less cost-effective. Lectures are often used for more academic or detailed information that may include questions and answers but limited discussion. Discussions are best with small groups so that people can actively participate. Discussion is good for problem-solving.

101. A: A BMI of less than 18.5 kg/m^2 is underweight. A BMI of 18.5–24.9 kg/m^2 is normal weight. A BMI of 25–29.9 kg/m^2 is overweight. A BMI of 30 kg/m^2 and above is obese, with over 40 kg/m^2 being extremely or morbidly obese.

102. C: The best solution for an older adult who has difficulty filling insulin syringes with the correct dosage is to arrange for the client to receive prefilled insulin syringes. This allows the person to remain independent in diabetic management by simplifying insulin preparation and preventing incorrect dosage. Further instruction in filling syringes may not be helpful if the problem is physical, such as poor vision or poor hand-eye coordination. Depending on family may be impractical in the long run and will decrease the person's autonomy.

103. D: An employment change is rarely a practical solution, and a person already stressed and overworked will not likely engage in activities that may take more time and increase his or her stress level. An initial lifestyle change that the CDCES should recommend is to engage in moderate exercise, such as taking a walk each day or practicing yoga or Tai Chi. In addition, the client needs to have a clear understanding about how diet affects blood glucose and should improve nutrition and aim to eat three balanced meals daily in order to help control blood glucose levels and lose weight.

104. D: For those who are housebound and have little opportunity to interact with others, message boards can be very helpful. Diabetes Daily provides a learning center with information about different topics related to diabetes, including blood sugar, diet and fitness, weight loss, treatments, technology, complications, and living with diabetes. It also provides forums in which users can pick topics of interest and interact with others with the same interests. General topics include the different types of diabetes, daily living, diabetes management, and challenges that people encounter.

105. C: High triglyceride levels (hypertriglyceridemia) are most closely associated with low HDL levels. High LDL, high glucose, and small-sized LDL particles are also common in those with type 2 diabetes, and are often seen in patients who also have high triglyceride levels. However, the correlation is not as strong.

106. C: Stress on the body usually results in an increase in hepatic glucose, thereby raising blood glucose levels. All of the other answer choices will lower blood glucose. Alcohol can cause a drop in blood glucose because the liver does not release as much glucose while it is metabolizing alcohol, but alcohol may raise blood glucose if the alcoholic beverage also contains substantial carbohydrates. Those at risk for hypoglycemia are encouraged to eat whenever they consume alcohol.

107. A: The social cognitive theory (SCT) maintains that individuals learn from their personal experiences as well as from observing the actions and experiences of others. SCT addresses psychosocial factors that influence health behavior and methods of stimulating behavioral change. The health belief model stipulates that a person's decision to change health behavior depends on several factors, including level of personal vulnerability, belief in seriousness of the problem, belief in effectiveness of the change, associated costs of the change, presence of action cues, and level of self-efficacy. The theory of planned behavior applies three major constructs: attitudes towards the desired behavior, perceived societal view of the behavior, and the knowledge/skill level of the person. The transtheoretical model (TTM) states that change is likely to occur only when the patient has reached a stage at which he or she is ready to change. The stages of the TTM are precontemplation, contemplation, preparation, action, maintenance, and termination.

108. C: Optimism is the attribute studied most extensively in terms of healthy adaptation to diabetes; it has proven to positively affect behavior change. Other common characteristics of those who adapt well to stressors such as a chronic disease are strong internal resources, a sense of purpose, high confidence levels, and overall hardiness, although these attributes have not been linked to success to the same extent as a sense of optimism. Stubbornness, affluence, and consistency may be viewed as assets in and of themselves but have not been identified in the literature as attributes common to those who adapt well.

109. A: Restriction of foods high in vitamin K, such as leafy green vegetables, is advised for those on warfarin (Coumadin) therapy, due to the effect of vitamin K on clotting mechanisms. It does not pertain to those with chronic kidney disease (CKD). General recommendations for those with mild to moderate CKD include good glycemic control, strict blood pressure control with an ACE inhibitor or ARB, and abstaining from NSAIDs. Other recommendations include optimal glycemic control, insulin adjustment as needed to prevent hypoglycemia due to longer action time, and treatment for anemia and osteodystrophy, which often accompany CKD.

110. A: Because there are no signs for medication names and many other proper nouns, a sign language interpreter would have to spell out the word each time it is spoken. Writing the name would make it simpler and more efficient for the interpreter because he or she could point to the name. While visual aids (including pictures) are very helpful for the hearing-impaired population, there is no reason to eliminate text based on a hearing disability alone. This modification would be more appropriate for those with a literacy deficit. Arranging chairs in a circle would be helpful if the group members were conversing with each other. In this case, however, all of the class members will need a clear view of the ASL interpreter. In a circle, some would be able to see the interpreter, but some would not. Because an interpreter has been secured, there is no essential need for paper and pens. If class members have questions, they can ask them via the interpreter. A paper and pen may be a nice touch for participants to take notes for themselves, but no more so than for a hearing audience.

111. B: Sugar alcohols are sugar substitutes that are lower in carbohydrates than sugar is, but they still contain carbohydrates. To calculate the impact that sugar alcohols have on blood glucose, the general rule is to subtract 50% of the grams of sugar alcohols from the total carbohydrate count. So, if a food item contains 15 grams of carbohydrates and 8 grams of sugar alcohols, the total carbohydrates would be 15 minus 4, or 11. Examples of sugar alcohols include mannitol, maltitol, xylitol, sorbitol, lactitol, isomalt, and hydrogenated starch hydrolysates. Erythritol, however, has no impact on blood glucose levels and can be completely subtracted from the total carbohydrate count.

112. A: The ADA National Standards for Diabetes Self-Management Education and Support advocate for the development of action-oriented behavioral goals and learning objectives. In addition, learning objectives should be demonstrative, or able to be witnessed. Words like "know" and "understand" are difficult to measure. One would ask, how can we verify that he or she knows or understands? Improving HbA1c is a worthy long-term clinical goal, but does not qualify as a behavioral objective. What action does the patient need to do to result in an improved HbA1c? Those actions would be more appropriate behavioral learning objectives.

113. C: When using an insulin pen device, the patient should prime the pen (perform an "air shot") before each use, whereas with a GLP-1 agonist medication, the priming is only done as part of new pen setup (before first use of each pen). The other choices do not accurately reflect the difference between insulin pens and GLP-1 agonist pens. Both pen types require a new pen needle with each use. With both types of medications, the injection site should be rotated. Both medications may be kept at room temperature for the approved in-use time period.

114. B: Testing only when the numbers are likely to look good misses the point of self-monitoring. The purpose of self-monitoring is to provide the patient with immediate feedback and data, enabling persons with diabetes to make changes in their management plans and current lifestyle behaviors if necessary. By only monitoring at times when the numbers look good, the patient misses the opportunity to make corrections at times that will ultimately improve overall glycemic control. On the other hand, it is appropriate for patients to monitor when they do not feel well, overnight when they are concerned about a change to basal insulin, and two hours postprandial.

115. A: According to the ADA, persons who are prediabetic or at risk for diabetes can lower their risk of developing diabetes by 58% by exercising for 30 minutes five times a week and by losing 7% of their body weight, or approximately 15 pounds if their beginning weight is 200 pounds. Online BMI calculators can help determine an ideal body weight; however, if persons need to lose a substantial amount of weight, they should be encouraged to initially set moderate goals because it can seem overwhelming to have to lose 50 or more pounds.

116. A: The normal range for alanine aminotransferase (ALT) varies according to age and sex, but for a male of 58, the range should be 13–40 U/L (this may vary slightly by laboratory). This client's ALT is 400 U/L, which indicates liver injury. ALT is found in liver cells and is normally found in small amounts in the blood. However, when hepatic cells are injured, ALT levels in the blood may rise markedly, making ALT measurement a sensitive test for liver function.

117. B: Food records provide the data by which the current nutrition plan and adherence to that plan may be evaluated by both the patient keeping the record and the educator or provider who reviews it with the patient. While a personal review of the record may encourage the patient, it is not the main purpose of recordkeeping. Insurance providers do not require a personal food log, as the RD notes are sufficient documentation. While recordkeeping is important in diabetes, development of this habit is not the main purpose of keeping a food log, nor is forcing the person to pay more attention to what he or she eats, although that is certainly an added benefit.

118. A: Direct observation during which the person talks through (i.e., explains what he or she is doing) and demonstrates tasks is the best method to use for evaluating if someone has developed adequate skills. One may be able to answer questions but still be unable to carry out tasks, and records may be inaccurate if someone is not carrying out tasks correctly. Additionally, people are not always objective when carrying out a self-assessment and may believe they are doing well when they are not, or vice versa.

119. B: Morbid obesity is defined according to the patient's BMI. Any BMI over 40 kg/m^2 is categorized as morbid obesity, and a BMI over 49 kg/m^2 is classified as super obesity. Therefore, a patient with a BMI of 41 kg/m^2 is morbidly obese. Choice A may not meet the criteria for morbid obesity, as we do not have the patient's height and cannot therefore calculate his BMI. Typically, someone with morbid obesity is at least 100 pounds overweight. Choice C says nothing about the patient's weight or BMI. The fact that the patient is considering bariatric surgery does not automatically indicate morbid obesity. Choice D only includes information about the patient's weight; his BMI could be normal if he is 6'9", overweight if he is 6'3", obese if he is 5'8", or morbidly obese if he is 5'3". Without the height information, the patient described in choice D cannot be classified.

120. A: A person with depression and anxiety may find it very difficult to focus on managing diabetes, so the individualized education plan should focus on emotional support and small, achievable goals that are not overwhelming and that can improve management. Physical exercise may benefit the client's emotional status and diabetes, but engaging in an exercise program requires some motivation, which may be lacking if he is depressed and anxious. It is important to collaborate to determine what the person decides is an achievable goal rather than having a goal imposed upon him or her.

121. A: With remote learning, the biggest challenge is typically maintaining the motivation to learn. Learners often start out enthusiastically but lose focus and become bored, especially if the remote learning is asynchronous and lacks interactivity. Other problems include the instructors' and learners' inability to correctly use the technology, especially those with low computer literacy. In some places, unreliable internet connections can interfere with remote learning, and dealing with distracting environments (e.g., children, background noise) can interfere with learning.

122. C: Approximately 50% of children and 60% of adults diagnosed with type 1 diabetes undergo a honeymoon phase after their diagnosis because their pancreases are still producing small amounts of insulin, which allows for lower insulin requirements and better and more stable control of glucose levels. This period typically lasts for 3–12 months, and persons can develop a false sense of security and believe that their diabetes is under control and needs less close monitoring; therefore, they must be cautioned to continue to carefully monitor their blood glucose levels.

123. B: Reaching out to referring providers is the most reliable source of patients. Although it usually requires an investment of time and effort, it often yields excellent and consistent results, especially once a trusting relationship has been established. Radio ads (as well as print ads, etc.) and word of mouth are also valuable and sometimes effective marketing strategies, but have not been shown to produce such consistent results. Finding previously hospitalized hyperglycemic patients may constitute a HIPAA violation if potential candidates are discovered through accessing protected health information for marketing purposes. Referral to a program by the hospital physician as part of hospital discharge process is of course a valid method to add participants, but this falls under the category of outreach to referring providers.

124. C: Flexibility exercise, or stretching, should be considered in the fitness plan, as it can provide fitness benefits such as increasing joint range of motion and stability for older adults. However, flexibility exercise should not take the place of aerobic and resistance exercise. It has been questioned whether flexibility training may decrease injury, but this has not been proven. The other types of exercise include aerobic exercise for cardiovascular health and resistance exercises for muscle strength and core conditioning, which improve glycemic control and increase mobility. Both are being addressed in the patient's current plan. Toning exercise is not an official exercise category.

125. D: The patient should prime the needle before dialing the dose for each and every injection. This is to expel any air in the pen and to "prime" the pen tip with insulin. There is no need to clean the skin with alcohol, as long as the skin is clean. Likewise, pinching of the skin is not necessary unless the patient is very thin or a child. Even then, with the small length of pen needle, pinching is not usually needed. After injecting the insulin, the patient should leave the needle in the skin for about 10 seconds to ensure that all of the insulin has been delivered. This is a step that many patients forget or were never taught because it is different from administration with a syringe.

126. D: A person with diabetes may be eligible for Social Security disability benefits if the complications prevent the person from working. However, if the complications can be managed, the person is typically not eligible. Persons with type 1 diabetes who are insulin-dependent and whose HbA1c runs 10% or greater are more likely to qualify than persons with type 2 diabetes. Complications that increase the chance of receiving disability benefits include comorbidities (e.g., heart disease; arthritis; open, unhealing wounds) and repeated hospitalizations for ketoacidosis.

127. B: The patient's sample meal has close to 60 grams of carbohydrate. The amount of carbohydrate in bread can vary by quite a bit; however, 15 grams per slice can be used for a rough estimate. In addition, half a grapefruit is also estimated at 15 grams. One cup of milk has approx. 12 grams of carbohydrate. Added together, this is reasonably close to 60 grams. A person that is counting carb servings (estimated at 15 grams per serving) would count 4 servings for a total of 60 grams. If a patient needed an exact amount, he or she would need to consult bread labels, measure the milk, etc. Some patients may be advised (or may prefer) to count exact carbs, but many will estimate and can benefit from practicing with estimation exercises.

128. C: Gastroparesis is a form of neuropathy that can occur in persons with diabetes when there is damage to the autonomic nervous system and the vagus nerve, which stimulates the production of digestive enzymes and gastric juices, regulates peristalsis, controls the pyloric sphincter, and promotes feelings of hunger and satiety. With gastroparesis, the emptying of the stomach slows, resulting in symptoms of bloating, fullness, nausea, and vomiting. There is no treatment to reverse the nerve damage, but management may include modifying one's diet, controlling blood glucose levels, and taking medications to relieve symptoms.

129. C: The situation that describes driving while experiencing hypoglycemia symptoms is the best choice to assess a patient's ability to deal with a glucose emergency. Hypothetical situations are excellent ways to assess a patient's diabetes knowledge; however, the diabetes educator must construct situations that will test the type of knowledge they are trying to assess. Choice A would assess a patient's ability to make appropriate food choices. Choice B deals with problem-solving related to travel and how to acquire medication, and choice D addresses the healthy coping skill of dealing with friends who mean well but are misinformed.

130. D: Misplacement of small items, such as glucose meters, was not one of the barriers reposted by patients in a recent survey (Tenderich, 2013). Common barriers do include cost, discomfort, lack of proper instruction and ongoing support, as well as others such as physical limitations (dexterity/visual disability), cognitive deficits, time constraints, and inconvenience, along with emotional components such as stress or anxiety.

131. A: Studies on the health effects of marijuana with diabetes vary, but there is some evidence that its use by a person with type 1 diabetes may increase the risk of DKA. In addition, because marijuana use has been linked to increased risk of cardiovascular events, this is a special concern for persons with type 2 diabetes because they are already at increased risk. A study by the National Survey on Drug Use and Health showed that, between 2021 and 2022, 9% of people with diabetes reported using marijuana, and the figure is probably higher since many states have legalized its use.

132. D: Demonstration is an active-learning instructional strategy in which the educator has a good amount of control over content because he or she first performs the demonstration. Choices A and B are active-learning instructional strategies that enhance learning, but over which the educator has less control of content. These are participant-driven to a greater extent than demonstration. Choice C is a passive-learning instructional strategy. Although this strategy affords the educator a great deal of control over content, it does not involve the learner to a great extent, and therefore typically yields less retention and understanding than more active-learning instructional strategies.

133. A: With diabulimia, a person restricts the use of insulin in order to lose weight and prevent the weight gain that may occur when insulin is controlling blood glucose levels. Diabulimia can result in repeated episodes of hyperglycemia, diabetic ketoacidosis (DKA), and HbA1c levels of 9.0% or higher. Persons may only withhold insulin, or they may exhibit other unhealthy eating patterns, such as binging and purging. Diabulimia can occur at any age but is most common in adolescents and young adults. Studies indicate that up to 40% of females with type 1 diabetes will, at some point, withhold insulin in order to lose weight.

134. B: Thiazolidinediones (TZDs) are generally contraindicated for patients with CHF. Use of TZDs may lead to fluid and sodium retention, which would worsen CHF symptoms. Other classes of medications, including DPP-4 inhibitors, alpha-glucosidase inhibitors, sulfonylureas, meglitinides, GLP-1 receptor agonists, biguanides, and amylin analogs, are not summarily contraindicated for use with CHF, but may need to be adjusted and carefully monitored according to manufacturers' indications.

135. D: The ADA's most recent Standards update states that there is no recommendation for ideal percentage (or number) of calories, or number of grams, from carbohydrates, protein, or fat that can be applied to *all* patients with diabetes. Instead, they recommend that nutrition plans should be individually tailored to the patient's preferences, activity level, and metabolic goals. The ADA recommends following the tenets of the Mediterranean diet, which includes healthy fats, over a low-fat diet.

136. C: The social worker is the team member that is best trained to address issues related to financial, familial, physical, transportation, or social barriers of many kinds. He or she will know of resources or can recommend referral to the necessary specialties for follow-up care. In addition, the social worker can make recommendations to the prescribing physician based on a focused, thorough assessment of the patient's capabilities and resources.

137. C: Social determinants of health have a critical effect on people's access to healthcare. Those who lack insurance often do not have enough income to pay for their treatments. Other social determinants of health include food (in)security, transportation availability (i.e., public, private), housing (e.g., adequate, substandard, homeless), education, employment status, neighborhood (e.g., affluent, crime-ridden), exposure to violence (e.g., domestic, community), social attitudes (e.g., racism, inclination toward conspiracy theories, ageism, homophobia), language and literacy, and health literacy.

138. B: It is important to provide factual information, but the focus for persons with diabetes should be on preventive care and measures to avoid complications; therefore, if a person is fearful that diabetes will result in blindness, the fact that good management of diabetes and preventive eye care reduce risk by 95% is essential information to share to help reduce the client's fear and also to encourage him to manage blood glucose and cholesterol levels effectively and have yearly eye examinations.

139. C: Annual influenza vaccination and hepatitis B vaccination series for adults less than 60 years old is an ADA-recommended Standard of Care in Diabetes; for influenza, the Standards specifically recommend that patients with diabetes receive a trivalent vaccine, not a live attenuated vaccine. For those unvaccinated adults who are 60 years or older, the hepatitis B vaccination should be administered at the discretion of the patient's physician. The other answer choices are only partially correct. An echocardiogram is not recommended annually as a Standard of Care. A dilated eye exam is recommended at diagnosis for those with type 2 diabetes, and within 5 years of onset for those with type 1 diabetes. Repeat exams should be performed annually (more often if needed), rather than every six months. The C-peptide exam is sometimes used to differentiate type 2 from type 1 diabetes, to assess endogenous insulin production, or to qualify a patient for insulin pump therapy (if it is an insurance provider requirement), but is not recommended as a Standard of Care.

140. A: The most important lifestyle change for this person is a diet change and exercise:

- Reducing saturated fats (e.g., red meats, processed foods) can lower LDL and reduce risk of plaque buildup.
- Reducing trans fats (e.g., fried foods, baked goods, margarine) can lower LDL and increase HDL.
- Eating foods high in fiber (e.g., oats, beans, lentils, fruits, vegetables) can lower LDL and slow absorption of carbohydrates.
- Exercising can lower LDL, increase HDL, and reduce BMI, reduce stress, and lower blood glucose levels.

141. A: All of the options are prerequisites for continuous subcutaneous insulin infusion (CSII) therapy *except* a diagnosis of type 1 diabetes. Candidates for CSII must be insulin-requiring, with little to no endogenous insulin production, but there are many patients with type 2 diabetes who also meet this criterion. Patients should be proficient at counting carbohydrates, as the pump delivers bolus doses based on the carbohydrate information entered by the patient. Clinical indications, as recommended by the ADA and ADCES, include failure to obtain optimal glycemic control on multiple daily injections of insulin. The patient should also demonstrate motivation and consistent blood glucose monitoring. Other prerequisites include being able to calculate bolus insulin doses and having good problem-solving skills. In addition to these prerequisites, other skills will need to be mastered before pump therapy is initiated.

142. B: A low-interest medical loan from her local bank would be the *least* helpful option on the list for this patient. The patient's budget is already stretched thin and a loan, even a low-interest loan, would add an extra cost burden. When the loan money runs out, she would likely require the same or greater resources for her medications and would also need to repay the loan. The first thing to do would be to see if anything can be done to reduce her cost burden from the perspective of requirements. For example, is it possible that a different testing regimen (one requiring fewer tests per day) may work? Can she use a generic meter that uses less-expensive test strips? Once all regimen options have been exhausted, the patient can check with programs and organizations that help those in need, specifically those who are uninsured with low income. Such organizations include Partnership for Prescription Assistance, local and state health department programs, and Needymeds.

143. B: Virtual reality gaming systems became popular and widespread during the 2010s, so most adolescents and young adults have grown up with and feel comfortable with this technology. Therefore, this age group is the most likely to want to engage in this type of education.

144. B: GLP-1 agonists, such as semaglutide, tirzepatide, and liraglutide, promote the greatest loss of weight for persons with diabetes. GLP-1 agonists mimic the hormone glucagon-like-peptide 1 (GLP-1) and stimulate the pancreas to produce insulin in response to elevated blood glucose levels and decrease appetite so people feel less hunger and feel full on a smaller amount of food. Weight loss with semaglutide averages 5–10%, and can be >15% with high doses. Weight loss with liraglutide averages 5–8% of body weight.

145. C: According to the American Diabetes Association, those with specific co-morbidities should have a thorough medical evaluation. These co-morbidities include proliferative retinopathy or severe non-proliferative retinopathy, as well as autonomic and peripheral neuropathy. An ECG stress test should be performed (especially since the patient is sedentary and has a history of a cardiac issues), as well as an updated retinopathy exam. Adjustments may need to be made to reduce further injury, including no vigorous aerobic exercise or resistance training and possible limitation of weight-bearing activities. Beyond cardiac stress testing and retinopathy, additional referrals listed in choice D are probably not necessary, since she has already been diagnosed and is being managed. A treating physician or other provider should be able to perform the rest of the pre-exercise medical evaluation and help develop an appropriate exercise plan.

146. A: Evaluation is defined as the systematic process by which the worth or value of something, teaching/learning in the case of DSMES, is judged. This is part of the fifth step in the DSMES process: assessment, goal setting, planning, implementation, and evaluation and monitoring.

147. C: According to Endocrine Society practice guidelines, adult and pediatric patients on basal-bolus therapy with a high risk of hypoglycemia should use rapid-acting insulin rather than short-acting (regular) for their boluses. The use of rapid-acting insulin has been shown in studies to reduce episodes of hypoglycemia compared to short-acting insulin, although most data are derived from studies of adults. Additionally, the Endocrine Society recommends that those who are at risk for hypoglycemia receive structured education on strategies to avoid it.

148. A: Assessment is the first step in the process of diabetes self-management education. The proceeding steps in the DSMES process (in order) are: goal setting, planning, implementation, and evaluation/monitoring. Diagnosis and referral, while necessary, are not considered official steps in the diabetes self-management education process.

149. C: Metformin reduces the production of glucose by the liver and increases the production of lactate and absorption of bile salts in the small intestines, resulting in gastrointestinal problems such as nausea, cramping, and diarrhea. Therefore, metformin should be taken with food because the food helps to slow the absorption of the drug, helping minimize its adverse effects. If rapid-acting metformin is used, it is typically taken with breakfast and dinner; however, extended-release metformin should generally be taken with the evening meal because this helps reduce adverse effects and allows for consistent blood glucose control during the night.

150. B: If a person with diabetes drinks excessive amounts of alcoholic beverages, such as vodka and whiskey, and fails to have an adequate intake of food, this can result in hypoglycemia because the alcohol inhibits gluconeogenesis (the process by which non-carbohydrates are converted into glucose) and it inhibits the liver's ability to release glucose, so the glucose level that is circulating in the bloodstream is inadequate for the usual dosage of insulin. Alcoholic beverages should be limited to two drinks daily for males or one drink daily for females and should always be ingested along with food.

151. D: Persons who smoke more than 10 cigarettes daily are likely to experience cravings when trying to stop smoking, so combination therapy is often the most successful. Combination therapy includes nicotine replacement therapies, such as nicotine patches or nicotine gum, in decreasing dosages as well as prescription medications, such as varenicline and bupropion, to help reduce cravings and withdrawal symptoms. People who are quitting smoking may also benefit from behavioral support, such as support groups (in-person or virtual), cognitive behavioral therapy, or counseling.

152. C: Each 1% of hemoglobin A1c (HbA1c) greater than 5% represents approximately 28–30 mg/dL. Therefore, if the person's hemoglobin increased from 7% (i.e., an average blood glucose of 154 mg/dL) to 8%, one can estimate that the average blood glucose level increased to approximately 182–184 mg/dL. HbA1c (glycated hemoglobin) measures the average blood glucose over the course of 2–3 months. Normal is less than 5.7%, prediabetes is 5.7–6.4%, and diabetes is 6.5% and higher.

153. D: Anxiety is manifested by taking extreme measures to avoid a feared outcome. In this case, the patient is cutting her medication, eating ice cream, and avoiding morning blood sugar as ways to deal with her anxiety over nocturnal hypoglycemia. Depression is usually associated with patients stating that they feel down and have a lack of interest or energy to do the things they need to. Eating disorders are mental health concerns, but his patient does not display the typical signs of an eating disorder. She has stated no weight obsessions or body image issues and she admitted that she eats ice cream every night and explains why she does it. While eating the ice cream is not recommended for her due to her high morning blood sugars, her rationale (that she does not want a low blood sugar) is sound. Denial is an emotional stage (not so much a mental health issue) that is characterized by the patient refusing to admit that there is a problem and therefore taking no steps to address it. Clearly, this patient senses a problem and is actually going farther than she should to address it.

154. D: National Standards for Diabetes Self-Management Education and Support do not specify which outcomes should be tracked. However, the ADCES states that programs must set behavioral goals with their participants in order to evaluate the effectiveness of the education and interventions provided by the program. Programs must also collect clinical outcome measures in order to evaluate the effectiveness of the change in behavior. Programs must have a system in place to collect behavioral/clinical outcomes in order to aggregate and evaluate the effectiveness of the education and interventions. While the other answer choices may be useful to evaluate the effectiveness of a specific program or intervention, they are not ADA- or ADCES-required aggregate objectives.

155. D: Medical waste disposal laws do indeed vary from state to state, and so patients and educators need to determine specific policies for their respective areas. It is true that in some states (California, for example), sharps must be discarded in official biohazard sharps containers. Likewise, some states (Texas, for example) allow people to put their needles and lancets in a hard-plastic container, then tape the lid on and throw it away with regular trash. There are a variety of policies that are somewhere in between. A good place to check for the local policy on medical waste disposal is safeneedledisposal.org.

156. D: Steroid-induced diabetes can occur when persons receive high dosages of glucocorticoids, such as after a craniotomy. The steroids cause increased insulin resistance and increase the production of hepatic glucose, resulting in hyperglycemia. Unless there are underlying diabetes risks, damage to beta cells from the steroids, or the steroids are continued at a high dose for a prolonged duration, the hyperglycemia decreases as the dosage of steroids is reduced. In most cases, there is resolution of the hyperglycemia and there is no further need for treatment once the steroids are discontinued.

157. B: Asian Americans tend to accumulate more visceral fat than other ethnic groups at lower waist sizes; therefore, although the standard risk factor is a waist circumference (in inches) of >35 for females and >40 for males, in Asian Americans, risks increase with a waist size of >31 for females and >35 for males. Additionally, Asian Americans are at a greater risk of developing insulin resistance and metabolic syndrome at BMIs that are generally considered healthy for other populations.

158. B: Kinesthetic learners (also referred to as tactile learners) are often movement-oriented and dislike sitting still for long periods, so they benefit from short teaching and learning sessions. They learn best by handling and manipulating items and prefer hands-on experience to reading, watching videos, or listening to audio recordings. Kinesthetic learners often have very good motor memory, so they can easily recall the steps to using a device and prefer trial-and-error approaches to learning. While learning styles do vary some from person to person, all people do need learn from visual information, auditory information, and by hands-on learning. Different materials lend themselves to a different format, but where possible, the best practice when presenting information to others is to use a mixture of formats, including hands-on materials, visual, and auditory information to keep the materials engaging to all learners.

159. A: Diabetic ketoacidosis (DKA) is characterized by hyperventilation, nausea, vomiting, weight loss, abdominal pain, lethargy, excessive thirst and urination, hunger, and a fruity odor of the breath (caused by acetone, a type of ketone). With DKA, the blood glucose level is typically greater than 250 mg/dL (13.88 mmol/L). DKA can lead to altered mental status, coma, and death if not promptly treated with insulin infusion and fluid and electrolyte replacement.

160. B: Although the general ADA recommendation for HbA1c is <7%, higher targets should be set for those patients with "history of severe hypoglycemia, limited life expectancy, advanced microvascular or macrovascular complications, extensive comorbid conditions, and those with long-standing diabetes in whom the general goal is difficult to attain." In cases such as these, the ADA recommends a target of <8%. An HbA1c closer to 9.5% may cause the patient discomfort from hyperglycemia and may exacerbate her already debilitating complications. More aggressive targets (<6.5%) may be appropriate for patients with short duration of diabetes, long life expectancy, and no significant CVD according to ADA Standards of Care. To set a target this low would increase this patient's chances of a fatal cardiac event.

161. A: Many over-the-counter medications may have an adverse effect on diabetes control. Decongestants, especially those containing pseudoephedrine or phenylephrine, can cause blood glucose levels to spike. Decongestants contain ingredients that mimic epinephrine, resulting in a sympathetic nervous response in which the liver releases more glucose to provide energy. Additionally, decongestants result in vasoconstriction, which can raise blood pressure and interfere with insulin sensitivity. Aspirin use may result in kidney damage and an increased risk of bleeding. Most antihistamines, such as diphenhydramine, have minimal effects on blood glucose. The use of laxatives may result in hypoglycemia.

162. C: The recommendations for alcohol intake are as follows: for males, no more than two drinks daily; and for females, no more than one drink daily. One drink equals 12 ounces of regular or light beer, 5 ounces of wine, or 1.5 ounces of distilled spirits.

Beverage	Carbohydrates (g)
Beer (12 oz)	Light, 6–12; regular, 13–17; craft, 20–30
Wine (5 oz)	Dry, 4–5; sweet/dessert, 15–25
Distilled alcohol (1.5 oz)	Pure, 0; flavored, 2–25; liqueurs, 10–20
Mixed drinks (1 oz)	5–30+

163. A: Staggering testing times by testing before and after different meals on different days can provide enough data to identify and manage blood glucose patterns within a few weeks. In the stated time frame of two to three weeks, this patient should have a least four readings before and after each mealtime, which may be enough to see where the problem lies. This pattern will not exceed his allotment of test strips and even leaves him some extras for emergencies such as when his blood sugar feels low or on sick days. Choice B will offer little insight, especially if his fasting values are close to normal. The diabetes educator would not be able to identify which meal(s) may be contributing to his high HbA1c. Choice C is only partially correct. Patients who take insulin do require more frequent self-monitoring, but this patient does not take mealtime insulin (or even mealtime oral meds) at this point. Furthermore, dismissing the financial concern because monitoring is important is not sensitive to the patient's barriers; if he cannot afford the test strips, he may not have a choice.

164. C: Preparation is the stage represented by this patient's words and actions. He has not yet actively engaged in the behavior change he needs, the action stage, but is no longer unaware of the problem, which is the precontemplation stage. He has even moved beyond just acknowledging there is a problem that he may want to do something about—the contemplation stage—to actually making plans that will facilitate behavior change—the preparation stage.

165. C: The bargaining stage is characterized by inaccurate explanations and/or erroneous cures. The patient "makes a deal" with self, provider, God, or others to get rid of the diabetes. Extremes of compulsive behavior often accompany this stage. Denial is characterized by disbelief in the diagnosis; anger is characterized by irritation, rage, anxiety, or guilt. Frustration and depression can occur at any time and are characterized by feelings of hopelessness and trouble establishing or maintaining good self-care habits. Acceptance is the stage at which the patient becomes involved in his or her care and requests information and help to improve.

166. A: Nonalcoholic fatty liver disease is associated with insulin resistance, which is when the body becomes less responsive to insulin so that more insulin is required to maintain normal blood glucose levels. With insulin resistance, the liver does not respond well to insulin's signal to stop producing glucose, so it is overproduced. Lipid metabolism is impaired, so free fatty acids are released from adipose tissue and accumulate to form fatty deposits in the liver (hepatic steatosis), which in turn increases insulin resistance and leads to type 2 diabetes mellitus.

167. B: An interpersonal barrier may include struggles with family, peers, or healthcare team members. In this case, that patient's interpersonal struggles relate to her ability to eat healthfully. Other types of barriers include personal (co-morbidities, physical disability, poor coping skills, and inaccurate health beliefs) and environmental (financial constraints, job-related issues, transportation issues, safety of environment, other priorities). These other types are represented in choices A, C, and D, but these are not the best choices for the scenario described because they do not focus on the patient's relationships with family members.

168. D: A serum creatinine of 2.8 mg/dL should raise a red flag, as it indicates likely renal impairment. Although estimated glomerular filtration rate (eGFR) is calculated with additional factors such as age, sex, race, and weight, the creatinine of this patient is not in the normal range for any demographic. Estimated GFR calculators are available online and typically use the MDRD Study Equation or the Cockcroft-Gault Equation. This patient should be referred to nephrology immediately. Although the HbA1c and LDL levels are considered slightly above ideal for most patients, they are not to the level of immediate concern. The HDL of 88 mg/dL is high, but for HDL the goal is to have a high value: above 40 mg/dL for men and above 50 mg/dL for women. Therefore, the HDL is not a concern.

169. D: To make sure that health information is protected in a way that does not interfere with a patient's healthcare, information can be used and shared (without written permission) with a patient's family, relatives, friends, or others the patient identifies who are involved with his or her healthcare or healthcare bills, unless the patient objects. Therefore, choices A and B are incorrect. However, some healthcare organizations have policies that go a step further to secure patient healthcare information, and so it is a good idea to know the organization's policies. Remember that HIPAA stipulates that patients have a right to their healthcare record, including lab results. It is dismissive to say that the result is not important and can wait.

170. B: Because celiac disease is an immune-mediated disorder, there is a greater prevalence among those with type 1 diabetes, as compared to the general population (1–16% of individuals with type 1 diabetes compared with 0.3–1.0% in the general population). It is not associated with insulin resistance and not more prevalent among the type 2 diabetes population. Gluten-free diets are not generally recommended as a meal plan option for those who have not been diagnosed with celiac disease, as whole grains provide energy, fiber, and other important nutrients. Screening for celiac disease shortly after diagnosis is recommended for all persons with type 1 diabetes, but screening is not recommended for those with type 2 diabetes in the absence of symptoms.

171. B: It is especially important when setting goals with a person with diabetes that the goals are achievable with reasonable effort because failure to achieve goals can lead the person to become frustrated and to lose motivation. The CDCES and the person's healthcare team should guide the person in setting attainable goals such as "I will decrease my HbA1c by 1% within 6 months." Losing 20 pounds in 30 days and lowering blood glucose levels to normal within 7 days are not realistic goals. An intake of carbohydrates of 50 g daily is very difficult to maintain and may be inadequate.

172. C: The "talk test" is used to determine if a person can tolerate a level of exercise and to assess the intensity of that exercise. This test is often used for persons who must avoid overexertion. Exercise intensity levels:

- Light: Includes walking, household chores. Able to talk normally throughout the exercise.
- Moderate: Includes fast walking, swimming, cycling. Able to talk but may need to pause for breath.
- Vigorous: Includes running, high-intensity interval training, fast cycling. Speaking more than a word or two is difficult because breathing is labored.
- Very high: Includes sprinting, very high intensity interval training. Unable to talk.

173. B: During adolescence, hormonal fluctuations may result in increased insulin resistance:

- Growth hormones can reduce sensitivity to insulin.
- Estrogen and testosterone affect how cells respond to insulin.
- Cortisol promotes production of glucose from protein and fat and decreases the insulin's effectiveness. High stress can increase cortisol levels.

Other factors in adolescence can also affect insulin resistance:

- Rapid growth requires energy that can change insulin sensitivity.
- Increased body fat can result in increased insulin resistance.
- A poor diet can lead to higher glucose levels that worsen insulin resistance.

174. B: The four Ds of dealing with food cravings are:

- Delay: Cravings often last for a short period of time—delaying for even 5 minutes may lessen cravings.
- Distract: Engage in an activity such as exercising, reading, messaging, or calling a friend.
- Deep breathe: Inhale slowly, hold for a count of five, and then exhale for a count of seven and repeat. Concentrating on breathing can help clear one's mind.
- Drink water: Studies have shown that some people mistake thirst for hunger and eat instead of drink. Additionally, drinking can help reduce a craving by altering sensations in the mouth.

175. C: While abandoning and revising objectives is part of the goal evaluation process, one must examine reasons why the objective was not achieved. It may be that the patient did not have enough time or that the pace was too aggressive for him, but these are only assumptions until the patient expresses them. It may be that the patient has not identified reasons why physical activity is personally meaningful and he is therefore lacking motivation. At times, it is important to acknowledge successes or ambitions in other self-care areas, rather than dwelling on failures, but without first discussing the physical activity goal in greater depth with the patient, one would not know his desires and obstacles associated with this specific goal. For example, it may be that the patient very much wants to exercise but has not been able to find a safe way to accomplish it.

CDCES Practice Test #2

1. Consider the following patient: male, age 46, previously sedentary, mild hypertension and hyperlipidemia (both adequately controlled with medication), type 2 diabetes, and a BMI of 26 kg/m^2. If this patient wishes to begin a moderate-intensity exercise regimen, what additional assessment is mandated?

a. Stress test with ECG (electrocardiogram)
b. DEXA scan to assess bone density and strength
c. Ankle-brachial index to rule out peripheral arterial disease
d. No routine testing is required. Clinical judgment should be used in the context of previous cardiovascular history.

2. For persons with diabetes, a 2-hour postprandial glucose goal is typically:

a. <130 mg/dL
b. <150 mg/dL
c. <166 mg/dL
d. <180 mg/dL

3. A patient with type 1 diabetes (on MDI) tells the diabetes educator that for religious reasons, he would like to fast one day each month (from after dinner until about 3 p.m. the next day—about 20 hours). Which response and action would be most appropriate?

a. Discuss possible challenges and the best way to address them, such as more-frequent monitoring, consideration of insulin pump therapy, and a plan to address high or low blood sugars.
b. Readdress the hazards of fasting with the patient, including hypoglycemia and DKA. Warn the patient that fasting is not advised for those with type 1 diabetes.
c. Offer to explain the health concerns to the patient's pastor in hopes that an alternative arrangement can be made.
d. Tell the patient that if he chooses to fast, he should take only half of his basal insulin and no bolus insulin. For hypoglycemia, he should use a glucagon injection.

4. Which of the following statements concerning treatment for peripheral arterial disease (PAD) is TRUE?

a. Reduction of blood pressure (by about 10/5 mmHg) has been shown to reduce the risk of amputation in PAD by 30%.
b. Control of blood glucose at an HbA1c of 7% or lower has been shown to significantly slow the progression of existing PAD.
c. Lowering lipids has been associated with nearly 40% reduction in new or worsening symptoms of PAD.
d. Casual (unsupervised) exercise programs have been shown to have excellent benefits for those with PAD, including reduction of PAD symptoms, increased circulation, and improved balance.

5. Which of these statements regarding obstructive sleep apnea is NOT accurate?

a. Treatment of sleep apnea has been proven to significantly improve blood pressure control.
b. Treatment of sleep apnea has been conclusively proven to improve glycemic control.
c. Treatment of sleep apnea has been shown conclusively to improve quality of life.
d. Persons who are obese are four to ten times more likely to have obstructive sleep apnea than people who are not obese.

6. Which of the following entities is NOT an organization that accredits or officially recognizes diabetes self-management education programs—a necessary requirement for Medicare reimbursement?

a. The National Certification Board for Diabetes Educators (NCBDE)
b. The American Diabetes Association (ADA)
c. The Association of Diabetes Care and Education Specialists (ADCES)
d. All of the above are organizations that can recognize or accredit DSMES programs.

7. Which of the following statements is NOT listed as a rationale for documentation of patient encounters (including assessment, education plan, and outcomes) under Standard 7 (Individualization) of the ADA National Standards for Diabetes Self-Management Education and Support?

a. Documentation provides proof of services rendered by the educator and can be used to verify practice hours for certification renewal.
b. Documentation is used to guide the education process.
c. Documentation provides evidence of communication among instructional staff and other members of the participant's healthcare team.
d. Documentation prevents duplication of services.

8. Which of the following mental health conditions that are commonly associated with diabetes can be addressed primarily by the diabetes educator and may NOT necessarily require a referral to a mental health professional?

a. Depression
b. Behavioral relapse
c. Eating disorder (e.g., bulimia)
d. Anxiety

9. Which of the following exercise precautions applies specifically to patients with unstable proliferative retinopathy?

a. Exercise beyond what is needed for activities of daily living (e.g., slow walking) is not advised, as increased blood flow may exacerbate retinal problems.
b. Swimming and other prone physical activities should be avoided because they increase pressure in the retinas.
c. Resistance training should not be included in the exercise regimen because the resulting excessive systolic blood pressure response may further damage the eyes.
d. Before beginning a moderate-intensity exercise program consisting of both aerobic and strength training exercises, patients should have a stress test and be cleared by a cardiologist.

10. When asked about his personal goal for diabetes education, a patient's reply is, "I don't know what you mean." What would be an appropriate response?

a. "What do you mean you don't know what I mean?"
b. "How do you hope that learning more about diabetes will help you?"
c. Do not say anything; allow him to think longer and then respond.
d. "Well, for example, would you like to achieve your ideal weight, or reach your target blood sugar? You know, things like that."

11. Which electrolyte level, frequently masked and appearing as normal, can be life threatening if not immediately corrected in diabetic ketoacidosis (DKA)?

a. Potassium
b. Phosphate
c. Sodium bicarbonate
d. Sodium

12. The following policies are part of a diabetes educator's DSMES program: asking patients if there are any dietary preferences or restrictions, inviting family members to participate, and being sensitive to one's rate of speech and tone of voice. These policies address which specific type of consideration?

a. Readiness for change variation among patients
b. Potential low literacy/numeracy levels among patients
c. Cultural characteristics/barriers of the population
d. Poor family and social support

13. For how long following intense, extended exercise should a person with diabetes be concerned about the possibility of activity-related hypoglycemia (assuming the person uses insulin)?

a. Up to 24 hours after the activity
b. Up to 8 hours after the activity
c. Up to 4 hours after the activity
d. Up to 2 hours after the activity

14. According to ADA/European Association for the Study of Diabetes guidelines, a solution to therapeutic inertia in medical management of type 2 diabetes is using:

a. Better diabetic education
b. Multidisciplinary teams
c. Specialist care
d. Strict glycemic targets

15. A diabetes educator discovers that the middle school her patient attends does not permit him to carry his blood glucose meter or insulin with him. What step below would the educator take to advocate for his patient?

a. Teach the patient how and when he should check his glucose to stay within the school guidelines (i.e., before and after school).
b. Show the patient ways he can hide his testing and insulin supplies and perform the necessary skills in the bathroom, so as not to get in trouble.
c. Contact the school principal, school nurse, and head district nurse to get clarification on the policy and explain the need for modification for the patient.
d. Encourage the parents of the patient to contact the school board or her legislator if necessary.

16. When meeting with a patient who has type 2 diabetes and is pregnant (26 weeks), the patient reports that her fasting and postprandial blood glucose values have been within the target range and that she is taking insulin before each meal as advised. However, she also reports that almost every day of the last two weeks, she has had a small to moderate amount of ketones in her urine. Of the options below, which management plan would best address this problem?

a. As long as ketones are not consistently present in large amounts and her blood glucose values are within range, there is no need to adjust her regimen at this time.
b. The patient's bedtime long-acting insulin dose should be increased to eliminate the ketones.
c. Since ketones are a byproduct of the breakdown of fat, the patient should increase the amount of fat eaten throughout the day so that she will gain weight instead of lose it.
d. The patient should add a substantial snack at bedtime, coupled with a dose of prandial insulin to cover the snack.

17. A patient states that he has the goal of getting his HbA1c to below 7% by the end of the year. He worries that having it high as it is now (7.9%) puts him at risk for complications. The diabetes educator notices that the patient's weight has been increasing. He admits that with his new job, he has not had time to work out at the gym and has been snacking a lot due to stress. Which of the actions below would be the BEST next step with this patient?

a. Discuss the increased risks of having an HbA1c level above 7%.
b. Ask open-ended questions that may help the patient identify some short-term goals that will help lower his HbA1c.
c. Lay out a daily schedule for the patient that facilitates his return to exercising, which will be sufficient to lower glucose levels without increasing his medication.
d. Explore why he eats when stressed and suggest some stress-reduction exercises that he can do at work.

18. Modifiable risk factors for the development of diabetes include:

a. Genetic predisposition
b. Family history
c. Hyperlipidemia
d. Ethnicity

19. Acute sensory neuropathy and chronic sensorimotor distal polyneuropathy (DPN) are characterized by severe burning pain in the lower extremities that is often worse at night. What is considered the key to effective management of these conditions?

a. Confirmation of diagnosis and ruling out other causes through neurologic testing
b. Pain management with medication and referral to a pain management specialist
c. Graded supervised aerobic exercise to safely improve circulation
d. Blood glucose control and stabilization

20. At a visit last month, a patient committed to quit smoking. When the diabetes educator calls to see how he is doing (four weeks later), he admits that he has had two relapses, but then "re-committed" to stop smoking each time. He asks if the educator has any tips to help him avoid these relapses. Which suggestion below is NOT a recommended relapse prevention strategy?

a. Be aware of risky behavior or situations that may lead to a relapse and try to avoid them.
b. Have a plan to combat negative thoughts or temptations.
c. Employ stress management techniques, such as cognitive reframing, turning to a support person, or others that the patient has used to help manage stress.
d. Acknowledge and repeat the mantra that the bad behavior is gone and will not come back (i.e., "I am not a smoker; I do not want or need to smoke").

21. Regarding communication among all members of a patient's healthcare team, which of the following statements is TRUE, according to the National Standards for Diabetes Self-Management Education and Support?

a. Because of HIPAA restrictions, providers and educators are limited in sharing patients' health information with team members without permission from the patients.
b. Sharing information among healthcare team members increases the likelihood that all the members will work in collaboration.
c. Patients report greater satisfaction when their information is shared among team members, and it saves them the time of having to repeat assessments.
d. Communicating with members of a patient's healthcare team under recent guidelines has resulted in additional costs in terms of time, money, and work burden.

22. The dawn phenomenon is caused by:

a. An excessive dosage of basal insulin
b. A surge of hormone production
c. Inadequate control of blood glucose
d. Dehydration due to inadequate fluid intake

23. A person with diabetes is a devout Muslim and plans to fast for the month of Ramadan even though Islam allows exemptions for illness. The person should be taught that the fast must be broken and glucose ingested if the fasting blood glucose level falls to:

a. ≤60 mg/dL (3.3 mmol/L)
b. ≤70 mg/dL (3.9 mmol/L)
c. ≤80 mg/dL (4.4 mmol/L)
d. ≤90 mg/dL (5.0 mmol/L)

24. A 29-year-old Hispanic female patient tells her diabetes educator that her goal is to lose 15 lb by her wedding day in three months. What element of the nutrition assessment is most important to focus on to help her meet her goal?

a. Composition of nutrients (protein/fat vs. carbohydrates)
b. Energy balance (total calorie intake vs. expenditure)
c. Type and amounts of carbohydrates consumed (i.e., glycemic index)
d. Total grams of fiber per day

25. Which of the following behaviors is the MOST likely indication that a patient is at a very low level of readiness to change?

a. The patient becomes tearful as the diabetes educator explains how to keep a food diary.
b. The patient watches a demonstration but does not say anything.
c. The patient volunteers to answer a review question at the end of class but gets the answer totally wrong.
d. The patient denies that they have diabetes and disagrees with the doctor's referral for DSMES.

26. What is the GREATEST risk for persons with small-nerve-fiber neuropathy, a subcategory of chronic sensorimotor distal neuropathy?

a. Injury from falls due to Charcot foot syndrome
b. Decrease in overall wellness due to limited mobility
c. Risk for sudden cardiac death due to cardiac denervation
d. Foot ulceration and subsequent gangrene and amputation

27. According to the ADA and the American College of Sports Medicine, those with diabetes should break up sedentary time by standing and walking around or performing some type of light physical activity every:

a. 30 minutes
b. 45 minutes
c. 60 minutes
d. 90 minutes

28. Which of the four types of readiness to learn includes consideration of past coping mechanisms and cultural background?

a. Emotional
b. Physical
c. Knowledge
d. Experiential

29. What is the ultimate goal of diabetes self-management education and support (DSMES)?

a. Optimal glycemic control
b. Imparting knowledge and skills needed to make important lifestyle (behavioral) changes
c. Reducing diabetes-related complications
d. Reduced incidence, cost, and effects of diabetes through improved prevention, diagnosis, and management

30. In a multidisciplinary team care approach to diabetes management, which of the individuals below is "central to the team," according to the National Standards for DSMES?

a. The patient
b. The diabetes educator
c. The case manager
d. The primary care physician

31. A 24-year-old with type 1 diabetes for three years manages his diabetes with multiple daily injections of basal and rapid-acting insulin. He reports a trend of high morning blood sugars and hypoglycemia just before meals during the day. The patient agrees to wear a continuous glucose monitoring (CGM) system for three days. Upon examination of the report, the diabetes educator notices two occurrences where the patient's blood glucose dropped below 60 mg/dL overnight. On the one night when this did not occur, fasting morning blood sugars were within target range. What is the likely explanation for what this patient is experiencing?

a. Somogyi phenomenon
b. Dawn phenomenon
c. Inappropriate nutrient balance at night (needs more protein)
d. Fluctuations in the honeymoon period

32. A client with type 1 diabetes takes a basal dose of long-acting insulin as well as mealtime insulin on a sliding scale. His glucose readings (in mg/dL) before meals and at bedtime vary widely:

Day	Fasting	Lunch	Dinner	Bedtime
Day 1	110	64	304	188
Day 2	107	288	298	163
Day 3	112	178	302	150

The most likely solution is to:

a. Increase the basal dosage of insulin.
b. Increase the basal and mealtime dosages of insulin.
c. Decrease the carbohydrate intake at meals.
d. Adjust the carbohydrate intake and mealtime insulin dosages.

33. Mrs. M is a 65-year-old Hispanic female with type 2 diabetes and a diagnosis of congestive heart failure. At this time, she takes no medication for her diabetes, and states that she follows a fairly strict carb-consistent diet. Her HbA1c values have steadily increased over the past year and have now reached 8.4%. In addition, her serum creatinine has also been increasing and is now at 2.1 mg/dL and her eGFR has decreased to 40 mL/min/1.73 m^2. She states that she is not willing to consider insulin at this time. Which medication would her provider likely prescribe?

a. Glucophage (metformin)
b. Actos (pioglitazone)
c. Lantus insulin (insulin glargine)
d. Jardiance (empagliflozin)

34. A diabetes educator is preparing to teach an introductory course at a community center on nutrition intervention as part of diabetes care. Which of the following materials would be MOST appropriate for the class the educator will be teaching?

a. Copies of ADA guidelines on nutrition
b. Models of foods, nutrition labels, and sample restaurant menus
c. Graphs showing rates of diabetes complication for different HbA1c levels
d. Props to demonstrate personal foot care (mirror, file, socks, types of shoes, etc.)

35. For patients with type 2 diabetes, the target range for BMI is:

a. <30 kg/m^2
b. <25 kg/m^2
c. 18.5–24.9 kg/m^2
d. 18.5–30 kg/m^2

36. A client complains that his smart insulin pen does not always synchronize with his mobile app. In order to synchronize properly, the pen must usually be within how many meters of the mobile app?

a. 5 meters (16.4 feet)
b. 10 meters (32.8 feet)
c. 15 meters (49.5 feet)
d. 20 meters (65.6 feet)

37. Hypoglycemia unawareness is the decrease or absence of the typical counterregulatory responses to low blood glucose. Which of the following options is the PRIMARY recommendation for addressing this phenomenon?

a. More-frequent blood glucose monitoring, including use of continuous glucose monitoring
b. Less-stringent glucose targets, at least for several weeks
c. More-stringent blood glucose control to restore autonomic responses to hypoglycemia
d. Increased precautions, including cessation of driving and limits on high-risk activity

38. For a 45-year-old who is newly diagnosed with diabetes and has reasonable health literacy, which instructional methods are usually the most appropriate?

a. Problem-solving and group education
b. Simple, clear instruction and hands-on learning with assistance
c. One-on-one coaching and demonstrations/practice
d. Simplified materials and visual aids and diagrams

39. Which of the following methods is LEAST recommended as a valid way to perform an initial patient DSMES assessment?

a. Talking to the nurse of the referring provider and using the information to complete the assessment form
b. Meeting with the patient face-to-face and asking questions of the patient and their spouse (if they have one)
c. Having patients complete an assessment form online before the first appointment and then following up with a few questions in person
d. Observing patients in a group setting while having each member of the group complete personal information on a standardized assessment form

40. Which of the following dietary interventions has NOT been shown to be an effective weight-loss strategy?

a. Four or five small meals/snacks throughout the day
b. Omitting breakfast to reduce total daily caloric intake
c. Emphasis on portion control
d. Meal replacements (such as liquid meals or pre-packaged weight loss meals)

41. A diabetes educator receives a referral for a patient, Mr. B, from his primary care provider for "medication consult and education related to history of non-compliance." Which of the following strategies would provide the diabetes educator with the most accurate and comprehensive assessment on Mr. B's medication knowledge, habits, and associated challenges?

a. Prepare a written knowledge assessment in which he will match the name of a medication he takes with the appropriate common side effect.
b. Spend extra time reading through the patient's chart notes written by the referring provider to get a better sense of the diabetes medication, education, and adherence history.
c. Ask the patient to bring a written list of what he is taking and when, then compare it to the list of what is currently prescribed.
d. Have the patient bring all the medication he currently takes, in the original containers, then have him describe for what purpose, when, and how he takes each medication.

42. An adolescent has recently been diagnosed with type 1 diabetes. The adolescent is slightly overweight but active in sports and social activities and resists staying on a low-carbohydrate diet. Which of the following is the most important consideration when educating the adolescent about diabetic management?

a. Preventing long-term complications
b. Adjusting insulin for exercise, diet, and illness
c. Adhering to a low-carbohydrate diet
d. Maintaining a low body weight

43. Which of the following nutrition modifications is NOT recommended for patients who suffer from gastroparesis?

a. Increased dietary fiber
b. Frequent small meals
c. Decreased dietary fat
d. Soft (e.g., over-cooked vegetables) or liquid foods

44. Which of the following disorders increases the risk that a woman who is pregnant will develop gestational diabetes?

a. Endometriosis
b. Hyperthyroidism
c. Celiac disease
d. Polycystic ovary syndrome

45. Which of the following foot care recommendations is NOT appropriate for a person with diabetes, assuming there are no physical limitations, loss of protective sensation, or lower extremity injuries or infections?

a. If foot odor is noticed, soak feet in a warm Epsom salt bath for 15–20 minutes per day.
b. If you notice dry skin, moisturize the area daily with lotion, except between the toes.
c. Wash your feet frequently. Pat skin dry and dry between the toes thoroughly.
d. If toenails are long enough to bump the inside of the shoe, trim straight across and file any sharp corners.

46. Which life transition poses the most challenges for the management of diabetes?

a. Infancy to childhood
b. Childhood to adolescence
c. Adolescence to adulthood
d. Adulthood to older adulthood

47. A new patient reports that she is not sure what type of diabetes she has because no one has ever given her a clear answer. She is 46 years old and Caucasian, with a BMI of 20. She states that she has always been thin and active, and that no one in her family has diabetes that she knows of. With the exception of her father, who has rheumatoid arthritis and psoriasis, her family history is unremarkable. She was diagnosed with diabetes two years ago and claims she is able to keep her blood sugar in the normal range with a careful low-carb diet. Her last HbA1c was 6.4%, and her most recent C-peptide level was on the low end of normal. Labs are also positive for GAD and islet cell antibodies. What type of diabetes does this patient MOST likely have?

a. Type 2 diabetes
b. Type 1 diabetes
c. Latent autoimmune diabetes of adulthood (LADA)
d. Maturity-onset diabetes of the young (MODY)

48. Read the patient statement below and select the response by the educator that is the BEST example of "developing discrepancy," one of the guiding principles of motivational interviewing.

Patient: "I just can't stand testing my blood sugar, although I have to admit that when I do and the number is high, I act on it right away."

a. Educator: "Just be glad that we have the meters we do today. Back in the day, it took more than a minute to get the result and you needed a much bigger drop of blood, which meant a much more painful finger poke!"
b. Educator: "It sounds like you are dealing with some serious obstacles when it comes to self-monitoring; yet, I also sense that when you do test, you are able to use the information to help you correct high blood sugars when needed. What effect do you think those corrections will have on your health in the long run?"
c. Educator: "It is just one of those things that people with diabetes have to deal with. Trust me, you are not alone—almost none of my patients enjoy testing their blood sugar, and I tell them the same thing I am telling you."
d. Educator: "Great job coming in with your meter and log book today. Let's see how you did over the last two weeks on correcting for highs and treating lows."

49. During the initial assessment process, a patient answers the question, "How important is it for you to make this change right now?" with a 9 out of 10 (very important) and answers the question, "How confident are you that you will be able to make this change?" with a 2 out of 10 (not very confident). In customizing this patient's DSMES plan, what should the focus be?

a. Providing materials and experiences to enhance knowledge and provide psychosocial support
b. Assisting the patient in managing stress levels
c. Highlighting the benefits of good diabetes management as a way to encourage behavior change
d. Explaining the two questions further to confirm understanding, as it is very uncommon for a patient to rate the readiness-to-change elements this far apart

50. All of the suggestions below are appropriate strategies to address financial barriers associated with self-monitoring of blood glucose, except one. Which suggestion is NOT a recommended cost-cutting strategy?

a. Obtain a generic meter with corresponding test strips from a big-box store such as Wal-Mart, where test strips are only about half the cost as those from other sources.
b. If possible, back-date the meter so that it will accept recently expired test strips.
c. Select a monitoring schedule/strategy that conserves test strips but still provides information to identify trends.
d. Regardless of the meter the clinic prefers, contact the insurance carrier to determine which meter/strip brand is preferred and therefore least expensive to the patient.

51. A client with type 1 diabetes uses basal and bolus insulin to control his blood glucose levels. His diabetes is fairly stable, but he has had occasional episodes of hypoglycemia. Before driving, he should check his blood glucose level and only drive if it is at least:

a. 70 mg/dL (3.9 mmol/L)
b. 80 mg/dL (4.4 mmol/L)
c. 90 mg/dL (5.0 mmol/L)
d. 100 mg/dL (5.6 mmol/L)

52. Which of the following diagnostic tests is most valuable in evaluating dietary and treatment compliance for a 70-year-old patient with type 2 diabetes?

a. Fasting blood glucose
b. Diabetes autoantibodies
c. Ketones (urine)
d. HbA1c

53. Which of the following patient statements would be LEAST important to note in the health history section of the initial DSMES assessment?

a. "My mother believes I got diabetes from eating too much candy as a kid."
b. "I was hospitalized eight months ago for DKA."
c. "I experience low blood sugar episodes about twice a month."
d. "I have had diabetes for 4 years, but I am not sure what type I have."

54. Which statement below is characteristic of a "patient empowerment" approach to DSMES, as opposed to more traditional behavioral theories?

a. Patients must rely only on themselves to deal with the challenges of a chronic disease, such as diabetes.
b. Patients learn from their own experiences and from observing the experiences of those around them.
c. The choices that have the greatest effects on diabetes outcomes are made by patients, not by healthcare professionals.
d. A patient's perception of how the community/society views a behavior will have a great impact on their intentions to adapt it.

55. A 52-year-old male has recently been diagnosed with type 2 diabetes and takes lisinopril 10 mg daily for hypertension with a current blood pressure reading of 136/85 mmHg. His BMI is 30 kg/m^2. His fasting blood glucose level is 158 mg/dL, and his HbA1c is 7.8%. What first-line medication is he most likely to be prescribed?

a. SGLT-2 inhibitor (e.g., empagliflozin)
b. Biguanide (e.g., metformin)
c. GLP-1 receptor agonist (e.g., semaglutide)
d. DPP-4 inhibitor (e.g., glipizide)

56. A woman who is newly diagnosed with type 1 diabetes works the night shift from 11 p.m. to 7 a.m. and often eats food purchased from vending machines on an erratic schedule. She has had difficulty managing her diabetes, including repeated episodes of hypoglycemia. Her educational plan should focus on:

a. Eating larger meals and frequent snacks during working hours
b. Adjusting her insulin to a lower dosage
c. Learning about the physiology of diabetes
d. Monitoring her glucose and managing her diet

57. The primary vascular change that results from diabetes is:

a. Vascular hyperpermeability
b. Atherosclerosis
c. Angiogenesis
d. Vasculitis

58. What is the recommended breakdown of macronutrients, according to the current American Diabetes Association nutrition recommendations?

a. Approximately 70% of total calories should come from carbohydrates, 20% from protein, and 10% from fat.
b. Approximately 45–55% of total calories should come from carbohydrates, 25–40% from protein, and 15–20% from fat.
c. Approximately 35–40% of total calories should come from carbohydrates, 20–30% from protein, and 30–35% from fat.
d. There is no specific mix of macronutrients recommended by the ADA. The best mix of macronutrients depends on individual circumstances.

59. A patient in a DSMES group asks why a person cannot use oral medication to treat type 1 diabetes. Which is the most accurate and appropriate response?

a. "Because type 2 diabetes is brought on by weight, and weight gain is a side effect of insulin, we avoid using insulin in those with type 2 diabetes while we prefer it for those with type 1, who are typically underweight."
b. "Everyone needs insulin to live. In type 2 diabetes, the insulin–producing cells (beta cells) may still be working somewhat but not well enough to keep blood sugar normal. Oral medications help the body's insulin to work better. In type 1 diabetes, the body has destroyed its own beta cells and so we must use insulin from an outside source."
c. "Type 1 diabetes is a more severe form of diabetes, and therefore we go straight for the most potent medication. Type 2 diabetes, on the other hand, is less severe and can be minimized by lifestyle changes, and so there are less-drastic medication options."
d. "Because type 2 diabetes is characterized by insulin resistance, most oral medications for type 2 diabetes work by improving a body's sensitivity to insulin. Those with type 1 diabetes are very sensitive to insulin. If some of these oral medications were used to treat someone who has type 1 diabetes, they would likely cause severe hypoglycemia."

60. What is the main difference between process (or formative) evaluation and outcomes (or summative) evaluation in diabetes education?

a. Process evaluation deals with patients, and outcomes evaluation deals with the organization.
b. The purpose of process evaluation is to determine adjustments that are needed in the educational process; the purpose of outcomes evaluation is to determine the effectiveness of the education process.
c. The scope of process evaluation is small, as in a single session or class, whereas the outcomes evaluation encompasses a period of time (usually one year) and includes statistics on an organization's productivity (e.g., number of patients served, classes taught).
d. The object of process evaluation is to identify gaps or deficits and then make changes and adjustments as needed; the object of outcomes evaluation is to compile and summarize data for reporting purposes.

61. Which patient statement regarding medication administration would cause the diabetes educator to suspect that further education is needed?

a. "When I had to skip breakfast and lunch the day of my procedure, I took my Diabeta® (glyburide) but skipped my Levemir® (detemir)."
b. "I leave my Lantus pen on my nightstand all the time so I will remember to take it at bedtime."
c. "I take my metformin every morning, even if I will be skipping breakfast."
d. "I throw away the NovoLog® (aspart) vial of insulin I am using after four weeks, even if it is still half full."

62. Which of the following assessment findings is most likely to indicate poor circulation in the lower extremities?

a. Substantial hair on the tops of the toes
b. Ankle-brachial index of 1.0
c. Diminished dorsal pedal pulses
d. Positive pinprick sensation at the level of the ankle

Refer to the following for questions 63 - 64:

Nutrition Facts
Serving Size 1 cup (70 g)
Servings Per Container 3

Amount Per Serving	
Calories 400	Calories from Fat 150
	% Daily Value*
Total Fat 19g	26%
Saturated Fat 5g	14%
Trans Fat 3g	
Cholesterol 1mg	1%
Sodium 580mg	32%
Total Carbohydrates 51g	17%
Dietary Fiber 3g	10%
Sugars 2g	
Protein 8g	

Vitamin A 10%	Vitamin C 0%
Calcium 6%	Iron 15%

* Percent Daily Values are based on a 2,000 calorie diet. Your Daily values may be higher or lower depending on your calorie needs.

	Calories:	2,000	2,500
Total Fat	Less than	65g	80g
Sat Fat	Less than	20g	25g
Cholesterol	Less than	300mg	300mg
Sodium	Less than	2400mg	2400mg
Total Carbohydrate		300g	375g
Dietary Fiber		35g	30g

Calories per gram:
Fat 9 • Carbohydrate 4 • Protein 4

63. A patient states that he eats about half of the package of this product at one time. What is the approximate total amount of carbohydrates the patient consumes of this product?

a. 25 g
b. 51 g
c. 75 g
d. 102 g

64. The patient claims that this is an ideal food for him. He says that he is not worried about counting his carbs for this food because the package says that the food is listed as a low-glycemic-index food. The label also tells him that the sugars are pretty low and so based on that alone, this food is a good choice. Finally, the fiber is high, which means that he does not need to count some of the carbohydrates. Which of the following statements is NOT correct in this situation?

a. The amount of fiber in this food is not high enough to discount from total carbohydrates.
b. The total sugar is not important because the starches rapidly convert to glucose as well.
c. Even though the food may be a low-glycemic-index food, moderation and tracking of all carbs is still needed.
d. The patient is correct. The combination of low sugar, low glycemic index, and high fiber make this an ideal food choice, in any amount.

65. What is the FIRST treatment priority for a person experiencing a hyperosmolar hyperglycemic state (HHS)?

a. Decrease blood glucose by infusing insulin.
b. Rehydrate by providing adequate intravenous fluids.
c. Correct electrolyte imbalances by monitoring and providing supplementation when needed.
d. Address the background infection that precipitated the HHS.

66. An early indication of hyperglycemia is:

a. Increased perspiration
b. Increased thirst
c. Episodes of dizziness
d. Weight gain

67. As of 2026, the American Diabetes Association recommends that metabolic surgery be considered only for those patients with type 2 diabetes who meet which of the following criteria?

a. Patient has tried numerous dietary and/or behavioral options to lose weight without measurable success.
b. Patient presents with weight-related comorbidities that are potentially life-threatening.
c. Patient's BMI is ≥30 kg/m^2, and glycemic control through other means has proven difficult.
d. There are no criteria at this time, as the ADA does not recommend metabolic surgery as a treatment option due to cost and associated risks.

68. Which of the following examples would a diabetes educator assess to be the MOST appropriate example of individual BGM record keeping?

a. A patient records her BG values with time, date, medications, food intake, and other activities in a spiral notebook instead of the log sheet provided by the clinic. The book is tattered and stained with blood and food.
b. A patient simply allows the meter to record all of his BG readings, then he brings the meter to the clinic for each visit.
c. A patient does not bring her meter to the clinic but writes her BG values on the log sheet provided by the clinic. She lists only the values and no other information (e.g., food, activity, medication).
d. A patient writes his BG values in the logbook that came with his meter. He includes times, activity levels, and illnesses, but does not write dates, food intake, or medication doses on the pages. He admits that he just picks any blank page to start the week and that some are out of order.

69. For hospitalized patients with diabetes, discharge planning, including appropriate diabetes education (i.e., "survival skills" education) should begin when?

a. As soon as the patient is admitted
b. As soon as the provider has written the discharge order
c. As soon as the patient states that they are ready for instruction
d. As soon as the appropriate diabetes treatment plan (e.g., diet recommendations, medications, BGM schedule, and BG targets) has been decided

70. A person with diabetes has found managing the disease difficult and has become increasingly depressed and withdrawn. What type of psychotherapy may be the most helpful?

a. Psychoanalysis
b. Interpersonal therapy
c. Cognitive behavioral therapy
d. Dialectical behavior therapy

71. Diabetes is a risk factor for periodontal disease. Which of the following increases this risk?

a. Lack of water fluoridation
b. High-calcium diet
c. Dyslipidemia
d. Smoking

72. Despite attending all classes as well as one-on-one visits with the educator, a patient performs only the bare minimum self-care skills. Beyond basic survival skills education, he has not been receptive to any additional information about his diabetes. Which explanation below is the most likely, and what is the logical course of action for the educator?

a. He did not fully understand the information in the classes; he would likely benefit from a review of the self-management material.
b. His personality is more introspective; he likely uses the problem-focused coping style. This patient should be presented with printed information that he can process privately and provided with contact information should he need help.
c. The patient is likely experiencing the "depression and frustration" emotional stage of dealing with a chronic disease. The educator should emphasize positive changes and accomplishments, but recognize the sense of loss that comes with facing a lifetime disease.
d. The patient's actions represent an avoidant coping style, commonly associated with emotional discomfort. The educator should initiate a frank, honest discussion on what he is feeling, including validating his feelings. Pushing additional, more in-depth diabetes education at this point is not helpful.

73. Which two risk factors have the strongest correlation with a patient's risk for development and progression of diabetic retinopathy?

a. Type of diabetes and HbA1c
b. Blood glucose control and blood pressure control
c. Blood glucose variability and smoking status
d. Blood pressure control and family history of eye disease

74. A diabetes educator is visiting with a patient who has type 1 diabetes and uses an insulin pump. The patient tells the diabetes educator that she is confused about the sick day instructions she has been given and asks why she should increase her basal rate when she is rarely able to eat anything when she feels sick. Which explanation below is MOST appropriate?

a. "You are correct to question these instructions. You should never take more insulin when you are not eating, as insulin will drop your blood sugar. Instead of increasing the basal rate, you should actually decrease it. Once you are feeling better and eating normally again, you can resume your regular basal insulin schedule."
b. "Food is needed to fight the illness and prevent diabetic ketoacidosis (DKA). Extra basal insulin will slowly lower your blood sugar. As your blood sugar drops, you will begin to feel hungry. So, in this case, the extra basal insulin actually acts as an appetite stimulant."
c. "During times of stress such as illness, your liver puts extra glucose into your blood. Your basal insulin covers the glucose from the liver, as opposed to glucose from the carbs you eat. Therefore, extra basal insulin is needed to address the extra liver sugar when you are sick. When you eat or drink something with carbohydrates, you would bolus accordingly."
d. "We know that because of dehydration, insulin does not get absorbed as well when you are sick. Therefore, in addition to drinking at least 8 oz of fluid every hour, you must also increase the basal insulin rate to compensate for the decrease in insulin absorption."

75. Which of the following options is a modifiable risk factor for type 2 diabetes?

a. Weight/obesity
b. Family history
c. Race/ethnicity
d. Age

76. A certified diabetes care and education specialist (CDCES) is providing education about self-care to a patient with diabetes. The first step in educating the patient should be to:

a. Establish goals and expected outcomes.
b. Review the person's medication schedule.
c. Discuss dietary restrictions.
d. Assess the person's readiness to learn.

77. According to the American Diabetes Association (ADA), the recommended blood pressure for persons with diabetes and additional risk factors, such as albuminuria or high cardiovascular risk, is a systolic blood pressure goal of:

a. <140 mmHg
b. <135 mmHg
c. <130 mmHg
d. ≤120 mmHg

78. The most efficient way for a person with diabetes to track physical activity is to:

a. Maintain a written record.
b. Use a wearable fitness device.
c. Prepare a schedule of activities.
d. Wear a pedometer.

79. A woman with type 1 diabetes wants to become pregnant and is undergoing preconception counseling. She has been advised to maintain her HbA1c at the target level for a few months prior to conception. The target level for preconception HbA1c is typically set at:

a. <7.5%
b. <7.0%
c. <6.5%
d. <6.0%

Refer to the following for questions 80 - 81:

A diabetes educator works at several different diabetes care centers across the state. In preparation for individualizing her interventions for the needs of each center's population, she is conducting population needs assessment for each of the centers.

80. Which geographic areas are most underserved in terms of access to diabetes education?

a. Inner cities
b. Suburban areas
c. Rural areas, particularly in the South
d. States with the highest population density

81. Which of the following statements relating to barriers to diabetes education is true?

a. Most primary care providers do not agree that their patients need more education and support for diabetes.
b. Patients over the age of 65 are more likely to seek diabetes education than their middle-aged counterparts are.
c. Reflecting the makeup of the diabetes population, the majority of participants in DSMES programs are minorities.
d. Tension and disagreement between primary care providers and diabetes educators regarding self-care recommendations has been found to be a barrier to patients' access to diabetes education.

82. The ADA recommends that all adults, regardless of BMI, be screened for type 2 diabetes and prediabetes by age:

a. 35
b. 40
c. 45
d. 50

83. Why does the American Diabetes Association recommend the development of standardized procedures for documentation, training health professionals to document appropriately, and the use of structured standardized forms based on current practice guidelines in the National Standards for Diabetes Self-Management Education and Support (DSMES)?

a. Such documentation practices and attributes are required by TJC (The Joint Commission).
b. Such documentation practices and attributes have been shown to improve documentation and may ultimately improve quality of care.
c. Such documentation practices and attributes will facilitate smoother clinic operations and reduce administrative costs.
d. Such documentation practices and attributes assist in the reimbursement process and are preferred by most insurance carriers.

84. A client's glucose levels remain high even though the insulin pump indicates that it is delivering insulin appropriately. The initial action should be to:

a. Check the reservoir.
b. Reposition the cannula.
c. Reassess the client's insulin-to-carbohydrate ratios.
d. Check the client's ketone levels.

85. Identify the statement below that is TRUE with regard to recommended lab values.

a. Someone with an HDL of 31 mg/dL is not at risk for CVD as long as their total cholesterol is not above 200 mg/dL.
b. A serum creatinine of 3.6 mg/dL in a 55-year-old female indicates probable renal impairment.
c. Regardless of regular BGM values, someone with type 1 diabetes with an HbA1c of 5.9% is well-controlled.
d. A patient who has a creatinine level of less than 56 IU/L does not have fatty liver disease.

86. The ADA recommends that persons with diabetes:

a. Visit a dentist twice yearly
b. Brush their teeth three times a day
c. Floss their teeth twice daily
d. Brush their teeth for at least 1 minute each time they brush

87. Like sulfonylureas, DPP-4 inhibitors stimulate the production of insulin. Unlike sulfonylureas, DPP-4 inhibitors:

a. Do not cause hypoglycemia
b. Causes severe hypoglycemia
c. Cannot be taken with metformin
d. Can have severe adverse effects

88. If a person has cognitive impairment or learning disabilities that interfere with learning, it is essential to:

a. Break information down into small, manageable steps.
b. Limit repetitions to prevent them from becoming bored.
c. Wait for the person to ask questions if they do not understand.
d. Avoid the use of visual aids, as these may overwhelm the person.

89. Which statement best describes how steroid use MOST affects blood glucose?

a. Steroid use induces insulin resistance and affects glucose metabolism, which is manifested especially in postprandial glucose levels.
b. Steroid use decreases the rate of insulin metabolism and therefore increases the risk for hypoglycemia.
c. Steroid use increases insulin resistance and is specifically manifested in fasting glucose levels.
d. Steroids suppress the immune system and deactivate a portion of both endogenous and exogenous insulin. Therefore, blood glucose typically rises with steroid use.

90. An adult male patient who is 6'1", 215 lb, and has type 2 diabetes, completes a 24-hour dietary recall. Which of his meals, reported below, does the diabetes educator assess to be the one MOST in need of modification?

a. Breakfast: 1 cup of Raisin Bran cereal with 1 cup skim milk, 12 oz orange juice, $\frac{1}{2}$ bagel.
b. Lunch: Large taco salad (tortilla bowl, chicken, cheese, lettuce, tomato, salsa, refried beans, sour cream), 16 oz Diet Coke.
c. Dinner: 2 cheeseburgers (with lean beef), side salad with light Italian dressing, 1 cup green beans, black coffee.
d. All meals are equally inappropriate and in need of modification.

91. A person with type 1 diabetes has had repeated episodes of severe hypoglycemia, exhibits a lack of hypoglycemic awareness, and has had difficulty achieving HbA1c goals. What is a reasonable HbA1c goal for this individual?

a. 6.0–6.5%
b. 6.5–7.0%
c. 7.0–7.5%
d. 7.5–8.0%

92. Which of the following labs require the patient to fast for a minimum of 8 hours?

a. Lipid profile
b. HbA1c
c. Microalbumin
d. ALT/AST

93. A patient with poorly controlled type 2 diabetes and hypertension has a history of falling in the home and complains of increasing problems with balance, leading the patient to become increasingly housebound. With whom is it most appropriate for the CDCES to coordinate when developing the plan of care?

a. Social worker
b. Occupational therapist
c. Psychotherapist
d. Physical therapist

94. Which of the following diabetes medications should NOT be omitted for a patient who is fasting in preparation for surgery?

a. Metformin
b. Sulfonylurea
c. Short-acting insulin
d. Long-acting (basal) insulin

95. A patient arrives late for his appointment. The diabetes educator notices that his HbA1c is higher and that his adherence to self-care skills (specifically monitoring, exercising, and taking medication) has decreased since his last visit 6 months ago. When the educator asks, "Over the last month or so, have you lost interest in doing things that usually bring you pleasure?" he replies, "Yes, I have to admit that I have." What implication does this have and what should the response be?

a. His answer suggests that the patient is in a "slump" (or "burnout"), which many people with diabetes experience. Assure him that it is normal and encourage him to think back to how he felt when he was faithfully performing self-care behaviors.
b. His answer is expected, for when a person neglects self-care behaviors, it negatively affects glucose levels, which then decreases one's ability to participate in pleasurable activities. Discuss this cycle with the patient and encourage him to be more diligent with his monitoring, exercise, and medication.
c. The patient's answer suggests that he may be experiencing diabetes-related anxiety. Stress, the body's response to the anxiety, is manifested in his increased HbA1c and neglect of self-care activities. Discuss ways to reduce anxiety and stress, such as medication or breathing exercises.
d. His response is a strong indicator of depression. Encourage the patient to meet with a mental health professional, then make the referral and offer to help schedule the appointment. Follow up with the patient by phone to ensure that he attended the appointment and schedule a follow-up visit for diabetes care in one month.

96. Which of the following assessment items is NOT considered a component of the "knowledge" area of a patient's readiness to learn?

a. Literacy/numeracy
b. Level of family support
c. Previous diabetes self-management education
d. Proficiency of self-care skills

97. A person who is learning to manage type 2 diabetes speaks English with a very strong Spanish accent. When teaching the person, the CDCES should:

a. Ask what language the client prefers instruction in.
b. Provide written, video, and audio materials in Spanish.
c. Arrange for an interpreter to be present.
d. Speak slowly in English and use simple vocabulary.

98. More than 50% of men notice the onset of erectile dysfunction within ten years of the diagnosis of diabetes. Various treatment options are available. Which patient below would NOT be a candidate for a phosphodiesterase type 5 inhibitor (PDE5 inhibitor) such as sildenafil (Viagra®), vardenafil (Levitra®), or tadalafil (Cialis®)?

a. A man with stage 3 chronic kidney disease
b. A man with moderate liver impairment
c. A man with mild ischemic heart disease who uses nitroglycerine spray PRN for chest pain
d. All of the above

99. A patient who has identified himself as a visual learner would likely most prefer which method of instruction?

a. Role-playing a scenario in which he orders a balanced meal at a restaurant.
b. Seeing pictures of food portions followed by booklets on meal planning.
c. A spoken explanation of how to adjust insulin depending on pre-meal glucose.
d. Group discussion on challenges relating to dealing with the stress of diabetes.

100. According to the principles of the American Association of Clinical Endocrinology Comprehensive Type 2 Diabetes Management Algorithm, persons with diabetes should reach target goals of their therapy and adjust the therapy as needed within a time period of:

a. 2 months
b. 3 months
c. 6 months
d. 12 months

101. Which of the following laboratory results may be an indication of kidney disease?

a. UACR 28 mg/g
b. eGFR 78 mL/min/1.73 m^2
c. Serum creatinine 0.89 mg/dL (0.5 mmol/L)
d. BUN 18 mg/dL (1.0 mmol/L)

102. What are the ADA-recommended cholesterol goals for adults with diabetes and no history of cardiovascular disease?

a. LDL <100 mg/dL, HDL >40 mg/dL (men) or >50 mg/dL (women), triglycerides <150 mg/dL
b. LDL <150 mg/dL, HDL >40 mg/dL (men) or >50 mg/dL (women), triglycerides <180 mg/dL
c. Total cholesterol <200, HDL >40 mg/dL, triglycerides <100 mg/dL
d. LDL <150 mg/dL, HDL >50 mg/dL (men) or >40 mg/dL (women), triglycerides <100 mg/dL

103. Standard 10 of National Standards for Diabetes Self-Management Education and Support states that DSMES providers will measure the effectiveness of the education and support and look for ways to improve any identified gaps in services or service quality. As a FIRST step in the continuous quality improvement process, the educator should ask which of the following questions?

a. What are we trying to accomplish?
b. What programs or initiatives should be implemented to improve outcomes?
c. How will we know if a change is an improvement?
d. What resources will be needed to implement changes to our current practice?

104. A 25-year-old person is newly diagnosed with type 1 diabetes and will be taking a basal dose of long-acting insulin and mealtime and bedtime doses of short-acting insulin on a sliding scale. The person plans to use an insulin pen and needs to learn to monitor their blood glucose levels. The person identifies as a visual learner. What approach should the CDCES use when instructing this client?

a. Demonstrate a procedure, explain each step, and ask the client to repeat and explain the steps.
b. Allow the client to handle the equipment and learn by doing.
c. Provide the client with a video, written directions, and illustrated instructions.
d. Wait and allow the client to ask questions.

105. In an area with a large Mexican immigrant population, which population health strategy is most likely to be successful in identifying and treating persons with diabetes?

a. Free screenings in churches, schools, and shopping areas
b. A radio-based public awareness campaign
c. Mailings of educational pamphlets
d. Internet-based interactive educational programs

106. Which of the following medications may react with glipizide (Glucotrol®) in a way that may result in an increased risk for hypoglycemia?

a. Corticosteroids (i.e., Deltasone®)
b. Protease inhibitors (i.e., indinavir)
c. Estrogen products (i.e., Premarin®)
d. Sulfonamides (i.e., Bactrim®)

107. What is a food source for monounsaturated fats?

a. Butter
b. Salmon
c. Avocados
d. Flaxseeds

108. The CDCES has explained to a parent of a child with type 1 diabetes that it is an autoimmune disorder. If the parent responds that the child got diabetes because of eating too much candy, this suggests that the parent lacks:

a. Literacy
b. Health literacy
c. Nutritional awareness
d. Critical thinking skills

109. The provider for a patient added pioglitazone (Actos®) to the patient's regimen one month ago. The patient visits his diabetes educator today and says that he is dissatisfied with the new medicine, as it "has not done one thing to help my blood sugar." After acknowledging his frustration, how should the educator respond to his complaint?

a. Suggest that he discontinue the medication and ask the provider to try something else.
b. Suggest that a higher dose may be needed and offer to consult with the provider to authorize a higher dose.
c. Suggest that the medicine may not be working because he is likely eating more, as evidenced by his weight gain since the last visit.
d. Explain that medications in this class can take up to 12 weeks to work.

110. A patient has a history of heart failure and chronic kidney disease. Which of the following medication types provides the most cardiorenal protection and so might be considered for this patient?

a. Sulfonylureas
b. GLP-1 agonists
c. SGLT-2 inhibitors
d. DPP-4 inhibitors

111. Which stage of diabetic retinopathy is characterized by neovascularization (new vessel growth) and/or vitreous or preretinal hemorrhage?

a. Proliferative diabetic retinopathy
b. Severe nonproliferative diabetic retinopathy
c. Moderate nonproliferative diabetic retinopathy
d. Mild nonproliferative diabetic retinopathy

112. A 24-year-old patient was diagnosed with type 1 diabetes after presenting with a glucose level of 468 mg/dL (26 mmol/L), polyuria, polydipsia, and weight loss. His condition has stabilized since starting insulin injections, and he now appears to be able to manage the diabetes with very little insulin and therefore believes that diabetic management will be simple and that no further instruction is needed. The CDCES should explain to him that:

a. His insulin needs will increase again.
b. He will no longer need to take insulin.
c. He was misdiagnosed and has type 2 diabetes.
d. His condition will remain stable at this level.

113. A diabetes educator receives the lab results for his next patient and sees that the HbA1c is 9.6%. When the patient enters the room, she tells the educator that she forgot her meter but brought her log book. The educator sees that for the past two months, she has not missed a single pre-meal or bedtime blood glucose test. All numbers are within target range. What is the most likely explanation for the discrepancy?

a. The patient likely has some type of anemia or hemoglobinopathy which results in her HbA1c not closely correlating with actual average estimated glucose.
b. The patient likely had a brand of BG meter that is inaccurate.
c. The patient is likely making up blood glucose values.
d. The patient is probably using improper testing technique.

114. To reduce the risk of complications from diabetes, such as heart disease, it is recommended that persons with diabetes aim for moderate aerobic exercise for a minimum of:

a. 60 minutes weekly
b. 90 minutes weekly
c. 120 minutes weekly
d. 150 minutes weekly

115. When asked to explain why he takes a specific oral diabetes medication, the patient does not look at the label. Instead, he opens the bottle and takes out a pill before answering. Which possible barrier should the diabetes educator investigate further?

a. Financial
b. Cognitive
c. Health literacy
d. Fear of side effects

116. A patient with type 2 diabetes is committed to exercising faithfully to both improve her glycemic control and lose weight. However, whenever she exercises for more than 30 minutes (at moderate intensity), her blood glucose drops below 80 mg/dL and she has to consume some type of sugary snack to bring it up. She is very discouraged that she is not able to lose weight due to having to supplement with extra sugar and calories when she exercises. Which of the following possible adjustments would be the best choice to make to the patient's regimen to prevent hypoglycemia and address her concern about weight loss?

a. She might consume a small amount of fat-free fruit before the activity (i.e., half a glass of orange juice).
b. She could omit her breakfast dose of repaglinide (Prandin®) on the mornings she will exercise.
c. She could skip her morning dose of metformin on mornings she will exercise.
d. She should not be concerned about the weight at this point, as exercise has many other benefits and she needs to treat low blood sugar.

117. If a person with diabetes intends to use nicotine gum to aid in smoking cessation and thereby reduce cardiovascular health risks, they should plan to use the gum for:

a. 6 weeks
b. 10 weeks
c. 12 weeks
d. 16 weeks

118. A client uses an insulin pump to manage his type 1 diabetes. He is training for a marathon and runs for prolonged periods three times weekly but experiences episodes of postexercise delayed-onset hypoglycemia during the night. On a day of exercise, he should:

a. Eat high-carbohydrate snacks before and after exercise
b. Decrease his basal insulin by 20% for 12 hours beginning the morning of the exercise
c. Exercise in the evening rather than in the morning and skip the evening insulin bolus
d. Decrease his basal insulin by 20% for 6 hours after exercise and eat snacks before and after exercise

119. An adolescent is diagnosed with type 1 diabetes and must learn to manage the condition, but his parents hover over him and repeatedly interfere, giving advice and critiquing while the adolescent is trying to learn. The adolescent wants the parents to leave, but they refuse to do so. The most appropriate solution is to:

a. Tell the parents to leave so the adolescent can concentrate.
b. Provide the parents with guidelines on more appropriate support.
c. Tell the adolescent to concentrate and ignore the parents.
d. Tell the parents directly that they are interfering with learning.

120. Which of the following statements regarding HbA1c is accurate in relation to persons with diabetes?

a. Regardless of age or other factors, an HbA1c greater than 7% represents a medically unacceptable risk.
b. HbA1c was adopted by the American Diabetes Association as a diagnostic tool for diabetes because there is almost no variation among race, gender, or age, and it remains largely unaffected by other medical conditions.
c. Screening for diabetes by using the HbA1c has been shown to identify more cases of previously undiagnosed diabetes than either the fasting plasma glucose or the 2-hour glucose tolerance test.
d. The ADA recommends that the HbA1c test should be performed at least twice annually, and more often in some cases.

121. A person takes metformin and glimepiride to control type 2 diabetes. Which of the following herbal supplements should be avoided?

a. St. John's wort
b. Milk thistle
c. Chamomile
d. Peppermint

122. In healthcare, evidence-based research is the basis for:

a. All processes and procedures
b. Routine administrative procedures
c. Individual judgment
d. Standard practices

123. The most common autoimmune disorder associated with type 1 diabetes mellitus is:

a. Hashimoto's thyroiditis
b. Addison's disease
c. Rheumatoid arthritis
d. Celiac disease

124. The primary goal of the Lifestyle Change Program of the CDC's National Diabetes Prevention Program is to prevent:

a. Complications of type 1 or 2 diabetes
b. Type 2 diabetes
c. Gestational diabetes
d. Diabetic ketoacidosis

125. A client has type 2 diabetes. Her HbA1c was 7.4% on diagnosis but it has decreased to 6.3% with metformin, a low-carbohydrate diet, and weight loss. Her fasting blood glucose levels are in the 90–126 mg/dL (5.0–7.0 mmol/L) range. According to the CDC, how often should this client's HbA1c be monitored?

a. Every month
b. Every 3 months
c. Every 6 months
d. Every 12 months

126. If a person with diabetes has peripheral neuropathy and adheres to a vegan diet, what dietary supplement may be recommended?

a. Vitamin C
b. Vitamin E
c. Vitamin B6
d. Vitamin B12

127. Which of the following methods is NOT recommended as an effective way to obtain information for tracking behavioral objectives?

a. Group classes
b. Email messaging
c. Phone consultation
d. Any of the above are legitimate ways to track patient progress of behavioral goals

128. A client who was recently diagnosed with type 1 diabetes is learning to manage his condition. He admits to being moderately anxious but has studied the materials that the CDCES provided and has done an internet search regarding diabetes. What is the most likely effect that his anxiety will have on his ability to learn?

a. It will likely have no effect.
b. It will likely lead to inaction and failure to follow through.
c. It will likely increase his ability to learn.
d. It will likely make it difficult for him to learn.

129. How frequently should most patients with diabetes receive a pneumonia vaccine in order to reduce the risks associated with pneumonia, according to recommendations of the American Diabetes Association?

a. One time for those ages 19-64, then a one-time revaccination for those ages 65 or older, at least 5 years after their prior vaccination
b. Every year
c. Every five years, unless the person has had pneumonia, and then vaccination is unnecessary
d. Every ten years until age 80, at which time revaccination is not recommended

130. A person with type 1 diabetes was recently diagnosed with celiac disease and reports switching to gluten-free foods, including gluten-free breads and pastas. The person should be advised to be especially diligent about:

a. Monitoring protein intake
b. Reducing the portion sizes of gluten-free products
c. Increasing dietary fat
d. Carbohydrate counting

131. According to the ADA consensus statement on managing preexisting diabetes in pregnancy, what is the optimal glycemic target for pregnant women with preexisting diabetes (assuming the target may be reached without excessive hypoglycemia)?

a. Pre-meal/fasting glucose <90 mg/dL and either one-hour postprandial glucose <120 mg/dL OR two-hour postprandial glucose <100 mg/dL; HbA1c <5.5%
b. Pre-meal/fasting glucose <95 mg/dL and either one-hour postprandial glucose <140 mg/dL OR two-hour postprandial glucose <120 mg/dL; HbA1c <6%
c. Pre-meal/fasting glucose <90 mg/dL and either one-hour postprandial glucose <120 mg/dL OR two-hour postprandial glucose <100 mg/dL; HbA1c <6%
d. Pre-meal/fasting glucose <100 mg/dL and either one-hour postprandial glucose <140 mg/dL OR two-hour postprandial glucose <120 mg/dL; HbA1c <7%

132. The Diabetes Prevention Program demonstrated that progression from prediabetes to type 2 diabetes can be delayed or even prevented through lifestyle modifications and weight reduction. Based on the results of this large-scale study, what does the American Diabetes Association recommend as a target weight reduction for those with prediabetes?

a. 10–20 pounds
b. 5–7% of body weight
c. Weight loss to within 10 pounds of ideal body weight
d. Body mass index (BMI) of 22 kg/m^2 or less

133. Which of the following does NOT need to be noted on the medication regimen portion of the initial DSMES assessment?

a. Daily multi-vitamin with iron
b. Two cinnamon capsules with each meal
c. Emergency albuterol inhaler for asthma (but has not used in three years)
d. All of the above should be noted.

134. Which of the following food options is the best example of an appropriate treatment option for a patient with a blood glucose level of 58 mg/dL?

a. 8 oz whole milk
b. 15 grapes
c. 2 Tbsp peanut butter
d. 2 Tbsp peanut butter on a slice of bread

135. Lipohypertrophy can be described as a thickened tumor-like swelling of the subcutaneous tissue or a mild swelling or lump under the skin at injection sites. When insulin is injected into these spots, insulin absorption is significantly decreased. What counsel should be given to a patient who exhibits signs of lipohypertrophy?

a. Begin antibiotic therapy under the direction of a dermatologist to reduce the swelling.
b. Apply warm compresses twice daily until the swelling is significantly reduced.
c. Avoid injecting insulin into those areas until the swelling is gone; rotate injection sites to prevent recurrence.
d. These swollen masses must be removed surgically, but this can typically be done as an outpatient procedure in a dermatology office.

136. Persons with diabetes should have emergency preparedness kits that are easily and quickly accessible in the event of an emergency or disaster and contain medical supplies that will last for at least:

a. 3 days
b. 5 days
c. 7 days
d. 14 days

137. If a person with type 2 diabetes has a high triglyceride level and a low HDL level, which of the following cholesterol-control drug types may be most indicated?

a. Omega-3 fatty acid supplements
b. Bile acid sequestrants (e.g., cholestyramine, colestipol)
c. Fibrates (e.g., fenofibrate, gemfibrozil)
d. Proprotein convertase subtilisin/kexin type 9 inhibitors (e.g., alirocumab, evolocumab)

138. Type 2 diabetes differs from type 1 diabetes in that persons with type 2 are NOT generally at risk for:

a. Hyperosmolar hyperglycemic nonketotic syndrome
b. Diabetic ketoacidosis
c. Erectile dysfunction
d. Acanthosis nigricans

139. To determine a patient's level of mastery of self-care skills such as insulin administration, which of the following evaluation methods should be used?

a. Return demonstration
b. Having the patient explain the process
c. Having the patient verbally acknowledge understanding of the skill
d. Completion of a short post-test (which can be quantified/scored)

140. A 56-year-old client diagnosed with type 2 diabetes has no health insurance, a history of drug abuse, and is homeless and lives in an encampment, scrounging and begging for food and often eating erratically. This client's individualized education plan should first focus on:

a. Diet and exercise
b. Community resources
c. Prevention of complications
d. Glucose testing and medications

141. According to ADA Standards, which statement regarding medical nutrition therapy and diabetes is NOT true?

a. Medical nutrition therapy is recommended for only those persons with diabetes who are underweight, overweight, or obese.
b. Medical nutrition therapy is recommended for anyone who has diabetes, regardless of nutritional status.
c. Children with diabetes and celiac disease should consult with a registered dietitian familiar with both conditions.
d. Because nutrition in the hospital setting is complex, a registered dietitian should be part of the inpatient diabetes care team to provide medical nutrition therapy.

142. The most significant risk factor for the development of type 2 diabetes in children is:

a. Family history
b. Obesity
c. Inactivity
d. Malnutrition

143. According to Medicare guidelines, which of the following patient characteristics or situations is NOT justification for individual sessions of diabetes education rather than group sessions?

a. The patient prefers one-on-one education because he does not get along with others.
b. No group classes are available within two months of the referral.
c. The patient has visual and/or language limitations.
d. The physician has a documented rationale for individual education, based on the educator's assessment and recommendation.

144. A patient takes insulin glargine (Lantus®) and has a treat-to-target self-adjustment scale, with a fasting morning glucose target of ≤120 mg/dL. It has been three months since his last visit. Since his last visit, his basal insulin dose has been self-increased by 18 units (to 48 units QHS). Today, his BG meter shows that his fasting glucose levels are still usually above target, sometimes within target, with an occasional hypoglycemic reading. Most bedtime glucose readings are well above target. The diabetes educator also notices that his weight has increased by 4 kg (about 9 pounds) since his last visit. What is the most likely explanation for these findings?

a. The patient requires additional basal insulin since most of his fasting morning readings are still above target. He should increase his dose according to the algorithm.
b. He requires additional basal insulin, but because he is taking more than 40 units, he may benefit by having a split dose (e.g., 25 units in the morning and 25 units at night).
c. Because he has some low readings (although few), he should decrease the dose and add bolus (mealtime) insulin during the day.
d. As evidenced by his weight gain and continued high readings, the patient is likely overeating. Help the patient evaluate current eating patterns and make adjustments.

145. For those who choose to consume alcoholic beverages, what guidelines do the American Diabetes Association provide in the Diabetes Standards of Care?

a. One drink per day or less for adult women and two drinks per day or less for adult men is what is recommended for those who use alcohol.
b. Two drinks per day or less for adult women and three drinks per day or less for adult men; abstaining from "hard liquor" is recommended.
c. Persons with diabetes should not consume alcohol due to the increased risk for hypoglycemia.
d. Persons with diabetes may consume alcohol without restriction as long as they account for carbohydrates and plan accordingly.

146. A man with type 1 diabetes became hypoglycemic and very confused and combative. He was initially detained by police before a friend reported that he was diabetic, and then he was transported to a hospital for treatment. The most appropriate preventive measure for such an experience is to:

a. Tell friends and associates about the condition.
b. Wear diabetes jewelry.
c. Carry a medical information card.
d. Rely on smartphone apps to alert medical authorities.

147. When evaluating a client's self-management skills, the CDCES observes her carrying out a foot examination. The client lifts her feet and briefly looks at their tops and bottoms. She reports that she examines her feet in that way after every bath. The CDCES should:

a. Remind the client to examine her feet daily.
b. Advise the client that her foot examination process is adequate.
c. Suggest the use of a mirror for the client to better examine her feet.
d. Review the correct foot examination procedure.

148. How frequently should a diabetes educator assess a patient's tobacco/nicotine use status and readiness-to-quit status?

a. At every visit for those patients who smoke and only at the initial assessment for those who do not
b. Annually, unless the patient mentions their status or readiness to quit without being prompted
c. At every visit
d. Whenever the educator notes signs that indicate a possible change in status

149. Which of the following choices would be the MOST appropriate method for screening for patient numeracy challenges?

a. Ask the patient about the highest grade they completed and how well they did in math.
b. Ask the patient if they have any trouble doing math problems.
c. Give the patient a standardized assessment test to be completed at home and have the patient bring it to the next appointment.
d. Present applicable hypothetical situations, such as choosing a menu with specified total grams of carbs or calculating a mealtime insulin dose using a correction scale.

150. Which of the following is NOT considered a critical skill needed by the diabetes educator to assess patients' abilities to plan goals?

a. Interpreting information gathering (i.e., assessing attitude, knowledge, and skill related to goal-setting ability)
b. Facilitating engagement (i.e., using skills to build a trusting relationship)
c. Reporting progress (i.e., documenting past and present progress, or lack thereof, in achieving set goals)
d. Analyzing problems (i.e., developing an understanding of factors related to a patient's self-management problems)

151. Which of the following examples violates infection control principles?

a. A patient uses soap and water instead of alcohol to clean the skin before administering an insulin injection.
b. A clinic uses one blood glucose meter to perform all point-of-care glucose tests for patients.
c. An inpatient diabetes educator trains all patients on pen use with a single pen, but changes the pen needle each time.
d. Parents who have two children with type 1 diabetes withdraw insulin from the same insulin vial but with a separate and new sterile insulin syringe for each child's dose.

152. National Diabetes Month presents an annual opportunity to promote diabetes advocacy through community outreach activities. What month is National Diabetes Month?

a. January
b. April
c. September
d. November

153. A diabetes educator for a clinic assesses and instructs patients on a variety of self-care skills. Which teaching strategy provides the best opportunity to both assess and instruct on self-administration of insulin?

a. A written quiz in which the patient puts insulin administration steps in order
b. A demonstration and return demonstration of insulin administration
c. A video on proper insulin administration technique that can be viewed multiple times
d. A printed handout with pictures depicting steps of insulin administration, followed by verbal acknowledgement of understanding

154. Which statement regarding dental disease and diabetes is FALSE?

a. Treatment of periodontal disease has been shown to reduce HbA1c levels.
b. Children with diabetes have significantly more dental caries than their non-diabetic counterparts.
c. Elevated glucose increases the frequency, progression, and severity of periodontal disease.
d. Medication such as diuretics and antidepressants may contribute to tooth decay and periodontal disease.

155. Which of the following is NOT information to be gathered as part of the initial individual DSMES assessment, according to the ADA National Standards for DSMES?

a. Financial status
b. Emotional response to diabetes
c. Cultural and religious practices that could affect diabetes
d. Sexual orientation

156. A member of the DSMES class group asks a specific question about food choices during session 1. The diabetes educator typically addresses healthy eating in session 2. What is the BEST way to handle the situation?

a. In order to capitalize on the apparent interest, abandon the planned order of classes. Talk about food today and discuss session 1 material next time.
b. Take a few minutes to briefly answer the question; acknowledge that many in the group likely have questions about food, and promise that this will be addressed in greater detail as part of the next session.
c. Tell the client that if he will be patient and remember his question for next session, you will promise to address it first thing.
d. Politely explain that there is a specific order in which the information needs to be presented to make the most sense. Ask him to limit his questions to the topic at hand but let him know that he may ask you one-on-one after class if he needs an immediate answer.

157. When educating an 18-year-old who is newly diagnosed with type 1 diabetes, which definition of diabetes is most appropriate initially?

a. A group of metabolic disorders that occur because of defects in insulin secretion and action
b. A disorder that prevents the body from using food effectively
c. A disorder that results in too much sugar in the blood
d. A disorder that can result in damage to the heart, eyes, kidneys, and blood vessels

158. The CDCES is teaching a 10-year-old child with type 1 diabetes about the disease and disease management. Which instructional approach is most likely to be effective?

a. Family-based education and interactive, hands-on activities
b. One-on-one coaching and visual aids and diagrams
c. Group education and interactive games
d. Family education and group education

159. A diabetes educator is conducting a seminar for family members and significant others of those with diabetes. In the educator's advice for this group, what would be described as the primary question a support person should ask themself?

a. "What will help the person with diabetes gain greater control of their chronic disease?"
b. "What can I do that will result in better blood sugars for the person with diabetes?"
c. "What does the person with diabetes want in the way of support?"
d. "What can I do or say that will result in a longer, complication-free life for the person with diabetes?"

160. Physiologic changes in aging are associated with an increased risk for diabetes and many diabetes-related complications, which may warrant the need for adjustments to the diabetes management plan. Which of the following changes is NOT commonly associated with advanced age?

a. Reduced metabolic rate that can alter digestion
b. Increased insulin resistance and decreased insulin effectiveness
c. Altered pain perception
d. Decreased renal function

161. A client with long-term diabetes who underwent amputation of his right leg is in an extended care facility and has recently been refusing meals, causing episodes of hypoglycemia; he also had an episode of DKA after eating a full box of chocolates that he had asked a friend to bring in. The CDCES recognizes that these behaviors may be indicative of:

a. Dementia
b. Passive-aggressive behavior
c. Inadequate education
d. Suicidal ideation

162. The first indication of early kidney damage is:

a. Difficulty initiating urine flow
b. Flank or lower back pain
c. Increased urinary frequency
d. Protein in the urine

163. A 62-year-old client with a long-term history of type 2 diabetes has recently begun complaining of blurry vision, floaters, and dark spots in her vision. She should be examined for:

a. Cataracts
b. Glaucoma
c. Macular degeneration
d. Diabetic retinopathy

164. According to the ADA Standards of Care, what is the recommended blood pressure target for most adults with diabetes who are being treated for hypertension?

a. <120/80 mmHg
b. <130/80 mmHg
c. <130/90 mmHg
d. <140/90 mmHg

165. Which of the following patient statements represents a situation in which specialty care provider resources are NOT being used according to ADA recommendations?

a. "I see a dentist twice a year even though I do not have, and have never had, gum disease."
b. "I see my ophthalmologist every 1-2 years even though he says that I have no signs of retinopathy."
c. "I had my cholesterol checked when I was diagnosed with diabetes, and because I did not require any medications to treat high cholesterol, I will have a lipid profile taken every 5 years."
d. "I see a nephrologist annually even though my BP is normal and I have no diagnosed kidney problems."

166. A patient who uses insulin is planning to travel. In terms of health and safety, which item below would be the LEAST important for the patient to include in his carry-on luggage?

a. Snacks such as nuts and string cheese
b. Insulin and syringes
c. Blood glucose meter and extra testing supplies
d. Diabetic ID and provider contact information

167. A 22-year-old female with type 1 diabetes (diagnosed three years ago) visits with the diabetes educator while home on summer break from college. She reports enjoying college but realizes that perhaps she has not been as responsible with her diabetes self-care as she really needs to be. Which of the following interventions below is the greatest priority for this patient?

a. Referral to a nephrologist to check for kidney problems
b. Referral to an ophthalmologist for an annual dilated eye exam
c. Referral for MNT for a review of good eating practices, including alcohol consumption
d. Pre-conception counseling to prevent unplanned pregnancy

168. If a patient does not have a puncture-proof sharps disposal container and needs to dispose of lancets and syringes, they can generally be:

a. Placed in a glass jar with a lid
b. Placed in a heavy-duty plastic container
c. Placed in a standard plastic food container
d. Wrapped in newspaper and placed in the trash

169. Most educators instruct patients to obtain a blood sample from the side of the finger when self-monitoring. What is the reason for this advice?

a. There are more capillaries on the sides of the fingers than the tip, and therefore it is easier to get a sufficient sample.
b. The sides of the fingers have fewer germs, since they do not come in contact with surfaces as much as the tips.
c. There is less pain when lancing the sides of the fingers, compared to the tips.
d. Studies have shown that drops obtained from the sides of fingers produce a more accurate whole blood sample result than alternative sites, including fingertips.

170. According to recently revised Medicare guidelines, a referral for medical nutrition therapy (MNT) by a registered dietitian can be made by whom?

a. Any credentialed or certified member of the diabetes care team, including the certified diabetes educator
b. A member of the diabetes care team with any of the following credentials: physician, qualified non-physician practitioner (NP or PA), or pharmacist
c. Only a primary care provider, including the treating physician or qualified non-physician practitioner (NP or PA)
d. Only the treating physician

171. Which of the following is the primary role of the diabetes educator regarding depression and diabetes?

a. Using a reliable, valid tool to diagnose patients who exhibit symptoms
b. Teaching patients depression prevention strategies, including stress management techniques
c. Screening patients and assisting them in getting access to care from a mental health professional
d. Conferring with a mental health professional to know how to appropriately counsel depressed patients on diabetes self-care

172. Alpha-glucosidase inhibitors help control diabetes by:

a. Reducing insulin resistance
b. Reducing the release of glucose from the liver
c. Increasing excretion of glucose through the urine
d. Slowing the absorption of carbohydrates by the gastrointestinal system

173. Of the choices below, what is the strongest predictor of health status?

a. Ethnic group
b. Literacy skill
c. Income level
d. Age

174. Which instructional strategy is likely to be MOST effective in terms of patient retention?

a. Slide show presentation with funny visuals and bullet list of main points
b. Current, well-referenced booklets with colorful diagrams, written at a patient's optimal reading level, that can be reviewed as desired
c. One-on-one conversation over the phone where the educator presents information and then rephrases the information using analogies to ensure understanding
d. Small group discussion around a table where patients teach each other a skill after seeing it explained and demonstrated by the educator

175. Which of the following behavioral objectives is an example of an immediate outcome?

a. Demonstrating proper technique for self-monitoring blood glucose
b. Reducing the number of missed doses of medication
c. Improving HDL to target level
d. Being 100% compliant on all recommended screenings

Answer Key and Explanations for Test #2

1. D: Routine testing is not mandated prior to exercise programs for patients with diabetes and cardiovascular disease, but the ADA recommends that clinical judgment be used based on the patient's comorbidities and history. A stress test with ECG may be warranted (but is not mandated) in this case, as this person is over 40, previously sedentary, has risk factors for CVD, and is beginning a program that is more intense than brisk walking, which is mild in intensity. The DEXA scan and the ankle-brachial index are not necessary based on the information given.

2. D: With diabetes, the person's blood glucose level is usually at its highest 2 hours after ingesting a meal. Typically, goals for blood glucose levels are 80–130 mg/dL when the person has fasted for 8 hours or more and <80 mg/dL at 2 hours postprandial. The goal for bedtime blood glucose may be individualized for an individual in order to prevent episodes of hypoglycemia, but it is usually in the 90–150 mg/dL range. Women with gestational diabetes have stricter guidelines: fasting, 95 mg/dL or less; 1-hour postprandial, 140 mg/dL or less; and 2 hours postprandial, 120 mg/dL or less.

3. A: A patient's social, cultural, and religious preferences should always be accommodated when possible. Several studies have shown that fasting, even with type 1 diabetes, can be accomplished safely. Recommendations include good baseline control, more-frequent monitoring, minor adjustment of basal insulin if needed (which is easier with an insulin pump), and prompt treatment of hypoglycemia. Patients in good control do not typically need to reduce basal insulin and should be prepared to end the fast with oral glucose if they experience hypoglycemia. Readdressing the hazards of fasting or talking to the pastor to find an alternative may be perceived as dismissive of the patient's wishes—like trying to "talk the patient out of" the idea. While the patient should be made aware of potential risks, the educator must respect his religious preferences and then present options and information that can help him decide on the best course of action.

4. C: Of the choices listed, only decreasing lipids has been shown to reduce PAD risks, progression, and/or symptoms. The UK Prospective Diabetes Study demonstrated that a reduction in blood pressure of 10/5 mmHg (systolic/diastolic) had no effect on the risk of amputation in PAD. As in other atherosclerotic diseases, glycemic control has not been shown to have an effect on the progression of PAD. Only supervised exercise training programs have been shown to be of benefit in improving walking for those with PAD. Unsupervised exercise programs have not yielded such results, nor any of the other results listed in choice D.

5. B: The evidence for a treatment effect of sleep apnea on glycemic control is mixed and inconclusive. Sleep apnea can be life-threatening and is a risk factor for cardiovascular disease. Treatment of sleep apnea significantly improves quality of life and blood pressure control. It is true that persons who are obese, particularly those with central adiposity, are four to ten times more likely to have obstructive sleep apnea. In fact, the rate of sleep apnea in obese participants enrolled in the Look AHEAD trial exceeded 80%. It is estimated that the prevalence in general populations with type 2 diabetes may be as much as 23%.

6. A: The National Certification Board for Diabetes Educators (NCBDE) does not accredit or recognize programs. Rather, they "promote the interests of diabetes educators and the public at large by granting certification to qualified health professionals involved in teaching persons with diabetes, through establishment of eligibility requirements and development of a written examination." The American Diabetes Association and the Association of Diabetes Care and Education Specialists both recognize diabetes self-management education programs. Each has a list of specific requirements and stipulations, although they are similar and both incorporate the National Standards for DSMES.

7. A: Providing proof of services rendered by the educator for use as verification of practice hours for certification is *not* listed as a purpose of documentation of a patient's assessment, education plan, and documentation in the ADA National Standards for Diabetes Self-Management Education and Support. Standard 7 states, "Documentation of participant encounters will guide the education process, provide evidence of communication among instructional staff and other members of the participant's healthcare team, prevent duplication of services, and demonstrate adherence to guidelines."

8. B: When a patient has changed behavior to adopt self-care strategies, they could relapse into old habits. The diabetes educator can assist in the prevention, recognition, and addressing of behavioral relapse. Teaching the patient to be self-aware and to have a plan to deal with stressful situations is an appropriate educator strategy to prevent relapse. The American Diabetes Association recommends intervention by a health professional when a patient exhibits signs of gross disregard for the medical regimen, depression, possibility of self-harm, debilitating anxiety, indications of an eating disorder, or cognitive functioning that significantly impairs judgment.

9. C: Patients with unstable proliferative retinopathy should not include strength training, weight lifting, or high-impact activities in the exercise regimen because the resulting excessive systolic blood pressure response may further damage vessels in the eyes. Patients with proliferative retinopathy will have significant restrictions to exercise, although some physical activity beyond activities of daily living is still recommended. Swimming, walking, low-impact dancing, and stationary cycling are some examples of recommended activities. While a stress test is recommended before beginning an exercise program for those of high risk, this test mainly assesses risks related to coronary artery disease, peripheral vascular disease, and autonomic neuropathy. Passing a stress test would not necessarily indicate safety of exercise for someone with proliferative retinopathy.

10. B: The diabetes educator should rephrase the question to "How do you hope that learning more about diabetes will help you?" The patient may need clarification on what is meant by diabetes education-related goals. Choice A is belittling and will put the patient on the defensive. Choice C is incorrect because the patient is awaiting information from the diabetes educator. While silence is appropriate while the patient thinks, it is not appropriate when he has expressed that he needs more information. Choice D is not the best choice because the educator is suggesting options ("putting words in his mouth"), rather than allowing the patient to state what really matters to him.

11. A: Potassium will almost always need to be given to a patient with DKA. Although potassium levels often appear normal or even high, hypokalemia is masked by dehydration. When fluids and insulin are given, potassium levels fall. This can result in heart arrhythmias and eventually death. Serum potassium levels should be checked frequently until they are stable. Serum phosphate may also be low, but research does not support supplementation because oral intake of food can correct this. Sodium bicarbonate is typically low as well (<15 mEq/L) in acidosis, but supplementation is controversial. Serum sodium levels may vary, and low levels are sometimes masked by dehydration, but this level is not as critical or as problematic in DKA as potassium.

12. C: Cultural characteristics/barriers of a population are addressed in many ways, among them asking about food preferences and restrictions, inviting family participation, and moderating speech rate and tone. Keep in mind that what may be culturally sensitive to one culture could be offensive to another. This underscores the importance of knowing the patient population. While readiness for change, low literacy/numeracy, and poor support are important considerations, they are not addressed by the policies described in the scenario.

13. A: Activity-related hypoglycemia may occur up to 24 hours after an intense activity is stopped. With intense or prolonged activity, the glycogen stores are depleted. In these situations, the patient may need to consume a moderate amount of carbohydrates during and/or within two hours after the activity to restore muscle glycogen. While all other choices are certainly within the window of concern, they do not cover the entire time span in which exercise-related hypoglycemia can occur.

14. B: Therapeutic inertia occurs when a person is maintained on dosages of medications that are not appropriate, such as when there is a delay in intensifying treatment when goals are not met or decreasing treatment when it is excessive. Causes may include inattention of the prescribing physician, failure of the patient to monitor adequately or to correctly report findings and symptoms, and failure of healthcare systems to provide adequate monitoring. ADA/European Association for the Study of Diabetes guidelines emphasize the importance of using **multidisciplinary teams** to address therapeutic inertia.

15. C: Responsibilities of a diabetes educator include promoting diabetes advocacy. Contacting the principal, nurse, and head district nurse to explain the situation and suggest reasonable options is the best way the educator can advocate for the patient in this case. The American Diabetes Association position statement on Diabetes Care in the School Setting states: "Federal laws that protect children with diabetes include Section 504 of the Rehabilitation Act of 1973, the Individuals with Disabilities Education Act, and the Americans with Disabilities Act. State and local laws may provide additional protections. It is illegal for schools to discriminate against students with disabilities, including diabetes. Any school that receives federal funding (i.e., public, charter, private, and parochial schools and postsecondary institutions) and any facility considered open to the public must reasonably accommodate the needs of students with diabetes. Indeed, federal law requires an individualized assessment and plan of care for any student with diabetes. The required accommodations need to be documented in a written plan developed under the applicable federal law, such as a 504 plan (named from Section 504), or Individualized Education Program (IEP), and should be based on the student's individualized Diabetes Medical Management Plan (DMMP)." The position statement goes on to state that is it is responsibility of the school to "grant permission for the student to check glucose, administer insulin, and treat hypoglycemia and hyperglycemia anywhere in the school, including their classroom, near their school activity, or in a private location, if desired, as indicated in the student's DMMP; to carry equipment (which may include a smartphone or smartwatch), supplies, medication, and snacks; and to perform diabetes management tasks." The other answer choices would be circumventing the student's rights or would be shirking the advocacy responsibility of a diabetes educator by suggesting that the parents handle it all.

16. D: Ketones cross the placenta and are harmful to the fetus, so maternal ketosis should be avoided. The patient's regimen should change to eliminate the ketones entirely. Because ketones represent starvation, when the body must burn fat reserves to meet energy needs, the remedy is usually an increase in dietary intake. However, good blood glucose levels must also be maintained, and therefore the patient will likely need to take insulin with the extra food. Increasing insulin without increased food intake will cause nocturnal hypoglycemia, and adding fat to the diet during the day is not likely to address the patient's needs overnight and may even increase ketosis.

17. B: Asking open-ended questions to help the patient identify immediate strategies will directly address the patient's desire to accomplish his long-term goal. He has expressed his willingness to make changes. He has already defined the main problem, identified his feelings, and set a long-term goal. The next step is to identify short-term goals that will contribute to the realization of the long-term goal. Patient empowerment models of care affirm that ideas and choices generated by patients will have the greatest effect on metabolic control. Choice A is redundant since the patient is already aware and convinced that he needs to lower his HbA1c to minimize his risks. Choice C is not a bad option, but it is a goal that comes from the educator, not the patient. If given the chance, the patient might suggest the same strategy. If he doesn't, it is likely not something he is prepared to do. Choice D does not address what the patient wants help with right now. His goal is to lower his HbA1c, not reduce his stress level at work. Of course, this topic is a worthwhile discussion, but right now the diabetes educator should focus on the immediate concern of the patient.

18. C: Modifiable risk factors are those over which the person can exercise some control. These include controlling hyperlipidemia through diet and medications, eating a healthy diet, managing overweight and obesity, managing hypertension, stopping smoking, and reducing or eliminating alcohol consumption. Nonmodifiable risk factors are those the person cannot control and include age, genetic predisposition, family history, ethnicity (e.g., Native Americans, Hispanic/Latino Americans, African Americans, Asian Americans, and Pacific Islanders have higher risks), history of gestational diabetes, and polycystic ovary syndrome ([PCOS] which increases risks because of hormone imbalances).

19. D: The key to management of both acute and chronic sensorimotor diabetic neuropathies is blood glucose control and stability. Several observational studies have suggested that neuropathic symptoms improve not only with optimization of control but also with the avoidance of extreme blood glucose fluctuations. Many patients will require pharmacological treatment for painful symptoms. Several medications, including tricyclic antidepressants (e.g., amitriptyline), anticonvulsants (e.g., gabapentin), SSRIs, and opioids (e.g., tramadol) have shown some success in managing symptoms; referral to pain management is also recommended in some cases. Appropriate diagnosis is through clinical findings, including pinprick, temperature, and vibration perception (using a 128-Hz tuning fork); 10-g monofilament pressure sensation at the distal halluces; and ankle reflexes, as well as the exclusion of non-diabetic causes. Consideration of non-diabetic causes typically include serum B12, thyroid function, blood urea nitrogen, and serum creatinine. This is part of the assessment and diagnosis process, however, and would not be considered key to the management of sensorimotor neuropathies. Finally, graded supervised aerobic exercise is recommended for those with cardiovascular autonomic neuropathy (CAN).

20. D: When patients have changed their behavior and intend to continue with the change, they need to understand that the old behaviors do not just go away; they "lie in wait" for an opportunity to return. This requires knowledge of relapse prevention and preparation to deal with the temptation. Techniques that are effective in dealing with temptation and risky behavior (to prevent relapse) include being aware of the risky behavior or situations, having a plan to combat negative thoughts and temptations, and employing effective stress management techniques. Denying that the temptation is still there may prevent the person from avoiding or planning for such occasions; this lack of preparation may contribute to relapse.

21. B: Communication among team members is part of the person-centered DSMES guidelines (standard 5) of the National Standards for DSMES. Proper communication increases the likelihood that all team members will work in collaboration for the patient's benefit. Such practices also reduce duplication of services, which reduces cost, and guide treatment and education-related decisions. While patients are likely to be more satisfied when all team members are working in collaboration, it does not mean that each provider should not perform a thorough assessment pertaining to the purpose for which the patient is seeking treatment or services. HIPAA rules allow for information to be shared among healthcare team members for the purpose of treatment activities without express consent from the patient.

22. B: The dawn phenomenon can occur with both type 1 and type 2 diabetes. In the dawn phenomenon, the person experiences high blood glucose levels in the early hours of the morning, typically between 2 a.m. and 8 a.m. This occurs because of a surge of natural hormones, such as cortisol, epinephrine, and growth hormones, that occurs during the night. This surge stimulates the liver to release stored glucose. Because the pancreas does not produce enough insulin, it cannot compensate adequately. Additionally, insulin resistance can result in cells being less responsive to insulin during the night.

23. B: Ramadan, the ninth month of the Islamic lunar calendar, is considered holy by the Muslim faith. During this month, which is 29 or 30 days, observants fast from dawn until sunset. Islam generally allows exemptions from fasting for illness during Ramadan, but fasting is a matter of conscience and some Muslim individuals with diabetes choose to fast. They must be cautioned to check their blood glucose levels often and to break the fast if their blood glucose level drops to ≤70 mg/dL (3.9 mmol/L).

24. B: The calorie balance/surplus (total calorie intake vs. calorie expenditure) has proven to be the most important aspect of weight loss. Other important elements include adherence to diet and enthusiasm of the counselor. Composition of nutrients, glycemic index, and fiber have not been shown to affect weight loss as much as energy deficit.

25. D: A patient that denies that they have diabetes and disagrees with the doctor's referral for DSMES is the most likely to have a very low level of readiness for change. This is a sign that the patient is resistant to accepting the diagnosis and is not ready to make changes in light of it. A tearful patient may be feeling overwhelmed or sad because of a belief that giving up favorite foods may be required. It may also be that the patient is not ready to change, but not necessarily. Choice B is incorrect because, while not speaking may at times indicate an unwillingness to change, the patient may also be concentrating on the demonstration. Choice C, incorrectly answering review questions, may be an indication that the patient misunderstood or did not see or hear the material, but is not a sign that the they are necessarily unwilling to change. Any response at all indicates that the patient is at least engaged.

26. D: With small-nerve-fiber neuropathy, which usually presents with pain but without objective signs of nerve damage, the greatest risk is for foot ulceration and subsequent gangrene and amputation. More than 80% of amputations follow a foot injury. About 75% of foot amputations are thought to be preventable. Charcot foot syndrome, increased falls, and decreased mobility are also risks associated with sensorimotor neuropathies, but are not the greatest risks. Cardiac death due to cardiac denervation is the greatest risk associated with diabetic autonomic neuropathy (DAN), and specifically cardiac autonomic neuropathy (CAN).

27. A: For those with diabetes, the ADA and the American College of Sports Medicine recommend:

- Aerobic exercise: ≥150 minutes per week over at least 3 days, with no more than 2 consecutive days without exercise
- Resistance training: two to three times per week
- Flexibility and balance training: two to three times per week
- Breaking up sedentary time: standing and walking around or performing some type of light physical activity every 30 minutes of sitting

- Individualized exercise regimen: tailored to individual needs/health
- Weight management: loss of 5–7% of body weight can improve blood glucose control

28. D: The four types of readiness to learn are:

- Experiential: past coping mechanisms, cultural background, locus of control, orientation, and aspiration level
- Emotional: level of anxiety, support system, motivation, risky behavior, frame of mind, and stage of development
- Physical: measures of ability, task complexity, environmental effects, status of health, and gender
- Knowledge: current knowledge base, cognitive abilities, learning disabilities, and learning style

29. B: The essential outcome of DSMES is sufficient knowledge to perform necessary skills and make the lifestyle changes required for satisfactory quality of life. These behavior changes lead to positive clinical outcomes as well as fewer diabetes-related complications. Decreased healthcare costs are an eventual long-term outcome that comes from improved clinical indicators, which result from positive lifestyle changes.

30. A: According to the National Standards, it is crucial that the individual with diabetes is viewed as central to the team and takes an active role. Other persons on the team may include diabetes educators, case managers, and both primary care providers and specialty care providers such as endocrinologists. Other members of the multidisciplinary team may include nutrition specialists, psychologists and other mental health specialists, physical activity specialists, optometrists, podiatrists, and others.

31. A: The Somogyi phenomenon, while rare, is a rebound from hypoglycemia that results in high morning glucose due to an exaggerated counterregulatory response. The dawn phenomenon is elevated fasting glucose in the morning, likely due to overnight growth hormone secretion and increased cortisol. It is not usually preceded by hypoglycemia. The recommendation for those with type 1 diabetes is to adjust insulin to meet the carbohydrate intake, which should be kept to an appropriate amount. Adding a protein snack at bedtime is not the best approach for this patient; it is questionable whether a protein snack would help, since protein has not been shown to increase plasma glucose concentrations. In addition, it does not explain why the glucose would "rebound" in the morning after nocturnal hypoglycemia. The *honeymoon period* is a phenomenon that occurs in patients with type 1 diabetes shortly after diagnosis and can last up to 12 months. It is characterized by the need for very little insulin. While the end of the honeymoon period is characterized by greater fluctuation in blood sugars, it would not explain this patient's consistent pattern of nighttime fluctuations, especially since he has had diabetes for three years.

32. D: Basal insulin controls glucose levels when a person is fasting. In this case, the morning fasting glucose levels are good (107–112 mg/dL), which suggests that the problem lies elsewhere. However, the client's glucose levels fluctuate significantly around mealtime, suggesting that the mealtime insulin dosages and the carbohydrate intake for the meals need to be assessed and adjusted to ensure that they are properly balanced to achieve optimum glucose control. The mealtime insulin dosages may be inadequate, and the client's carbohydrate intake at mealtimes may be very inconsistent.

33. D: Jardiance (empagliflozin), an SGLT2 inhibitor, would most likely be recommended for this patient. 2026 ADA guidelines recommend that this class of drug be used as pharmacologic management for individuals with type 2 diabetes and heart failure, as it has been proven to decrease heart failure-related hospitalizations in this population in addition to providing effective glycemic management. Due to the increased creatinine levels, the patient would not be a candidate for metformin, as metformin relies on sufficient kidney function to metabolize appropriately. Metformin use in renal-impaired patients may lead to lactic acidosis. FDA guidelines recommend against initiating metformin in individuals with an eGFR below 45 mL/min/1.73 m^2. Likewise, pioglitazone is not a first-line drug and is not recommended for those with congestive heart failure. While basal insulin is generally a safe choice, is it not usually used as first-line treatment and the patient is not willing to consider it. Sitagliptin has been shown to be both effective and safe as a first-line diabetes medication and can be used in patients with impaired renal function and history of heart disease, although a reduced dose may be needed.

34. B: Models of foods, nutrition labels, and sample restaurant menus would be the most appropriate materials for this class. Copies of the ADA guidelines would not be appropriate because they are written for healthcare professionals, and the audience may contain people with low literacy levels. Likewise, graphs comparing HbA1c with rates of complications may be confusing to those with low literacy or numeracy, and such materials do not address issues of food. Similarly, foot care props do not relate directly to nutrition and would distract from the topic of the lesson. They would, however, be very appropriate for a class on reducing risk and preventing complications through good foot care.

35. C: The target BMI for those with either type 1 or type 2 diabetes is 18.5–24.9 kg/m^2, which is considered to be the normal range. With a BMI >25 kg/m^2, the person is at greater risk of cardiovascular complications. An initial weight loss goal for those who have a BMI above the target range is often 5–7% of the total body weight. Type 2 diabetes is commonly associated with obesity, so being underweight is rarely a problem for people with type 2 diabetes; however, a BMI <18.5 kg/m^2 may indicate a need to gain weight.

36. A: If a smart insulin pen does not always synchronize with its mobile app, the first thing to assess is whether the client is attempting to synchronize within 5 meters (16 feet) of the mobile device. Smart insulin pens are class 2 Bluetooth devices, which have a theoretical range of up to 10 meters (33 feet); however, the reality is that this distance range is rarely attained because walls, other devices, and battery strength can reduce the range.

37. B: The primary recommendation for those with hypoglycemia unawareness is relaxation of glucose targets. Less-stringent targets, resulting in several weeks with no episodes of hypoglycemia, have been demonstrated to improve counter-regulation and awareness to some extent in many patients. More-frequent monitoring is also advised, including the use of continuous glucose monitoring systems. However, this recommendation is secondary to preventing hypoglycemia through less-stringent glucose targets. Hypoglycemia unawareness is related to deficient counterregulatory hormone release and autonomic responses. Unlike autonomic neuropathy, these conditions are caused by hypoglycemia, rather than hyperglycemia. Therefore, more-stringent blood glucose control would not be appropriate.

38. C: When a person is first diagnosed with diabetes, they may be anxious and easily overwhelmed with information, even if their health literacy is good. The best approach is to use one-on-one coaching, which allows the CDCES to assess the person's knowledge base, immediately address concerns, and answer any questions that may arise. The CDCES should address basic skills, such as testing glucose levels, through demonstration and hands-on practice to help the client gain confidence in carrying out procedures. Instructions should be clear, and a step-by-step approach should be used.

39. A: Talking to the nurse of the referring provider and using the information to complete the assessment form is the least effective and least recommended way to complete the initial assessment. While gathering information from referring providers may be helpful, the bulk of the information assessment should come from the patient or from direct observation of the patient. All other answer choices—face-to-face meeting (with family members), completion of an electronic form prior to visit, and group assessment with individuals completing personal information on their own—are all acceptable methods of conducting initial DSMES assessments.

40. B: Omitting breakfast has *not* been shown to result in weight loss. Having more-frequent but smaller meals has been shown to be an effective weight-loss strategy, as has portion control and the use of premeasured meal replacements (liquid meals or prepackaged meals). It is worth noting that reducing overall energy intake to 500 to 1000 kcal less than that which is needed for weight maintenance has been shown to result in a one to two pound per week weight loss, but it is not recommended that this calorie reduction be achieved by skipping breakfast.

41. D: To accurately assess what patients are taking, as well as their understanding and habits of medication administration, it is best to have patients bring all of their medications in the original containers and describe what each is for, when they take it, and any problems they experience. This allows the educator to get a sense of the patient's medication knowledge and health literacy, and allows the educator to check prescription dates and other details. A written medication quiz will not provide all of the information needed, including an idea of patient habits, and would not be valid if the patient has a literacy deficit (which in and of itself can contribute to non-adherence). Similarly, studying the chart notes and comparing written lists may provide pieces of the picture but leave out important parts that reflect the patient's own experience and challenges.

42. B: Adolescents are often at increased risks of hyperglycemia and hypoglycemia, especially if they do not adjust their carbohydrate intake and insulin to account for physical activities such as participation in sports. Additionally, they are often inconsistent in their diet and resist rigid dietary restrictions. Adolescents usually want to fit in with their peers and engage in the same types of activities. Therefore, it is essential that adolescents learn to adjust insulin for exercise, diet, and illness so they can remain independent but decrease their risk of complications.

43. A: *Reduced* fiber intake is suggested for patients who suffer from gastroparesis. Other recommendations include: frequent small meals, decreased fat intake, and soft or liquid meals. Vegetables, for example, may still be included in the meal plan, but should be cooked until very soft to aid digestion. Therefore, choices B, C, and D are appropriate modifications and not the correct choices.

44. D: Polycystic ovary syndrome (PCOS) is a risk factor for the development of gestational diabetes. PCOS is associated with insulin resistance, which can lead to hyperglycemia, and the additional insulin resistance that occurs during pregnancy can compound this problem. Additionally, PCOS is characterized by overweight or obesity, which is also a risk factor for gestational diabetes. Hormonal abnormalities, such as elevated androgens, can increase metabolic abnormalities. Gestational diabetes is usually diagnosed between 24 and 28 weeks of pregnancy, and symptoms typically recede after delivery. Approximately 15% of women have PCOS.

45. A: Routine foot soaks should be avoided unless directed by a physician. Moisturizing dry skin (except between toes), washing and drying feet, and trimming long toenails straight across are all appropriate recommendations. Keep in mind that those with poor vision, unsteady hands, neuropathy, or current lower extremity problems may be advised to have a professional trim their toenails. Other foot care recommendations include: check all areas of the feet every day for wounds or signs of infection, inspect shoes for wear and tear and proper fit, avoid going barefoot, test water temperature before stepping into a tub, have regular foot exams, and seek medical care immediately for any potential problems.

46. B: The transition from childhood to adolescence poses the most challenges for management of diabetes because the increase in growth hormones, estrogen, and testosterone can cause increased insulin resistance, so insulin dosages may need to be readjusted. Additionally, adolescents face social pressure to fit in and may resist dietary restrictions and monitoring. They may skip doses of insulin and may engage in risk-taking behaviors, such as drinking and smoking, which can affect glucose levels. Adolescents may want increasing independence in diabetic care, but they need to be well-prepared with education for the complexities of that care.

47. C: Latent autoimmune diabetes of adulthood (LADA), a form of slow-onset type 1 diabetes, is the most likely diagnosis for this patient. It is characterized by positive GAD/islet-cell antibodies and a normal to low C-peptide level, and can often be managed with diet in the beginning months or years. Those with this type of diabetes are typically well into their adult years (over age 35) and not usually overweight (although they may be). Type 2 diabetes is not the best choice because the patient does not exhibit typically obvious signs of insulin resistance, such as excess weight and family history. In addition, persons with newly diagnosed type 2 diabetes often have a high C-peptide level and do not have positive GAD or islet cell antibodies. Type 1 diabetes is only correct if the diabetes educator categorizes LADA as a form of type 1 diabetes, which some organizations do. However, this patient is older than is typical, and maintains an HbA1c of 6.4% without insulin, even 2 years after diagnosis, so clearly there is a distinction. Maturity-onset diabetes of the young (MODY) typically occurs in persons under the age of 25 years (although it can also occur in those much older). MODY is a type of diabetes in which a single genetic defect causes a problem with the pancreas reacting to increasing glucose appropriately. Therefore, C-peptide levels may be normal (since endogenous basal insulin is not necessarily affected). Like with type 2 diabetes, cell islet antibodies are not found. Unlike type 2 diabetes, those with MODY are usually not obese and are usually quite sensitive to insulin or sulfonylurea medications.

48. B: This response is the best example of *developing discrepancy* in motivational interviewing. The idea is that the inconsistency between a behavior/belief and the desired outcome will spur the patient to conclude that it is worth the struggle to make changes. In this case, the educator acknowledges the struggle and the discrepancy between the two sides of the argument and then helps the patient focus on the long-term outcome of fewer complications and better health. Choice A does not validate the patient's struggles, but rather dismisses them. In addition, it does not highlight the positive outcome that may result if the patient does monitor. Choice C somewhat acknowledges the struggle by pointing out that many patients experience the same thing, but the response does not highlight the discrepancy. Choice D praises the patient, which is important, but skips over the patient's comments entirely. It does not acknowledge the struggle or point out the discrepancy between the current thought and desired outcome.

49. A: Providing materials and experiences to enhance knowledge and provide psychosocial support will best address this patient's lack of confidence of success. While managing any lingering stress is important, it does not address possible knowledge gaps or confidence issues that may be contributing to the discrepancy. Highlighting the benefits of good diabetes management is incorrect because this action would be more appropriate if the patient rated the importance to make the change as low. The patient is already convinced of the importance of the change, and highlighting its benefits is not the priority. Finally, it is not unusual for patients to believe it is very important to change but to have low confidence in their ability to do so. This may be due to a lack of knowledge, skill, or self-confidence.

50. B: Backdating the meter to accept expired test strips is *not* an appropriate cost-cutting strategy. Accuracy of results would be suspect, and with an incorrect meter date, both the patient and provider may easily become confused when examining data and making regimen changes. Appropriate cost-cutting strategies include using a less-expensive generic meter or test strips, testing less frequently but often enough and at the right times so that trends can be seen, and sticking with the brand of meter and strips most covered by the patient's insurance carrier. Sometimes, a clinic staff member will suggest a meter with which they are most comfortable and confident, but patient-centered care considers barriers to the patient and makes accommodations when possible. The equipment and monitoring approach that will allow the patient to monitor consistently will ultimately be best.

51. C: The general recommendation is that persons with type 1 diabetes should check their blood glucose levels before driving and only drive if their blood glucose level is at least 90 mg/dL (5.0 mmol/L). If the blood glucose is less than that, then the person should ingest a fast-acting carbohydrate and wait until the blood glucose level increases. Additionally, the person should keep fast-acting glucose (e.g., glucose tablets, hard candy) in the vehicle and be aware of signs or symptoms indicating hypoglycemia and pull over and stop driving immediately if they occur.

52. D: HbA1c provides information about the average glucose content of the blood over the previous 2- to 3-month period, so it is useful for monitoring compliance with diet and treatment, although it cannot be used alone for diagnosis. Fasting blood glucose provides the glucose level after 8–12 hours of fasting, but this can be affected by recent diet changes and may fluctuate. Ketone testing is used for screening but is not sensitive enough for monitoring or diagnosis. Diabetic autoantibodies are tested to differentiate type 1 from type 2 diabetes.

53. A: "My mother believes I got diabetes from eating too much candy as a kid" is not part of the health history but rather may speak to the family dynamics and support. All of the other choices would be more important to note, including choice D, which gives the duration of diabetes.

54. C: "The choices that have the greatest effects on diabetes outcomes are made by patients, not by healthcare professionals" is a guiding principle of patient empowerment approaches to DSMES. Patient empowerment approaches also stipulate that patients are in control of their own self-management, and that the consequences of those choices rest first and foremost on the patient. Choice A is not a tenet of any DSMES theoretical approach, as support (family, healthcare team, peers, etc.) is recognized as a crucial element. Choice B is a characteristic of the social cognitive theory. Choice D is a tenet of the theory of reasoned action/planned behavior. The latter two theories are examples of traditional theoretical approaches to behavior change.

55. B: Metformin reduces the amount of glucose produced by the liver, increases insulin sensitivity, and decreases intestinal absorption of glucose, and has minimal risk of hypoglycemia; therefore, it is often recommended as the first-line drug for treatment of type 2 diabetes. Metformin may promote mild loss of weight and may have cardiovascular benefits that reduce the risk of heart attack, which would be beneficial for this person. Additionally, generic formulations are available, so the drug is of low cost. Adverse effects are generally minimal but can include gastrointestinal system upset such as loose stools, diarrhea, and nausea, although these symptoms are usually temporary.

56. D: A person managing type 1 diabetes while working the night shift (e.g., 11 p.m. to 7 a.m.) faces many challenges because their natural circadian rhythm is disrupted and this can affect blood glucose levels. Glucose monitoring and managing diet are critically important. The person may need to bring prepared meals from home and schedule regular mealtimes because having irregular mealtimes and intake make it difficult to plan one's insulin needs. Persons who work nights may benefit from insulin pumps and continuous glucose monitoring (CGM).

57. B: Atherosclerosis, a condition in which blood vessels become narrow and hardened because of plaque buildup, is a common effect of diabetes on the vasculature and can lead to cardiovascular disease (especially coronary artery disease), PAD, diabetic retinopathy, kidney disease, and stroke. The risk of atherosclerosis increases with diabetes and can affect both large and small blood vessels. Risk factors include poorly controlled blood glucose levels, chronic inflammation, high blood pressure, and dyslipidemia. Atherosclerosis is the underlying cause of death for up to 80% of persons with diabetes.

58. D: There is no specific mix of macronutrients recommended by the ADA. The best mix of macronutrients depends on individual circumstances. Studies thus far have not conclusively identified an optimal mix of macronutrients for persons with diabetes. Dietary Reference Intakes (DRIs) may be helpful for patients seeking guidance on an appropriate mix. Regardless of macronutrient mix, total caloric intake must be appropriate to the individual's weight-management goals. Choice A suggests a higher proportion of carbs than typically recommended. Choice B suggests a higher proportion of protein (and less fat) than typically recommended; this mix is the closest to the dietary reference intakes. Choice C suggests a lower proportion of carbohydrates than what is normally recommended.

59. B: This response is an accurate description of the difference between type 1 and type 2 diabetes, specifically why oral medications work on the latter but not the former. The other options are partially true, but also include fallacies. Choice A claims that insulin is used for type 1 diabetes primarily for weight gain. This is false. Choice C states that type 1 is more severe than type 2. This is a fallacy. Severity is a measure of level of control, not type. Choice D suggests that oral medications would be effective (if too drastic) for lowering blood glucose of someone with type 1 diabetes. This is not true. Oral medication would have little or no effect and would not sustain a person with type 1 diabetes.

60. B: The main difference between *process evaluation* and *outcomes evaluation* is in the purpose of each. The purpose of process evaluation is to determine and make needed adjustments to the educational process. The purpose of outcomes evaluation is to determine the effects, or outcomes, of education efforts. Both types evaluate the instruction; the educator is evaluating elements of the actual educational content and delivery (from different perspectives), not evaluating a patient. For both types of evaluation, the process involves gathering data, summarizing, interpreting, and making a judgment as to whether the action or program being studied was successful or if it is in need of adjustments. Both can be used to gather data for reports and/or to make changes. The scope of process evaluation is limited to a single learning experience, such as a class or workshop, and examines issues such as the appropriateness of timing, materials, logistics, etc. The scope of outcomes evaluation encompasses the whole education process but focuses on effectiveness in terms of patient learning and behavioral objectives.

61. A: Glyburide is a sulfonylurea, an insulin secretagogue with a comparatively high rate of hypoglycemia. This medication should not be taken if the person does not intend to eat that day. In addition, basal insulin is usually taken in a full or reduced amount even when the person is NPO, as basal insulin primarily addresses hepatic glucose. The other answer choices all indicate correct understanding. Lantus® (glargine) can be kept at room temperature for the duration of its use. Metformin does not require food, as it will not cause a drop in glucose to lower than a normal level. Insulin in a vial or pen should not be used beyond the recommended amount of time, which for NovoLog (as well as most insulins) is 28 days.

62. C: Diminished or absent dorsal pedal pulses (caused by the dorsalis pedis artery) indicate poor circulation. All of the other choices are normal findings for a lower-extremity assessment. Note that pulse palpation often has false positives and false negatives, so one must practice the technique in order to prevent erroneous assessment findings.

63. C: Approximately 75 grams of carbohydrates are consumed when the patient eats half of the package of this product. There are three serving per package; therefore, half of the package would be equivalent to 1.5 servings. Carbohydrates listed on the label are per serving, so 51 times 1.5 is about 75 g of carbohydrate.

64. D: The statement that is *not* applicable in this situation is that the patient has correct assumptions about this food. All of the other answer choices are correct. The fiber in this food is not high enough to discount from total carbs. The sugars are not as important as the total carbs, nor is the glycemic ranking (i.e., glycemic index) of the carbs. These are all common mistakes patients make when interpreting nutritional information on product packaging.

65. B: The first treatment priority in HHS is rehydration to expand intravascular volume and restore renal perfusion. Rehydration alone may cause glucose values to come down somewhat. Glucose values, often extremely high (>600 mg/dL), need to be addressed as well, but as a secondary or tertiary priority. Electrolyte (potassium, sodium, phosphorus, magnesium) imbalances likewise must be addressed but come after rehydration in terms of priority. Often, there is an underlying condition, such as infection, that precipitates HHS. This must be addressed to prevent relapse, but again, it is not as critical as rehydrating the patient.

66. B: Hyperglycemia is categorized as a fasting blood glucose level greater than 125 mg/dL (6.9 mmol/L) for nondiabetics and greater than 180 mg/dL (10.0 mmol/L) 1–2 hours postprandial for persons with diabetes. Signs of hyperglycemia include:

- Increased thirst and increased urination, resulting in dry mouth
- Blurred vision and headaches
- Fatigue
- Persistent hunger despite having eaten

Persons with long-standing type 2 diabetes may not show typical signs of hyperglycemia even when it is present, so monitoring blood glucose levels is important.

67. C: The ADA, in agreement with the American Society for Metabolic and Bariatric Surgery, states that metabolic surgery should be considered for adults with type 2 diabetes and BMI ≥30 kg/m^2 (BMI ≥27.5 kg/m^2 for Asian American adults), especially if the diabetes or associated comorbidities are difficult to control with lifestyle and pharmacological therapy. Patients should first try other methods, but if these are unsuccessful, metabolic surgery may be warranted if the patient's BMI is 30 kg/m^2 or greater.

68. A: The patient who records all information in her spiral notebook is the best example of good BGM record keeping, regardless of the condition of the book. The information she has recorded will enable her (as well as the healthcare team members) to get a complete picture of how her blood glucose responds to food, activity, medication doses, etc. By recording dates and times, she will be able to identify patterns more easily, as will the educator/provider. The other answer choices are each missing an important component. By not keeping a written record, the patient in choice B is missing the important factors (food, activity, medicine) that may help explain and ultimately improve his BG readings. The patient in choice C, who does not bring her meter to her appointment, is missing the opportunity to have the meter tested for accuracy, and does not allow the healthcare team the opportunity to download its data (to confirm that her recordings are accurate and complete and to view helpful summary report data), or to assess her BGM technique. A patient record that does not indicate the days on which the readings were taken, as in choice D, is at a great disadvantage because neither the patient nor the educator will be able to associate the readings with what was happening at the time, including food and medication (since he did not record those items with his readings).

69. A: An ADCES position statement on inpatient diabetes management clearly states that diabetes-specific discharge planning should begin upon admission and provide a smooth transition from hospital to home. There are several elements of a successful discharge from the hospital, including patient survival skills education (which can be accomplished without a provider order), gathering all patient supplies, and helping arrange follow up appointments. While some elements may require a provider order or prescriptions, many elements of the plan can and should be worked on as soon as it is known that the patient being admitted has diabetes. While educational activities should ideally be performed when the patient is most ready to learn, many things can be done to make the transition smoother for the patient, such as constructing a list of follow-up appointments or writing out instructions on how to use a monitor, etc. An inpatient diabetes educator can certainly facilitate this discharge planning, but other team members (floor nurse, inpatient dietitian, provider, social worker, patients' family members, etc.) can certainly be involved as well.

70. C: Depression occurs in 20–30% of people with diabetes. Those with type 1 diabetes often find management difficult because of the need for insulin and blood glucose monitoring. Those with type 2 diabetes often deal with obesity and chronic health problems associated with the disease. Cognitive behavioral therapy has been found to help individuals better cope with their disease because it focuses on identifying and changing negative thought patterns and behaviors and teaches effective coping strategies.

71. D: According to the CDC, smoking doubles the risk of developing periodontal disease; therefore, if a person with diabetes—already at risk for periodontal disease—smokes, this markedly increases the risk that the person will develop periodontal disease. Smoking impairs the immune system, so the bacteria in the mouth can invade the gums and cause infection that allows plaque and tartar to build up. Gingivitis occurs, and as it worsens and periodontal disease develops, the gums begin to recede and the bone and tissue deteriorate.

72. D: An avoidant coping style is characterized as doing only the bare minimum and ignoring or blocking additional information that is beyond survival skills alone. Avoidance is often associated with the emotional discomfort that comes with fear, anxiety, anger, shame, or other uncomfortable feelings the patient may be experiencing. An exploration and validation of these feelings should be the priority above reviewing or adding additional diabetes education. Conversely, in the "depression and frustration" emotional stage of dealing with chronic disease, a person will often express a loss of control and an inability to handle the expectations associated with diabetes self-care. The patient described in this question may have those fears, but he has not yet faced them.

73. B: The development and progression of diabetic retinopathy correlate strongly with both blood pressure and blood glucose control. These risk factors are both modifiable. The risk factor most closely associated with diabetic retinopathy is duration of diabetes. Other modifiable risk factors (although not as closely correlated) include lipid control and smoking status. Some possible risk factors may include age, glucose variability, clotting factors, renal disease, and use of specific medications, although these factors remain in question.

74. C: The most appropriate response to the patient's question about why she should increase her basal rate during a time of illness is to explain that stress increases hepatic glucose production, and therefore basal insulin needs increase as well. The other choices are incorrect, although each contains a small bit of truth. While insulin does lower blood glucose as stated in choice A, extra insulin is needed during times of illness, even if the person is not eating, to address increased hepatic glucose. Too little insulin in a person with type 1 diabetes can rapidly lead to diabetic ketoacidosis (DKA). Not taking enough insulin, including on sick days, is a major contributor to DKA. Choice B is correct in that food/calories are required for energy needed by the body to fight illness and to prevent DKA, but the purpose of insulin is not that of an appetite stimulant. Choice D is correct in that drinking at least 8 oz of fluid per hour is recommended for a person with diabetes who is sick, but the recommended increase in basal insulin is not due to poor absorption, but rather increased demand.

75. A: Weight is a modifiable risk factor for diabetes. A modifiable risk factor is one that can be changed by the person who is at risk for diabetes. A person can change their weight through managing diet and exercise. While family history, race, and age are risk factors for type 2 diabetes, they are not considered modifiable. Physical activity is another modifiable risk factor.

76. D: If a CDCES is to provide education about self-care to a person with diabetes, the first step in educating that person should be to assess their readiness to learn. There are four types of readiness that must be assessed: physical, emotional, experiential, and knowledge. Many different factors can affect readiness—for example, a patient whose pain is uncontrolled or who is very anxious may have difficulty concentrating and processing information. As another example, a patient who is hard of hearing or has impaired vision may not be able to benefit from available materials.

77. D: For most adults with diabetes, the ADA recommends that blood pressure be maintained at less than 130/80 mmHg; however, if someone has added risk factors—such as high cardiovascular risk or evidence of kidney disease, such as with albuminuria—then the goal is lowered to a systolic pressure of less than 120 mmHg, unless they suffer from orthostatic hypotension or dizziness and cannot tolerate a blood pressure this low. The American College of Cardiology/American Heart Association guidelines are similar.

78. B: Wearable fitness devices, such as the Fitbit and Apple Watch, can provide comprehensive information about a person's activities:

- Steps taken and estimated distance
- Heart rate monitoring to track the intensity of exercise
- Exercise tracking for different types of exercise
- Detailed logs that provide the duration of an exercise, heart rate zones, calories burned, and distances covered
- GPS and location tracking to show the person's route, speed, and distance
- Active and sedentary minutes and hourly reminders
- Fall detection and emergency SOS to alert first responders to falls

79. C: Maintaining adequate control of blood glucose levels is especially important for women with diabetes who want to become pregnant because high glucose levels increase the risk of birth defects. A person wanting to get pregnant should monitor blood glucose levels often and try to maintain levels as close to normal as possible, aiming for a target HbA1c of less than 6.5% if the person is able to tolerate that level without frequent episodes of hypoglycemia. CGM use may be recommended.

80. C: Recent survey data showed that rural areas, particularly in the southern states, are underserved by diabetes educators. These studies also found that a strong majority (75%) of diabetes education practices are located in urban or suburban areas, and a majority are in the most populous states.

81. D: It is true that tension and disagreement between primary care providers and diabetes educators regarding self-care recommendations has been found to be a barrier to patients' access to diabetes education, according to a national study. This can often be avoided or at least resolved with effective communication. The same study revealed that most physicians want their patients to have more diabetes support and also want patients to have easier access to diabetes education. Patients over the age of 65 have a much higher rate of diabetes than their middle-aged counterparts do. However, they are less likely to participate in diabetes education; only one-third of patients seen by diabetes educators were over the age of 65. Similarly, although rates of diabetes are highest among minority populations (Hispanic, African American, Native American, Pacific Islander, etc.), the majority of patients seen by diabetes educators are non-Hispanic white people.

82. A: The ADA recommends that all adults be screened for type 2 diabetes and prediabetes by age 35, regardless of BMI. However, adults ages 18–35 may be considered for screening if they are overweight or obese (BMI ≥25 kg/m^2 [or 23 kg/m^2 for Asians]) and have additional risk factors, such as a first-degree relative with diabetes, hypertension, dyslipidemia, PCOS, history of gestational diabetes, or signs of insulin resistance, or are of an ethnicity with high risk (i.e., Asian, African American, Latino, Native American, or Pacific Islander).

83. B: According to the ADA National Standards for Diabetes Self-Management Education and Support (DSMES), "evidence suggests that the development of standardized procedures for documentation, training health professionals to document appropriately, and the use of structured standardized forms based on current practice guidelines can improve documentation and may ultimately improve quality of care." While these documentation practices may facilitate smoother clinic operations and reduce administrative costs, this is not the reason for the ADA recommendation. It is not true that such practices and attributes are required by the Joint Commission or by insurance carriers.

84. D: If a client's glucose levels remain high even though the insulin pump indicates that it is delivering insulin appropriately, the client's ketone levels should be checked because hyperglycemia and increased ketones are indications of diabetic ketoacidosis (DKA), which is life-threatening. Ketones appear in the urine when the level of insulin is too low to allow glucose to enter cells, so fat is broken down for energy, producing ketones as a byproduct. If ketones are present, this may indicate that insulin dosages are too low, that the insulin pump is malfunctioning, or that the cannula is blocked and not delivering the recorded dose.

85. B: Serum creatinine is used to calculate glomerular filtration rate (GFR), a measure of kidney function. Any level above 1.3 mg/dL for men or 1.1 mg/dL for women is considered out of normal range and should be examined further. A serum creatinine of 3.6 mg/dL for a woman would translate to a GFR of 20% for an African American woman and 16% for those of other ethnicities, if using the MDRD formula. This would equate to stage 4 chronic kidney disease (CKD). Therefore, this statement is true. Choice A is false because someone with an HDL of 30 mg/dL is still at risk for cardiovascular disease (CVD), even with a total cholesterol of less than 200 mg/dL. Choice C is false because an HbA1c of 5.9% may be the result of many lows and some high glucose levels, just as it may indicate good control. The BGM values are needed to determine this. Choice D is false because creatinine is a measure of kidney function, not liver function. Liver function tests include ALT, AST, and alkaline phosphatase, among others. Less than 56 IU/L is the normal range for ALT, but still does not rule out fatty liver disease.

86. A: Dental care is especially important for persons with diabetes because of the increased risk of periodontal (gum) disease, xerostomia (dry mouth), tooth decay, candidiasis (thrush), and burning mouth syndrome. According to the ADA, persons with diabetes should:

- Use fluoride toothpaste and a toothbrush with soft bristles.
- Brush their teeth twice a day for 2 minutes each time.
- Floss their teeth once daily or use an interdental brush.
- Visit the dentist two times yearly for a dental checkup and teeth cleaning, more frequently if the dentist indicates that there is a need to do so.

87. A: In response to eating, the gut releases incretin hormones, such as GLP-1, that stimulate the pancreas to release insulin in response to increased blood glucose levels. The DPP-4 enzyme breaks down these incretins, reducing the duration of their effect. DPP-4 inhibitors block the action of the DPP-4 hormone so that the incretin hormones (primarily GLP-1) stay active for longer, resulting in increased secretion of insulin when blood glucose levels rise. Because insulin is released only in response to increased glucose levels, DPP-4 inhibitor use does not result in hypoglycemia, unlike insulin or sulfonylureas.

88. A: If a client has cognitive impairment or learning disabilities that interfere with learning, it is essential to break information and tasks down into small, manageable steps and wait until the client has mastered the initial steps before proceeding to the next. Too much information up front may overwhelm the individual and add to any confusion. A person with difficulty learning is often reluctant to acknowledge the problem or to ask questions. Visual aids, such as step-by-step illustrations that can be used as a guide, can be very helpful, especially if one cannot rely on memory.

89. A: Steroid effects on glucose metabolism include down-regulation of glucose transporter 4 (GLUT-4) in the muscle so that more insulin is needed for the uptake of glucose into cells. This results in hyperglycemia, specifically post–prandial hyperglycemia. Steroids do not decrease metabolism of insulin and do not increase risk for hypoglycemia. Steroids may also promote glucose production in the liver, reduce binding of insulin to the insulin receptor cells, and decrease insulin secretion from the islet cells, all of which may affect fasting glucose levels, but this is not the most pronounced effect. While steroids do suppress the immune system, it is inaccurate to say that steroids "deactivate" insulin.

90. A: The breakfast meal is definitely the most unbalanced. The meal consists of almost all carbohydrates, and total carbohydrates are over 120 grams (twice the normally recommended amount for most men). While lunch and dinner may be on the large side in terms of serving sizes and total calories, they are at least balanced between protein, fat, and carbs, and both have closer to the typically recommended amount of carbohydrates.

91. D: The usual HbA1c goal for persons with type 1 diabetes is less than 7%, but those who have had difficulty achieving their HbA1c goals and have had repeated episodes of severe hypoglycemia and exhibited lack of hypoglycemic awareness are at greater risk from hypoglycemia than from elevated HbA1c. For these individuals, the goal is often to maintain HbA1c in the 7.5–8.0% range. If persons have been able to control their diabetes without excessive hypoglycemia, the target goal may be less than 6.5%.

92. A: A lipid profile, or cholesterol testing, should be performed when the patient is in a fasting state because recently consumed food can affect the triglyceride level. An advantage of the HbA1c test is that it is not affected by recent food or drink. A urine microalbumin test checks the urine for protein and is a screening test for renal impairment. It can be performed randomly, with no fasting required. ALT/AST are parts of a liver function test. Some providers may order this test with fasting because some foods, medications, or alcohol may affect the test. However, this it is not typically necessary.

93. D: If an older person with poorly controlled type 2 diabetes and hypertension has a history of falling in the home and complains of increasing problems with balance, the CDCES should coordinate the plan of care with a physical therapist. The physical therapist can evaluate the patient's gross motor coordination and assist them with postural control and physical skills as well as recommend devices for safe ambulation, if necessary.

94. D: Patients who take basal insulin should not omit their dose if they are fasting before surgery. Omitting basal insulin will result in high blood glucose before, during, and after surgery, which can lead to surgical site infections. Metformin should be omitted, as taking it on an empty stomach can cause gastrointestinal upset; in addition, any situation that may result in a use of contrast dye, tissue hypoperfusion, or acute renal dysfunction (such as surgery) warrants holding the dose of metformin. Sulfonylurea medications should be omitted because they may cause a drop in glucose due to the mechanism of action on the pancreas. Short-acting insulin should be omitted as well (unless given by the surgical team to correct a high pre-operative glucose), as it is meant to be taken with food and could cause hypoglycemia in someone who is not eating.

95. D: This patient has answered in the affirmative to depression screening questions. Although the diabetes educator cannot confirm a diagnosis of depression, his answer is sufficient to warrant a referral to a mental health specialist. Depression affects 20–25% of the population of people with diabetes (twice that of the general population). Many people with diabetes who suffer from depression find adhering to the rigorous self-care activities very difficult, if not impossible. While "burnout" in those with diabetes is not uncommon, this patient's reply to the question indicates that it may be something more serious and that further evaluation is warranted. Neglect of diabetes self-care will result in poor control, but depression is not something that a person can always "snap out of." He may lack the energy and so the depression must be addressed. Anxiety, on the other hand, is typically characterized by irrational fears and avoidant or extreme behaviors.

96. B: Level of family support, while very important to assess, is not considered an element of patient knowledge. Literacy/numeracy, previous DSMES, and proficiency of self-care skills are all important elements to assess in order to gauge the patient's knowledge and ability to gain knowledge.

97. A: Some individuals retain their accents long after they have become fluent in reading, speaking, and understanding English, so one should never make assumptions about a person based on their accent. The best course of action is to ask what language is preferred. If the person lacks adequate English skills to understand, then an interpreter should be used, and written, video, and audio materials should be provided in the preferred language, if possible. Illustrated guides with minimal text may also be helpful.

98. C: Of the patients listed, only the man with ischemic heart disease who uses a nitrate-containing medication is contraindicated from using PDE5 inhibitor medications. This is due to a potentially serious, even fatal, drop in blood pressure that may occur. For patients with mild to moderate kidney disease and liver disease, the dose of the medications may need to be adjusted. For patients with severe hepatic or renal disease, such those on dialysis, some of these medications are contraindicated. Check detailed manufacturers' information for details before suggesting them to patients.

99. B: A visual learner is most likely to prefer and/or benefit from seeing, watching, or reading, including visual demonstrations and visual aids as well as reinforcement through reading materials. Choices C and D represent auditory and verbal instructional methods. While role-playing (choice A) has verbal, auditory, tactile, and visual elements, it is more action-oriented and may therefore be distracting to a strictly visual learner. While learning styles do vary some from person to person, all people do need learn from visual information, auditory information, and by hands-on learning. Different materials lend themselves to a different format, but where possible, the best practice when presenting information to others is to use a mixture of formats, including hands-on materials, visual, and auditory information to keep the materials engaging to all learners.

100. B: Principle 7 of the Principles of the American Association of Clinical Endocrinology Comprehensive Type 2 Diabetes Management Algorithm states that persons with diabetes should reach their target goals of therapy and adjust the therapy as needed within 3 months, and should adjust treatment as needed promptly rather than delaying. Healthcare providers should review client goals at each visit and make the changes needed to control lipids, glucose, and blood pressure. The American Association of Clinical Endocrinology also recommends that persons with diabetes use a CGM to monitor their blood glucose levels and help them safely reach their goals.

101. B: Tests that are especially important when assessing kidney function include:

- eGFR: Normal range is ≥90 mL/min/1.73 m^2, so a finding of 78 mL/min/1.73 m^2 is abnormal. This test shows how effectively the kidneys filter the blood.
- UACR: Normal range is <30 mg/g. Increased albuminuria is often an early sign of kidney damage.
- Serum creatinine: Normal range for males is 0.74–1.35 mg/dL (0.04–0.07 mmol/L); for females, the normal range is 0.59–1.04 mg/dL (0.03–0.06 mmol/L).
- BUN: Normal range is 7–20 mg/dL (0.39–1.11 mmol/L).

102. A: The American Diabetes Association recommends cholesterol goals of LDL <100 mg/dL, HDL >40 mg/dL (men) or >50 mg/dL (women), and triglycerides <150 mg/dL. In choice B, the LDL and triglyceride targets listed are both too high. Choice C focuses on total cholesterol, which is not emphasized as much as LDL; it omits LDL, which is the primary target; and also does not differentiate between men and women for HDL goals. Choice D has mixed up the LDL and triglyceride goals as well as the men's and women's targets for HDL.

103. A: The first step toward providing better quality DSMES programs is to reflect on the question, "What are we trying to accomplish?" This is often answered by systematically examining process and outcome data. Once the goal has been established, the data should be further analyzed to reveal the root of the problem. The next questions are, "How we will know a change is actually an improvement?" and "What changes can we make that will result in improvement?" Only once these questions are answered should one ask what programs or initiatives might improve effectiveness, followed by what resources will be needed to make the change and how the effectiveness of changes will be measured. By considering all of these questions in a systematic way, the continuous quality improvement process will result in ever-improving delivery of DSMES.

104. C: Visual learners remember what they read or see more than what they hear or handle, so if a client identifies as a visual learner, the CDCES should try to provide as much visual material as possible, including videos, written directions, and illustrated instructions and guides. Visual learners may also like to take their own notes. Clients may like to refer to these materials when carrying out procedures. Auditory learners learn best by listening and asking questions. The CDCES should explain each step in a procedure during a demonstration and ask the client to repeat back the procedure and explain its steps. While learning styles do vary some from person to person, all people do need learn from visual information, auditory information, and by hands-on learning. Different materials lend themselves to a different format, but where possible, the best practice when presenting information to others is to use a mixture of formats, including hands-on materials, visual, and auditory information to keep the materials engaging to all learners.

105. A: For immigrant populations, the most successful strategies are usually those that directly reach the population in the places they are comfortable and feel safe, such as churches, schools, and shopping areas, especially if some of the population members are undocumented. The CDCES can also work with employers to allow screenings in the workplace, stressing that persons who have diabetes will likely be more productive and take fewer sick days if they are properly treated.

106. D: Sulfonamide medications compete with sulfonylurea medications, such as glipizide, for protein binding sites, thereby keeping more of the glipizide acting in the blood stream. This can result in hypoglycemia. Corticosteroid medications tend to raise blood sugars, especially postprandial blood sugars. This effect is more on the intrinsic disease than on other medications. Likewise, protease inhibitors (antiviral drugs) such as indinavir, and estrogen products such as Premarin® tend to raise blood glucose through intrinsic effects.

107. C: Unsaturated fats are typically those that are liquid at room temperature. Two types of unsaturated (or healthy) fats that should be included in the diet:

- Monounsaturated fats (i.e., those with a single unsaturated carbon bond): Can help reduce LDLs and increase HDLs and help control blood glucose levels and insulin sensitivity. Found in olive oil, canola oil, peanut oil, nuts (e.g., almonds, pecans, hazelnuts), seeds (e.g., sesame, pumpkin), and avocados.
- Polyunsaturated fats (i.e., those with more than one unsaturated carbon bond): Include essential fatty acids (e.g., omega-3, omega-6) that are important for heart health. Found in fatty fish (e.g., salmon, sardines, mackerel), chia seeds, walnuts, soybeans, nuts, seeds, and vegetable oils (e.g., sunflower, safflower, corn).

108. B: An individual can be literate (able to read and write) and still lack health literacy, which refers to one's ability to understand, interpret, and apply health-related information. The parent has some nutritional awareness, realizing that candy may affect diabetes but does not understand the implications of an autoimmune disorder. In response, the CDCES should acknowledge the parent's concern about sugar but clarify, in simple terms, the difference between type 1 and type 2 diabetes and encourage the parent to ask questions if there is a lack of understanding.

109. D: Thiazolidinediones (TZD) medications, such as pioglitazone (Actos®) can take 12 to 16 weeks to reach maximum effect; many patients may notice no difference after only one month. At this point, neither a different medication nor a higher dose is warranted. It is possible that the patient may have gained weight with the medication, as it is a reported side effect. This does not necessarily mean that the patient is eating more, as often the weight gain is due to increased water retention. The educator should assess for edema in the lower extremities and consult with the provider on an appropriate diuretic or dose alteration if edema is present.

110. C: SGLT-2 inhibitors (e.g., empagliflozin, canagliflozin, dapagliflozin, and ertugliflozin) reduce the risk of heart failure and other cardiovascular events and slow the progression of kidney disease because they reduce the loss of protein in the urine. GLP-1 agonists also have cardioprotective benefits and some renal protection, but they are not as effective as SGLT-2 inhibitors. In some cases, SGLT-2 inhibitors and GLP-1 agonists may be given together to enhance their benefits. Metformin has milder cardioprotective benefits but does not have strong protective benefits for the kidneys.

111. A: Proliferative diabetic retinopathy is characterized by neovascularization (new vessel growth) and/or vitreous or preretinal hemorrhage. No stage of nonproliferative diabetic retinopathy includes neovascularization. Severe nonproliferative retinopathy will have more than twenty intraretinal hemorrhages in each of the four quadrants, definite venous beading in 2 or more quadrants, or prominent intraretinal abnormalities in at least one quadrant (but no neovascularization or preretinal hemorrhage). Mild nonproliferative retinopathy has microaneurysms only. Moderate nonproliferative retinopathy may have more than just microaneurysms but no signs as significant as with severe nonproliferative retinopathy.

112. A: If a 24-year-old client diagnosed with type 1 diabetes with a glucose level of 468 mg/dL (26 mmol/L), polyuria, polydipsia, and weight loss has stabilized since starting insulin injections and now appears to be able to manage his diabetes with very little insulin, the CDCES should advise him that his insulin needs will increase again. Symptoms of type 1 diabetes usually do not occur until destruction of approximately 90% of the pancreatic islet. Once stabilized, the person often experiences a "honeymoon" period, during which the remaining cells seem to produce enough insulin, but the process of cell destruction and increased blood glucose will continue.

113. C: While all of the answers are within the realm of possibility, the most likely explanation is that the patient is fabricating her BGM values. Four elements, when combined, suggest this explanation. First, the BGM values and HbA1c indicate very different levels of control. Second, she did not bring her meter (which could be downloaded), but somehow remembered her log book (which is usually kept with the meter). Third, she has every single number filled in; it is highly unlikely that a person would not have missed one test in three months; and fourth, there are no numbers out of target range (highly unusual for anyone with diabetes). Fabricating BGM values is not uncommon. Even though the patient only hurts herself by lying, many patients fear being lectured or letting down the provider/educator. The best way to avoid this is to establish a trusting, non-judgmental relationship with the patient from the beginning. Anemia and most hemoglobinopathies normally result in lower HbA1c values than fingerstick values would indicate. While no BG meter claims to be 100% accurate, the International Organization for Standardization (ISO) requires that 95% of readings to be ±20% of actual value; this variation would not explain the discrepancy between in-target BGM results and an HbA1c of 9.6%. Technique should be evaluated, but again, it is highly unlikely that any technique flaw could be responsible for such a discrepancy.

114. D: Persons with diabetes should have 30–60 minutes of moderate aerobic exercise daily for most days of the week, with an ultimate goal of at least 150 minutes per week. Ideally, the person should begin with 10 minutes of stretching and then 15–20 minutes of moderate aerobic exercise, which can include walking, bicycling, swimming, water aerobics, dancing, jog-walking, hiking, doubles tennis, rowing, Tai Chi, climbing stairs, and use of an elliptical machine.

115. C: Relying on the color of a medication, along with saying "I forgot my glasses," or using pictures drawn on the bottles, etc. are all signs of possible health literacy barriers. Financial barriers could be indicated by a patient skipping doses or cutting doses in half, or by delaying picking up prescriptions. Cognitive barriers would be indicated by a patient exhibiting confusion or forgetfulness; fear of side effects might be the cause of a patient not taking medication at all, or taking a lower dose than recommended. If any barrier or adherence issue is suspected, the educator should investigate further by using open-ended, non-judgmental questions.

116. B: Cutting back on repaglinide (Prandin®) on mornings she exercises will reduce the amount of insulin released by her pancreas for a short time. With less insulin, she is less likely to experience hypoglycemia, and therefore she may not need to consume extra glucose after her workouts. To test this, the educator should advise the patient to check her blood glucose before and immediately following exercise and at periodic intervals afterwards. Advise the patient that she should treat hypoglycemia whenever her glucose drops too low. Consuming a small amount of juice before the activity may prevent the hypoglycemia, but does not address the patient's concern about consuming extra calories. Telling the patient not to worry about the extra calories is dismissive of the patient's values and concerns. Patient-centered care recognizes that patients are likely to adhere to lifestyle modification recommendations when they foresee an outcome that matters to them. Skipping metformin is unlikely to prevent the hypoglycemia, as metformin does not cause an increase in circulating insulin.

117. C: Initially, smokers are advised to chew the gum every 1–2 hours, at least nine pieces daily for the first 6 weeks and then with decreasing frequency. Smokers are advised to chew the nicotine gum for the full 12 weeks for best results. The gum causes a tingling sensation in the mouth, and users are advised to chew the gum until the tingling sensation has stopped—usually after approximately 30 minutes.

118. D: Postexercise delayed-onset hypoglycemia often occurs 4–12 hours after exercise, but can be delayed for up to 48 hours. Exercise causes muscles to become more insulin-sensitive, thereby using more glucose from the bloodstream, and the muscles pull additional glucose to replenish glycogen stores. Exercise also increases the glucose-lowering effects of insulin and sulfonylureas. To prevent postexercise delayed-onset hypoglycemia, a person with an insulin pump should decrease their basal insulin dose by 20% for 6 hours after exercise, eat carbohydrate snacks before and after exercise, and eat a snack with protein and carbohydrates before bedtime.

119. B: Overinvolved parents can present a challenge when educating a child or adolescent, and adolescents especially strive for independence and autonomy. The best solution is to prepare in advance and have written guidelines to give to parents that outline how they can provide support to their adolescent and encourage the adolescent to independently manage their diabetes. The guidelines should stress the importance of providing positive reinforcement, waiting for the child to ask for help before offering it, and avoiding critiquing what the child is doing.

120. D: It is accurate to say that the ADA recommends that the HbA1c test should be performed at least twice annually, and more in some cases. For those who have had medication changes or have not reached their glycemic goal, quarterly tests are recommended. Some patients who require intensive management may need even more frequent testing. All other statements are false. A 7% target is a general recommendation for HbA1c. For those with hypoglycemia unawareness, comorbidities, or age concerns (i.e., young children or the elderly), the risk of a lower HbA1c outweighs the risks associated with a higher HbA1c. While it is true that the HbA1c has been adopted by the ADA as a valid diagnostic tool, the industry recognizes that there are significant variations in HbA1c results among races as well as in those with anemias and hemoglobinopathies. Similarly, the HbA1c test identified fewer cases of previously undiagnosed diabetes than either the fasting plasma glucose or the 2-hour glucose tolerance test.

121. A: St. John's wort (*Hypericum perforatum*) is a plant that is often used as a natural remedy for mild depression and sleep disorders. It interferes with many medications, including those used for the treatment of diabetes. St. John's wort may speed the metabolism of metformin and decrease the effectiveness of sulfonylureas such as glimepiride and glipizide. St. John's wort may increase the clearance of some drugs, such as DPP-4 inhibitors (e.g., sitagliptin, saxagliptin) and increase the hepatic breakdown of thiazolidinediones (e.g., pioglitazone, rosiglitazone).

122. D: Standard practices in healthcare are developed from evidence-based research. Evidence-based research uses the best available data from well-designed research studies, such as randomized controlled trials, as well as the clinical expertise of healthcare professionals in interpreting data. Steps to evidence-based practice include asking a clinical question (such as in the population, intervention, comparison, outcome, and time [PICOT] format), searching for evidence, appraising the evidence, applying the evidence, initiating change, assessing outcomes, and disseminating findings. Benefits include improved patient outcomes and quality of care.

123. A: Autoimmune thyroid disease, including Graves' disease and Hashimoto's thyroiditis, occurs in 17–30% of persons with type 1 diabetes mellitus. Hashimoto's thyroiditis is by far the most common autoimmune disorder associated with this condition. Because type 1 diabetes is an autoimmune disease, persons with the disease are more prone to developing other autoimmune diseases. In Hashimoto's thyroiditis, the immune system produces antithyroid antibodies that attack the thyroid gland, resulting in its inability to produce adequate amounts of thyroid hormones.

124. B: The CDC's National Diabetes Prevention Program offers the Lifestyle Change Program to guide persons with prediabetes or those at risk from developing type 2 diabetes. The year-long program meets weekly for the first 6 months and twice monthly for the remaining 6 months. The sessions are led by a lifestyle coach, and the curriculum includes lessons, handouts, other resources, and access to a support group of peers. Lessons cover healthy eating, exercise, and coping with stress and challenges. Some programs are free, but some charge a small fee. The costs may be covered by Medicare, Medicaid, and private insurance.

125. C: According to the CDC, if a person with diabetes has stabilized, their HbA1c is less than 7.0%, and blood glucose levels are within the target range, the person's HbA1c needs to be checked only every 6 months. However, if the person is not meeting target goals or the treatment has changed, the HbA1c should be checked every 3 months and the person's blood pressure and weight should be checked as well.

126. D: Vitamin B12 is almost exclusively found in animal products; therefore, vegans (who avoid all meats and dairy products) should generally take a vitamin B12 supplement. A deficiency of vitamin B12 can lead to nerve damage, which is especially concerning for a person with diabetes who already has peripheral neuropathy. Signs of vitamin B12 deficiency can include depression, changes in cognition, memory impairment, and generalized fatigue. Some diabetes medications, such as metformin, can also reduce vitamin B12 levels, resulting in deficiency.

127. D: There are many effective ways to track patient progress of behavioral goals, including individual visits, group classes, email or text messaging, phone consultations, regular mail, and other methods. The key is to make sure the method is standardized (i.e., collected consistently at predetermined time points) and convenient for the patient.

128. C: Studies have shown that moderate anxiety can be a positive factor in increasing a person's ability to learn because the person is motivated to take action to resolve the anxiety. However, if a person's anxiety is too low or too high, this can impact the ability to learn. If a person has low anxiety, that person may not take learning seriously and may fail to follow through. If anxiety is high, then the ability to learn may be seriously impacted. A person with high anxiety may need repeated explanations and practice and much encouragement to overcome their anxiety.

129. A: ADA Standards of Care advises to administer pneumococcal polysaccharide vaccine (Pneumovax specifically) to all diabetic patients 19-64 years of age. A one-time revaccination is recommended for individuals >64 years of age previously immunized when they were <65 years of age if the vaccine was administered >5 years ago.

130. D: Carbohydrate counting is especially important for persons with type 1 diabetes and celiac disease because most gluten-free substitutes for bread and pasta are higher in carbohydrates and have higher glycemic indexes than regular products. Persons with both disorders should work with a dietician to develop an individualized meal plan because celiac disease can lead to vitamin and other nutrient deficiencies because of malabsorption. Celiac disease occurs in 5–10% of persons with type 1 diabetes; therefore, all persons with one of the disorders should be tested for the other one.

131. B: According to the most recent ADA Standards updates, when managing pregnancy with pre-existing diabetes, optimal glucose targets are: pre-meal/fasting glucose <95 mg/dL and either one-hour postprandial glucose <140 mg/dL OR two-hour postprandial glucose <120 mg/dL and HbA1c <6%. Choices A and C are too stringent, and choice D is not stringent enough. Note that for pregnant patients, hypoglycemia is generally defined as a blood glucose level of less than 70 mg/dL, although this may need to be adjusted for each individual.

132. B: The ADA Standards of Care for Diabetes recommend that patients with prediabetes be referred to an effective ongoing support program targeting weight loss of 5–7% of body weight and increasing physical activity to at least 150 min/week of moderate activity such as walking. While other weight loss goals may be applicable or desired by some patients, the ADA target recommendations are based on the results of the Diabetes Prevention Program, which found that 7% body weight reduction and increased physical activity resulted in 58% less conversion to diabetes at 3 years and 34% less at 10 years, without medication.

133. D: All of the mentioned medications/supplements should be noted on the mediation regimen portion of the initial DSMES assessment. A medication regimen should include all prescription, over-the-counter medications, vitamins, and complementary and alternative therapies.

134. B: Fifteen grapes contain about 15 grams of carbohydrate and no significant protein or fat. When treating hypoglycemia (i.e., 58 mg/dL), a person should consume about 15 grams of carbohydrate that is *not* mixed with fat, for fat will delay the absorption of the carbohydrate. Whole milk, peanut butter, and bread with peanut butter all contain fat that will increase the amount of time it takes for the blood glucose level to rise.

135. C: By avoiding the area, lipohypertrophy can resolve itself in a few weeks to several months. Therefore, the best advice is to select alternative sites in which to inject insulin. Antibiotic therapy, warm compresses, and surgical removal are not recommended treatment options.

136. C: Persons with diabetes should have emergency preparedness kits that contain adequate medical supplies to last 1 week. Medical supplies should include all testing equipment, medications, syringes, quick-acting glucose, and extra batteries for their CGM. An insulated cooling container is essential for insulin, and frozen gel packs, phase-change material cooling packs, or vacuum-insulated containers should be ready to place in the kit. If ice is used to keep insulin cool, it should be made with salt water so it will melt more slowly.

137. C: Fibrates, such as fenofibrate and gemfibrozil, act by increasing lipolysis and clearance of triglyceride-rich particles. Fibrates are particularly effective for the treatment of high triglyceride levels and low HDL cholesterol levels. They are typically able to lower triglyceride levels by 20–50% and raise HDL levels by 10–20%. Persons taking fibrates must have their liver enzyme levels monitored because the drugs can elevate liver enzymes and increase the risk of gallstones. Additionally, fibrates may cause muscle pain in some persons.

138. B: In type 2 diabetes, because some insulin is still produced, lipolysis (i.e., the breakdown of fat into ketone bodies) does not occur; therefore, persons with type 2 diabetes generally do not develop DKA, although it may occur if the body is under extreme stress, such as with a severe infection that results in a marked fall in insulin production. Clients with type 2 diabetes are at risk for hyperosmolar hyperglycemic nonketotic syndrome, erectile dysfunction, acanthosis nigricans (i.e., darkened skin in the groin area, axillae, and around the neck), visual disturbances, and neuropathy.

139. A: Assessing a patient's mastery of a self-care skill should be accomplished by observing return demonstrations. This enables the educator to identify improper technique or areas for improvement. Return demonstrations with proper technique should be documented to establish proper evaluation. A verbal explanation of the skill does not allow the educator to witness the skill in action and may not reveal some problem areas, such as visual or dexterity issues. Verbal acknowledgement of understanding is the least valid, as it relies on understanding and mastery as *perceived* by the patient. The person with the skill expertise should evaluate the skill level and offer guidance. Verbal response/acknowledgement would be more appropriate for assessments relating to a patient's values and obstacles (information for which the patient *is* the ultimate authority). A post-education assessment is more appropriate for evaluating knowledge level, but may not necessarily translate into application or tactile skills. An advantage of written assessment tools, particularly pre- and post-education, is that change in knowledge or retention of knowledge can be quantifiably measured.

140. B: There is little chance that a homeless person with a history of drug abuse, living in an encampment, and scrounging or begging for food is going to adhere to a plan that focuses on treatment or prevention because that person does not have access to food, medications, supplies, or adequate facilities, Instead, the plan should first focus on community resources that are available, such as housing, Medicaid, rehabilitation programs, and food distribution centers. The social worker should determine what resources may be available.

141. A: It is *not* true that medical nutrition therapy (MNT) is recommended for only those persons with diabetes who are underweight, overweight, or obese. In fact, MNT is recommended for anyone who has diabetes, regardless of nutritional status. In addition, a registered dietitian should be closely involved with a patient's diabetes care plan to assist with individualized meal planning in many cases, such as if the patient is a child with celiac disease, is hospitalized, or is pregnant; if the patient has co-morbidities affected by diet; or if the patient has prediabetes.

142. B: The most significant risk factor for the development of type 2 diabetes in children is obesity, which may be related to diets high in simple carbohydrates and fats and lack of adequate exercise. Type 2 diabetes may be diagnosed as early as 4 years of age but is most commonly diagnosed during puberty, which is associated with an increased risk of developing hypertension. Generally, diet and exercise interventions need to be aimed at the entire family rather than just the child.

143. A: Medicare guidelines do not justify individual sessions for diabetes education simply because the patient prefers one-on-one education. There must be a documented rationale, such as unavailability of classes, physical or cultural barriers, or another physician-documented need to provide reimbursement for one-on-one classes.

144. D: As evidenced by his weight gain and continued high readings, the patient is likely overeating. This is further supported by the fact that occasionally the insulin is sufficient to keep his glucose within target range or even low. The educator should help the patient to evaluate his current eating patterns and make adjustments. His BG meter logs may at first indicate a need for more insulin, but the weight gain must also be taken into consideration. Decreasing the dose without addressing the nutritional aspects would leave the patient with high fasting glucose levels. However, once the patient is able to reduce intake, a lower dose of insulin may be needed. At some point, he may also require mealtime insulin, but the weight increase is the first clue that he is overeating; it is best to adjust one element at a time. A need for bolus insulin would be indicated by BG values that increase consistently after meals throughout the day.

145. A: If adults with diabetes choose to use alcohol, they should limit intake to a moderate amount (one drink per day or less for adult women and two drinks per day or less for adult men), according to the ADA Standards of Care. Choice B is more alcohol than the recommended limit for persons with diabetes. Choice C is incorrect because persons with diabetes may consume alcohol in moderation, although they should take precautions to prevent hypoglycemia, such as eating food if taking insulin or using sulfonylurea medications. Choice D is also incorrect, as it includes the words "without restriction," implying that any amount is acceptable.

146. B: Telling friends about the condition, carrying a medical information card, and using smartphone apps are all helpful preventive measures; however, wearing diabetes jewelry is especially important because it is easily seen. It should be worn by any persons at risk for hypoglycemia. Various types of medical jewelry are available, including wrist and ankle bracelets, pendants, necklaces, bag tags, and pins. Sources of this jewelry include the MedicAlert Foundation, Lauren's Hope Med ID Jewelry, and Medical ID Fashions. Colored silicone bracelets are available for children.

147. D: The person's foot examination is too cursory, so the CDCES should review the procedure. Persons with diabetes should do daily (not just after bathing) foot exams to look for any abnormalities, such as cuts, blisters, erythema, edema, nail changes, or skin changes. Neuropathy can impair the sensation of pain, so clients need to be aware that they may not feel an injury. The entire foot, including between the toes, should be examined carefully. If clients cannot adequately examine their feet, they can use a mirror or ask a family member to examine their feet.

148. C: According to 2026 ADA Standards, every patient's tobacco/nicotine use status, including readiness to quit if they use tobacco or nicotine in any form, should be discussed at every visit. Smoking cigarettes, along with exposure to secondhand smoke, has been proven to cause a large number of complications in people with diabetes, including cardiovascular disease, kidney disease, visual impairment, and premature death. Quitting smoking can reduce these risks, and in some case even reverse complications caused by smoking. Vaping nicotine products (e.g., e-cigarettes) and other forms of tobacco/nicotine use may not be as harmful as combustible cigarettes, but they do pose significant health risks. Patients should be encouraged to quit tobacco/nicotine entirely and given appropriate support to do so, including referral to counseling and pharmacologic therapy as needed.

149. D: Presenting a scenario that is applicable to the patient will give the clinician an opportunity to observe whether the patient has the capability to make the calculations necessary for safe and appropriate action. The patient's education level and math grades are not indicative of current skill or ability level. Asking the patient to self-report numeracy problems is unreliable because the patient may give an inaccurate self-assessment due to embarrassment or not realizing that they even struggle with numeracy. Assigning a take-home math test runs the risk that the patient will have someone else complete it or help with completing it, and it is likely to miss specific areas/topics that currently apply to this specific patient.

150. C: Reporting progress is not a critical educator skill when assessing a patient's ability to plan goals. Monitoring progress is an important part of the goals process, but not in assessing one's ability to *plan*. The four critical skills for assessing patients' planning skills are: interpreting information gathering, facilitating engagement, testing hypotheses, and analyzing problems.

151. C: To reduce the risk of transmitting blood-borne diseases, all efforts should be made to limit any possible contact with another person's blood. It violates infection control recommendations to use the same pen, which will come in contact with a patient's skin and possibly blood, for multiple patients, even with a new pen needle. If the educator wants to instruct with a training pen, then they should use a new pen each time, and properly discard it after use. An alternative to this would be to demonstrate with the pen, injecting into simulated skin, and then have the patient demonstrate injection technique using their own pen or a sterile disposable syringe. Cleansing with soap and water is now preferred over alcohol to prep fingers for blood glucose self-monitoring. Clinics are within infection control guidelines to use one meter to check blood glucose for many patients as long as a sterile, single-use lancet is used for each person. Finally, if parents use a sterile single-use syringe for each child, then withdrawing insulin from the same vial would not violate infection control principles.

152. D: National Diabetes Month (also referred to as American Diabetes Month or Diabetes Awareness Month) is observed in November each year. The first National Diabetes Week, which later evolved into National Diabetes Month, was observed in 1948. On its website, the National Institute of Diabetes and Digestive and Kidney Diseases (part of the National Institutes of Health) declares that National Diabetes Month is "a time for individuals, organizations, and communities across the country to shine a spotlight on diabetes." This annual national campaign presents great opportunities for local diabetes education outreach and advocacy activities.

153. B: Demonstrating a skill such as insulin administration allows the patient to learn by watching, listening, and then doing. The return demonstration also allows the educator to witness the patient's level of competency and then correct mistakes. This teaching strategy takes a bit more time than many others, and works best in one-on-one situations or in small groups, but is the most effective way to both teach and assess a clinical skill. A written quiz may be a way to assess knowledge but does not enable the educator to assess the patient's technique, nor does it provide the best opportunity to instruct. A video or printed handout can instruct to a certain extent, but neither provides a means of assessing the patient's ability to self-administer insulin. These tools are best used to reinforce the demonstration. While verbal acknowledgement of understanding may be part of the assessment, it is not sufficient to assess a patient's level of understanding and competency of a self-care skill such as insulin administration.

154. B: Children with diabetes do not have higher rates of dental caries than non-diabetic children do, but they do have more plaque and gingival inflammation, and more teeth with poor gum attachment. Dental care is very important for persons with diabetes, but it is often neglected. Only about 65% of persons with diabetes report seeing a dentist at least once a year. Hyperglycemia contributes to increased periodontal disease, and periodontal disease contributes to hyperglycemia and increased insulin resistance. Treatment of dental disease has been shown to improve glycemic control and vice versa. In addition to hyperglycemia, some medications for depression and hypertension (e.g., diuretics) frequently used by those with diabetes can also lead to increased dental problems because they contribute to dry mouth.

155. D: Sexual orientation is not information collected during the initial assessment, as stipulated in National Standards for DSMES. Although level of family support is assessed, this does not extend to the nature of sexual orientation. The other choices—financial status, emotional response, and cultural influences—are all part of the information gathered, along with many other factors.

156. B: When a group member asks a question that is "off topic," the best approach is to answer briefly and then redirect back to the topic at hand. Adult learning principles state that persons learn best when there is something they want to know. These "teachable moments" are a great opportunity to provide information that will be meaningful and memorable. However, it would not be appropriate to completely switch the curriculum plan based on one question. Others in the group may want to know about the material in session 1, and it is likely that each session's material is meant to build on what was presented previously. It would be dismissive to avoid answering at all; DSMES should be individualized, which means providing each individual with the knowledge they seek; therefore, choices C and D are not the best either.

157. B: The ADA's definition of diabetes is quite technical, describing diabetes as a group of metabolic diseases with hyperglycemia and problems with insulin: It can be incomprehensible for those with low health literacy or knowledge of medical terms, so the initial definition should be stated with simple and understandable wording that is still accurate (i.e., a disorder that prevents your body from using food effectively). Then, the CDCES can add more technical terms and information as the person begins to learn more about the disease.

158. A: Family-based education is especially important when educating a child about diabetes to ensure that the family is supportive and knows how to assist the child. However, children learn best when engaged, making interactive, hands-on activities especially effective. A number of games and apps are available for children and adolescents. One long-standing model is Rufus, the Bear with Diabetes, a plush toy and app in which children manage a bear's type 1 diabetes.

159. C: The key question that people involved in the role of social support should ask themselves is, "What does the person with diabetes want in the way of support?" The person with diabetes should verbalize their support needs clearly, and may require educator "coaching" to become comfortable with this. Sometimes well-meaning friends and family can be overbearing, which not only strains the relationship, but also does not usually result in improvement for the person with diabetes. By contrast, some family and friends may be disengaged or distant when it comes to supporting their loved one with diabetes. This can be frustrating for the person with diabetes, who may benefit from help from the educator in finding ways to involve loved ones to an extent that is both helpful and comfortable for all those involved.

160. B: Risk of severe hypoglycemia *increases* with age due to slower metabolism of insulin and other medications. Therefore, older adults will typically see a reduction in the needed insulin dose as age advances. Reduced metabolic rate, altered pain perception, and deceased renal function are all age-related physiologic changes that may require adjustments to the patient's diabetes treatment plan. Other concerns include decreased appetite, decreased sense of taste and smell, increased risk for falls and fractures, memory and cognitive deficits, and more.

161. D: This person is exhibiting signs of depression and suicidal ideation through actions such as refusing meals and eating a full box of chocolates. Approximately 25% of all suicides are committed by older adults, who may attempt it through practices that are contrary to their medical needs. Factors that contribute to suicidal ideation include chronic pain, physical limitations, emotional burdens, changes in body image and identity, social isolation, fear of dependency, and economic stress. This client needs psychological and psychiatric support to better cope and manage his diabetes.

162. D: Up to 40% of persons with diabetes develop some degree of nephropathy (kidney disease). With early kidney damage, persons typically have no symptoms; however, an early indication is when protein (albumin) is found in a urine sample. Protein is usually filtered by the kidneys and remains in the blood, but with damage to the glomeruli (the filtering units in the kidneys), the glomeruli become more permeable and proteins may leak into the urine. Nephropathy is common in persons with diabetes who have poorly controlled blood glucose levels and hypertension.

163. D: Blurring of vision, floaters, and dark spots in the vision are indicative of diabetic retinopathy. Persons may not notice symptoms in the early stage when small vessels in the retina become damaged, making regular eye exams essential. During the proliferative stage, new, fragile vessels grow and rupture, resulting in floaters and dark spots in the vision and blurring or even sudden loss of vision. Management includes strict control of blood glucose levels and can include invasive procedures such as focal laser treatment, pan-retinal photocoagulation, injections, and vitrectomy.

164. B: 2026 ADA guidelines, supported by the American College of Cardiology/American Heart Association, note that according to clinical trials, maintaining a blood pressure of less than 130/80 mmHg decreases cardiovascular events and microvascular complications. A blood pressure in the range of 130/80 mmHg to 150/90 mmHg requires pharmacologic intervention (generally an ACE inhibitor or ARB as the first-line treatment) in addition to lifestyle changes. A blood pressure greater than or equal to 150/90 mmHg requires the use of two pharmacologic agents.

165. D: Seeing a nephrologist annually in the absence of hypertension or kidney problems is not necessary, though annual screening of urinary albumin and eGFR is recommended to monitor kidney function. The primary care provider or endocrinologist can check blood pressure and kidney function and then refer if a problem is identified. According to ADA Standards of Care, regular dental visits and an annual dilated eye exam to check for retinopathy are both recommended components of comprehensive diabetes care. If there is no evidence of retinopathy in one or more annual eye exams, eye exams may be recommended for every one to two years. If lipid levels are not high enough to require pharmacologic treatment, lipid profiles are only required every 5 years after diagnosis.

166. A: While snacks are important, they should contain carbohydrates in case of low blood sugar or a delayed meal. Snacks such as nuts and cheese may be helpful if a person gets the "munchies," but for safety, he should bring hard candy, fruit, or some other form of carbohydrate. All other items listed should be included in carry-on baggage when traveling.

167. D: Preconception counseling should be provided on a regular basis to every woman of child-bearing age with diabetes. This counsel is particularly important to this patient because she is on her own at school and admits to "slacking" on her diabetes self-management, which may also mean that she is not being as careful in other areas. There is no indication that the patient has undiagnosed kidney problems, especially at a diagnosis duration of three years. Similarly, dilated eye exams are recommended at five years from onset for those with type 1 diabetes. Further MNT (assuming the patient received MNT at diagnosis) is not indicated unless there is some change in health status that warrants a different diet or need for more in-depth education, such as preparing for insulin pump therapy. The educator is capable of reviewing dietary principles, including alcohol consumption.

168. B: Persons with diabetes who use sharps should try to always have a puncture-proof disposal container to dispose of them, but if a sharps container is not available, then a heavy-duty plastic container (such as those that are used for laundry detergent) may be used. Lightweight plastic containers, such as those used to store food, are too easily punctured and should not be used. Sharps should never be placed in the trash without a puncture-proof container because they pose a risk to anyone who handles the trash.

169. C: Patients are usually instructed to use the sides of the fingers because there tends to be less pain due to fewer nerve endings. All of the other answer choices are false. There is no evidence to date that it is easier to obtain a drop of blood from the side than from the tip of the finger due to better blood circulation. Patients should clean their hands thoroughly, so germs are not the reason for this advice. Blood from the fingertip or the side of the fingertip is equally representative of whole blood. Some sites, such as the arm and leg, may not represent the true value as well. Keep in mind that while the side of the finger is suggested, if a patient prefers to lance the tip of the finger instead, the educator should accommodate their preferences.

170. D: Under current Medicare guidelines, only the treating physician can refer patients for medical nutrition therapy (MNT). Medicare will not accept a referral from a CDE, pharmacist, or qualified non-physician practitioner. Typically, Medicare covers three hours of MNT in the first year of diagnosis, then 2 hours per year in each subsequent year. This benefit is different from diabetes self-management training (DSMT), the referral for which may be made by a physician or a qualified non-physician practitioner. DSMT and separate MNT services may not be provided or billed on the same day but may be performed by the same person (if the CDE is an RD) on separate days. While Medicare and other insurance providers' coverage can be detailed and confusing to navigate, it is important to assist the patient by making sure that referrals are provided in a manner that provides maximum reimbursement to the patient.

171. C: The rate of depression for those with diabetes is about twice that of the general population. The role of the diabetes educator when it comes to depression is to screen when appropriate and assist those who may be depressed in obtaining help from a mental health professional. This may include helping the person with the referral and scheduling the appointment, as those who are depressed may lack the energy to accomplish these tasks. Of course, those who have clinical depression that is not treated will also find it very difficult, if not impossible, to perform the many self-care behaviors needed for good diabetes management. It is not within the diabetes educator's scope of practice to diagnose depression. Depression is not the same as stress. It is inaccurate to say that an educator can teach strategies that will prevent clinical depression. While communication with the patient's mental health professional may be helpful in helping the patient with diabetes to learn self-care strategies, it is not the priority intervention.

172. D: In the small intestines, carbohydrates are broken down into simple sugars such as glucose by digestive enzymes, including alpha-glucosidase. Alpha-glucosidase inhibitors (such as acarbose and miglitol) block the actions of alpha-glucosidase, slowing the absorption of carbohydrates and preventing postprandial spikes in blood glucose levels. Alpha-glucosidase inhibitors are often taken with other drugs, such as metformin or insulin. Alpha-glucosidase inhibitors by themselves do not cause hypoglycemia, but they may cause flatulence, abdominal distension and discomfort, and diarrhea.

173. B: Literacy skills are the strongest predictors of health status—stronger than ethnicity, income level, age, and other factors. Literacy dictates a patient's ability to understand important elements of health status, self-care, and care plans so that they can appropriately care for themselves across the continuum.

174. D: Small group discussion around a table where patients teach each other a skill after seeing it demonstrated by the educator is an instruction strategy that addresses visual, auditory, and tactile learning styles and, of the strategies described, is likely to be the most effective for patient retention. The interaction (teaching back) makes it memorable; studies show that people remember best when they not only see and hear something, but also when they say and do it. All of the other answer choices are good strategies, but are not likely to lead to the best retention.

175. A: The best example of an immediate outcome is one that can be measured at the time of the intervention, in this case demonstrating proper technique for self-monitoring. The other choices are examples of intermediate results over time, indicate behavioral change, and require more than one measurement. Reducing the number of missed doses of medication requires a pre- and post-assessment for comparison to show a reduction. Improvement in HDL is more a clinical indicator than a behavioral objective; the behavior associated with this clinical objective may be to increase exercise, change an element of the diet, or take medication. In addition, it also requires a pre- and post-assessment for comparison. Being 100% compliant on screenings is a goal that would be set and then require action; it is measured at a specified later date and time. It is an example of an intermediate objective.

How to Overcome Test Anxiety

Just the thought of taking a test is enough to make most people a little nervous. A test is an important event that can have a long-term impact on your future, so it's important to take it seriously and it's natural to feel anxious about performing well. But just because anxiety is normal, that doesn't mean that it's helpful in test taking, or that you should simply accept it as part of your life. Anxiety can have a variety of effects. These effects can be mild, like making you feel slightly nervous, or severe, like blocking your ability to focus or remember even a simple detail.

If you experience test anxiety—whether severe or mild—it's important to know how to beat it. To discover this, first you need to understand what causes test anxiety.

Causes of Test Anxiety

While we often think of anxiety as an uncontrollable emotional state, it can actually be caused by simple, practical things. One of the most common causes of test anxiety is that a person does not feel adequately prepared for their test. This feeling can be the result of many different issues such as poor study habits or lack of organization, but the most common culprit is time management. Starting to study too late, failing to organize your study time to cover all of the material, or being distracted while you study will mean that you're not well prepared for the test. This may lead to cramming the night before, which will cause you to be physically and mentally exhausted for the test. Poor time management also contributes to feelings of stress, fear, and hopelessness as you realize you are not well prepared but don't know what to do about it.

Other times, test anxiety is not related to your preparation for the test but comes from unresolved fear. This may be a past failure on a test, or poor performance on tests in general. It may come from comparing yourself to others who seem to be performing better or from the stress of living up to expectations. Anxiety may be driven by fears of the future—how failure on this test would affect your educational and career goals. These fears are often completely irrational, but they can still negatively impact your test performance.

Elements of Test Anxiety

As mentioned earlier, test anxiety is considered to be an emotional state, but it has physical and mental components as well. Sometimes you may not even realize that you are suffering from test anxiety until you notice the physical symptoms. These can include trembling hands, rapid heartbeat, sweating, nausea, and tense muscles. Extreme anxiety may lead to fainting or vomiting. Obviously, any of these symptoms can have a negative impact on testing. It is important to recognize them as soon as they begin to occur so that you can address the problem before it damages your performance.

The mental components of test anxiety include trouble focusing and inability to remember learned information. During a test, your mind is on high alert, which can help you recall information and stay focused for an extended period of time. However, anxiety interferes with your mind's natural processes, causing you to blank out, even on the questions you know well. The strain of testing during anxiety makes it difficult to stay focused, especially on a test that may take several hours. Extreme anxiety can take a huge mental toll, making it difficult not only to recall test information but even to understand the test questions or pull your thoughts together.

Effects of Test Anxiety

Test anxiety is like a disease—if left untreated, it will get progressively worse. Anxiety leads to poor performance, and this reinforces the feelings of fear and failure, which in turn lead to poor performances on subsequent tests. It can grow from a mild nervousness to a crippling condition. If allowed to progress, test anxiety can have a big impact on your schooling, and consequently on your future.

Test anxiety can spread to other parts of your life. Anxiety on tests can become anxiety in any stressful situation, and blanking on a test can turn into panicking in a job situation. But fortunately, you don't have to let anxiety rule your testing and determine your grades. There are a number of relatively simple steps you can take to move past anxiety and function normally on a test and in the rest of life.

Physical Steps for Beating Test Anxiety

While test anxiety is a serious problem, the good news is that it can be overcome. It doesn't have to control your ability to think and remember information. While it may take time, you can begin taking steps today to beat anxiety.

Just as your first hint that you may be struggling with anxiety comes from the physical symptoms, the first step to treating it is also physical. Rest is crucial for having a clear, strong mind. If you are tired, it is much easier to give in to anxiety. But if you establish good sleep habits, your body and mind will be ready to perform optimally, without the strain of exhaustion. Additionally, sleeping well helps you to retain information better, so you're more likely to recall the answers when you see the test questions.

Getting good sleep means more than going to bed on time. It's important to allow your brain time to relax. Take study breaks from time to time so it doesn't get overworked, and don't study right before bed. Take time to rest your mind before trying to rest your body, or you may find it difficult to fall asleep.

Along with sleep, other aspects of physical health are important in preparing for a test. Good nutrition is vital for good brain function. Sugary foods and drinks may give a burst of energy but this burst is followed by a crash, both physically and emotionally. Instead, fuel your body with protein and vitamin-rich foods.

Also, drink plenty of water. Dehydration can lead to headaches and exhaustion, especially if your brain is already under stress from the rigors of the test. Particularly if your test is a long one, drink water during the breaks. And if possible, take an energy-boosting snack to eat between sections.

Along with sleep and diet, a third important part of physical health is exercise. Maintaining a steady workout schedule is helpful, but even taking 5-minute study breaks to walk can help get your blood pumping faster and clear your head. Exercise also releases endorphins, which contribute to a positive feeling and can help combat test anxiety.

When you nurture your physical health, you are also contributing to your mental health. If your body is healthy, your mind is much more likely to be healthy as well. So take time to rest, nourish your body with healthy food and water, and get moving as much as possible. Taking these physical steps will make you stronger and more able to take the mental steps necessary to overcome test anxiety.

Mental Steps for Beating Test Anxiety

Working on the mental side of test anxiety can be more challenging, but as with the physical side, there are clear steps you can take to overcome it. As mentioned earlier, test anxiety often stems from lack of preparation, so the obvious solution is to prepare for the test. Effective studying may be the most important weapon you have for beating test anxiety, but you can and should employ several other mental tools to combat fear.

First, boost your confidence by reminding yourself of past success—tests or projects that you aced. If you're putting as much effort into preparing for this test as you did for those, there's no reason you should expect to fail here. Work hard to prepare; then trust your preparation.

Second, surround yourself with encouraging people. It can be helpful to find a study group, but be sure that the people you're around will encourage a positive attitude. If you spend time with others who are anxious or cynical, this will only contribute to your own anxiety. Look for others who are motivated to study hard from a desire to succeed, not from a fear of failure.

Third, reward yourself. A test is physically and mentally tiring, even without anxiety, and it can be helpful to have something to look forward to. Plan an activity following the test, regardless of the outcome, such as going to a movie or getting ice cream.

When you are taking the test, if you find yourself beginning to feel anxious, remind yourself that you know the material. Visualize successfully completing the test. Then take a few deep, relaxing breaths and return to it. Work through the questions carefully but with confidence, knowing that you are capable of succeeding.

Developing a healthy mental approach to test taking will also aid in other areas of life. Test anxiety affects more than just the actual test—it can be damaging to your mental health and even contribute to depression. It's important to beat test anxiety before it becomes a problem for more than testing.

Study Strategy

Being prepared for the test is necessary to combat anxiety, but what does being prepared look like? You may study for hours on end and still not feel prepared. What you need is a strategy for test prep. The next few pages outline our recommended steps to help you plan out and conquer the challenge of preparation.

Step 1: Scope Out the Test

Learn everything you can about the format (multiple choice, essay, etc.) and what will be on the test. Gather any study materials, course outlines, or sample exams that may be available. Not only will this help you to prepare, but knowing what to expect can help to alleviate test anxiety.

Step 2: Map Out the Material

Look through the textbook or study guide and make note of how many chapters or sections it has. Then divide these over the time you have. For example, if a book has 15 chapters and you have five days to study, you need to cover three chapters each day. Even better, if you have the time, leave an extra day at the end for overall review after you have gone through the material in depth.

If time is limited, you may need to prioritize the material. Look through it and make note of which sections you think you already have a good grasp on, and which need review. While you are studying, skim quickly through the familiar sections and take more time on the challenging parts.

Write out your plan so you don't get lost as you go. Having a written plan also helps you feel more in control of the study, so anxiety is less likely to arise from feeling overwhelmed at the amount to cover.

STEP 3: GATHER YOUR TOOLS

Decide what study method works best for you. Do you prefer to highlight in the book as you study and then go back over the highlighted portions? Or do you type out notes of the important information? Or is it helpful to make flashcards that you can carry with you? Assemble the pens, index cards, highlighters, post-it notes, and any other materials you may need so you won't be distracted by getting up to find things while you study.

If you're having a hard time retaining the information or organizing your notes, experiment with different methods. For example, try color-coding by subject with colored pens, highlighters, or post-it notes. If you learn better by hearing, try recording yourself reading your notes so you can listen while in the car, working out, or simply sitting at your desk. Ask a friend to quiz you from your flashcards, or try teaching someone the material to solidify it in your mind.

STEP 4: CREATE YOUR ENVIRONMENT

It's important to avoid distractions while you study. This includes both the obvious distractions like visitors and the subtle distractions like an uncomfortable chair (or a too-comfortable couch that makes you want to fall asleep). Set up the best study environment possible: good lighting and a comfortable work area. If background music helps you focus, you may want to turn it on, but otherwise keep the room quiet. If you are using a computer to take notes, be sure you don't have any other windows open, especially applications like social media, games, or anything else that could distract you. Silence your phone and turn off notifications. Be sure to keep water close by so you stay hydrated while you study (but avoid unhealthy drinks and snacks).

Also, take into account the best time of day to study. Are you freshest first thing in the morning? Try to set aside some time then to work through the material. Is your mind clearer in the afternoon or evening? Schedule your study session then. Another method is to study at the same time of day that you will take the test, so that your brain gets used to working on the material at that time and will be ready to focus at test time.

STEP 5: STUDY!

Once you have done all the study preparation, it's time to settle into the actual studying. Sit down, take a few moments to settle your mind so you can focus, and begin to follow your study plan. Don't give in to distractions or let yourself procrastinate. This is your time to prepare so you'll be ready to fearlessly approach the test. Make the most of the time and stay focused.

Of course, you don't want to burn out. If you study too long you may find that you're not retaining the information very well. Take regular study breaks. For example, taking five minutes out of every hour to walk briskly, breathing deeply and swinging your arms, can help your mind stay fresh.

As you get to the end of each chapter or section, it's a good idea to do a quick review. Remind yourself of what you learned and work on any difficult parts. When you feel that you've mastered the material, move on to the next part. At the end of your study session, briefly skim through your notes again.

But while review is helpful, cramming last minute is NOT. If at all possible, work ahead so that you won't need to fit all your study into the last day. Cramming overloads your brain with more information than it can process and retain, and your tired mind may struggle to recall even previously learned information when it is overwhelmed with last-minute study. Also, the urgent nature of cramming and the stress placed on your brain contribute to anxiety. You'll be more likely to go to the test feeling unprepared and having trouble thinking clearly.

So don't cram, and don't stay up late before the test, even just to review your notes at a leisurely pace. Your brain needs rest more than it needs to go over the information again. In fact, plan to finish your studies by noon or early afternoon the day before the test. Give your brain the rest of the day to relax or focus on other things, and get a good night's sleep. Then you will be fresh for the test and better able to recall what you've studied.

Step 6: Take a Practice Test

Many courses offer sample tests, either online or in the study materials. This is an excellent resource to check whether you have mastered the material, as well as to prepare for the test format and environment.

Check the test format ahead of time: the number of questions, the type (multiple choice, free response, etc.), and the time limit. Then create a plan for working through them. For example, if you have 30 minutes to take a 60-question test, your limit is 30 seconds per question. Spend less time on the questions you know well so that you can take more time on the difficult ones.

If you have time to take several practice tests, take the first one open book, with no time limit. Work through the questions at your own pace and make sure you fully understand them. Gradually work up to taking a test under test conditions: sit at a desk with all study materials put away and set a timer. Pace yourself to make sure you finish the test with time to spare and go back to check your answers if you have time.

After each test, check your answers. On the questions you missed, be sure you understand why you missed them. Did you misread the question (tests can use tricky wording)? Did you forget the information? Or was it something you hadn't learned? Go back and study any shaky areas that the practice tests reveal.

Taking these tests not only helps with your grade, but also aids in combating test anxiety. If you're already used to the test conditions, you're less likely to worry about it, and working through tests until you're scoring well gives you a confidence boost. Go through the practice tests until you feel comfortable, and then you can go into the test knowing that you're ready for it.

Test Tips

On test day, you should be confident, knowing that you've prepared well and are ready to answer the questions. But aside from preparation, there are several test day strategies you can employ to maximize your performance.

First, as stated before, get a good night's sleep the night before the test (and for several nights before that, if possible). Go into the test with a fresh, alert mind rather than staying up late to study.

Try not to change too much about your normal routine on the day of the test. It's important to eat a nutritious breakfast, but if you normally don't eat breakfast at all, consider eating just a protein bar. If you're a coffee drinker, go ahead and have your normal coffee. Just make sure you time it so that the caffeine doesn't wear off right in the middle of your test. Avoid sugary beverages, and drink enough water to stay hydrated but not so much that you need a restroom break 10 minutes into the test. If your test isn't first thing in the morning, consider going for a walk or doing a light workout before the test to get your blood flowing.

Allow yourself enough time to get ready, and leave for the test with plenty of time to spare so you won't have the anxiety of scrambling to arrive in time. Another reason to be early is to select a good seat. It's helpful to sit away from doors and windows, which can be distracting. Find a good seat, get out your supplies, and settle your mind before the test begins.

When the test begins, start by going over the instructions carefully, even if you already know what to expect. Make sure you avoid any careless mistakes by following the directions.

Then begin working through the questions, pacing yourself as you've practiced. If you're not sure on an answer, don't spend too much time on it, and don't let it shake your confidence. Either skip it and come back later, or eliminate as many wrong answers as possible and guess among the remaining ones. Don't dwell on these questions as you continue—put them out of your mind and focus on what lies ahead.

Be sure to read all of the answer choices, even if you're sure the first one is the right answer. Sometimes you'll find a better one if you keep reading. But don't second-guess yourself if you do immediately know the answer. Your gut instinct is usually right. Don't let test anxiety rob you of the information you know.

If you have time at the end of the test (and if the test format allows), go back and review your answers. Be cautious about changing any, since your first instinct tends to be correct, but make sure you didn't misread any of the questions or accidentally mark the wrong answer choice. Look over any you skipped and make an educated guess.

At the end, leave the test feeling confident. You've done your best, so don't waste time worrying about your performance or wishing you could change anything. Instead, celebrate the successful completion of this test. And finally, use this test to learn how to deal with anxiety even better next time.

Review Video: Test Anxiety
Visit mometrix.com/academy and enter code: 100340

Important Qualification

Not all anxiety is created equal. If your test anxiety is causing major issues in your life beyond the classroom or testing center, or if you are experiencing troubling physical symptoms related to your anxiety, it may be a sign of a serious physiological or psychological condition. If this sounds like your situation, we strongly encourage you to seek professional help.

Online Resources

Due to our efforts to try to keep this book to a manageable length, we've created a link that will give you access to all of your online resources:

mometrix.com/resources719/certdiabedu

It's Your Moment, Let's Celebrate It!

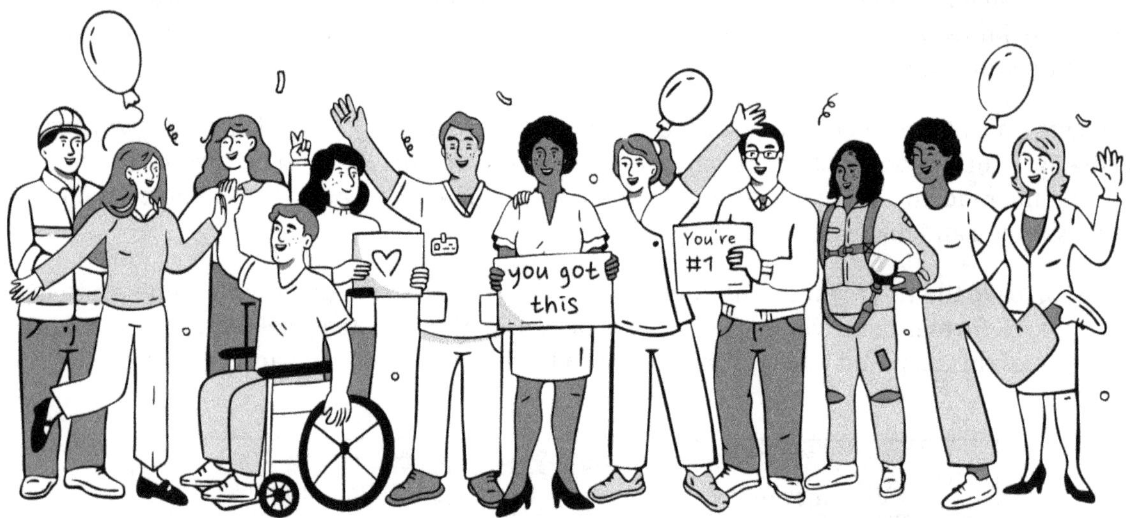

Share your story @mometrixtestpreparation